The Complete

Herbal
Tutor

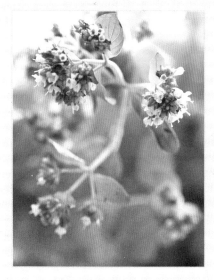
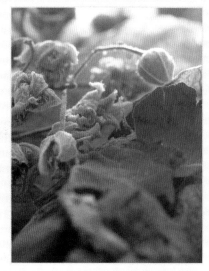
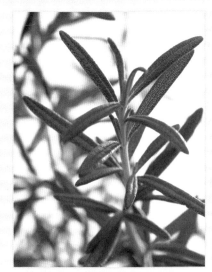
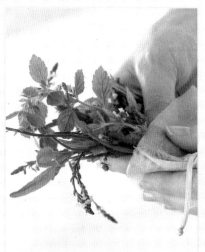
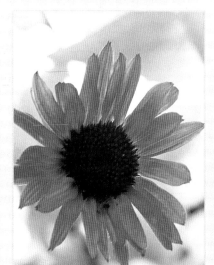
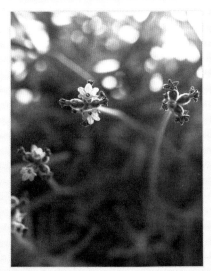
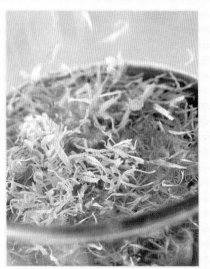
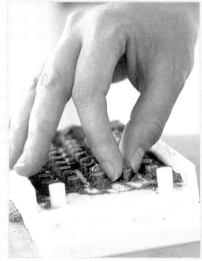
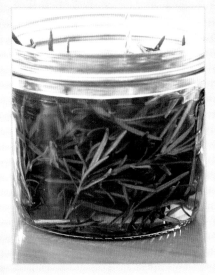

Contents

Introduction

Herbs are the most extraordinary plants. Their incredible ability to heal on all levels of our being never ceases to amaze and inspire me. I have been asked so many times during my years in practice as a herbalist how I came to be in this profession, and the story actually begins in my childhood.

Herbal roots

I have loved herbs ever since I was a child, intrigued by their delicious scents – all so unique – and their beautiful shapes and forms. I was brought up in the country and loved being surrounded by natural beauty, and have never been able to live in a town or city. My mother gave me a piece of her garden when I was little so that I could grow my own herbs and flowers, and this was my favourite occupation.

This 18th-century German engraving depicts a female herbalist at work.

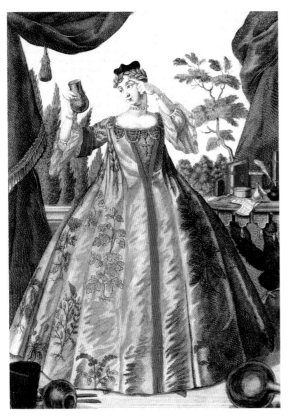

Studies in herbalism

In my early 20s, while living in a cottage on a small island off the east coast of England, growing my own food and harvesting as much from the wild as I could, I began to learn about the wild herbs that were growing around me. I realized that the earth provides all the raw ingredients for our health and wellbeing, and that herbs have the ability to keep us in balance in body, mind, emotion and spirit – if we could only understand their gifts to us to their fullest extent. After travelling in many parts of the world, looking for meaning in existence that would guide me to finding the right direction in my life, I resolved to find a place to study herbal medicine. After four years of studying I became a member of the National Institute of Medical Herbalists, a body of professional herbalists that has existed since 1864.

Once in practice I continued to study, constantly searching for more pointers towards understanding the human organism and the keys to health and harmony, so that I could better serve my patients as well as my family and myself. Over the next few years I studied homeopathy, aromatherapy, therapeutic massage and counselling, and then finally I found Ayurveda, the system of healing that resonated with me more than any other to date. Ayurveda is a body of knowledge and wisdom from India incorporating a complex system of medicine as well as guidelines for a way of living, the aim of which is not only freedom from suffering in mind and body but also enlightenment itself. Since then I have continued to study herbal medicine and Ayurveda, and to incorporate the wisdom of all I learn into my practice and my writing.

A holistic approach

The writing of *The Complete Herbal Tutor* was motivated by the growing interest in using herbal medicine in a practical yet informed way among healthcare practitioners and lay people alike. There is a great need for contemporary information encompassing a holistic view that acknowledges the intimate connection of mind and body, and promotes health and health education rather than solely addressing illnesses and how to treat the symptoms arising from them. The book provides a practical, accessible reference guide to the use of the 150 most common herbs in the modern practice of Western herbal medicine, and by doing so highlights the great contribution herbs can make to modern medical care. I have endeavoured to emphasize how herbs are used most effectively when they are prescribed after the taking of a full case history, with the intention of aiding innate homeostatic mechanisms while addressing the underlying problems that give rise to health problems, including diet and lifestyle.

Treatment advice

In describing the herbal treatment of over 100 common ailments, the book is not intended to replace proper medical care, which may require the greater knowledge and expertise of the professional medical herbalist or mainstream healthcare practitioner. The format of the ailments section follows a body-system approach, including the main systems affected by common illness, and the health problems covered in the text are those that I have frequently encountered in my practice of nearly 30 years as a professional herbalist and those that I consider to be most applicable to treatment using herbs.

Our herbal heritage

A conventional medical view might take some exception to aspects of herbal philosophy and approach to treatment that may follow some rather unorthodox lines. There may not be much scientific justification for, for example, the use of 'alterative' or cleansing herbs to clear the body of toxins, or cooling herbs to clear 'accumulated heat', but they are integral to the philosophies of ancient and respected systems, such as Chinese, Tibetan and Ayurvedic medicine, that have survived almost intact for at least 5,000 years, providing the framework for the healthcare of millions of people. I believe we can greatly benefit from their profound wisdom and insight, which gives us a background and context for understanding how herbs are used, and for this reason I have included a chapter on 'Global herbal traditions' (see pages 8–35).

Practical guidance

The hedgerows, our gardens and the shelves of health-food stores and pharmacies alike are lined with dazzling arrays of herbs that can be overwhelming to many who

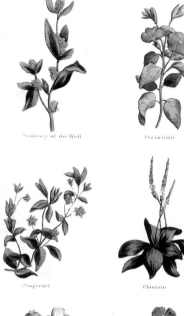
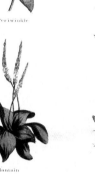
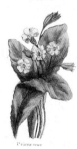

Plants and herbs profiled in Nicholas Culpeper's *Complete Herbal*, published in 1652, are still in use today.

feel they lack the necessary knowledge to choose those appropriate to their needs with confidence. The media presentation of herbs has shifted from extolling the virtues of herbs and their 'miraculous cures', declaring that everything natural had to be safe and free from the side effects of modern drugs, to the opposite view, which perhaps makes more exciting reading, alarming the public that herbs have potential side effects and may even be dangerous. Without sufficient real evidence it is easy for lay people and professionals alike to be susceptible to such hype, but with more information it is possible to have a more realistic view. I hope that this book will serve all those using herbs for themselves, their friends and family or their patients, who wish to learn more about the safe and effective use of herbal medicines and navigate themselves through questions regarding dosage, interactions and contraindications so that they can use herbs with the confidence they deserve.

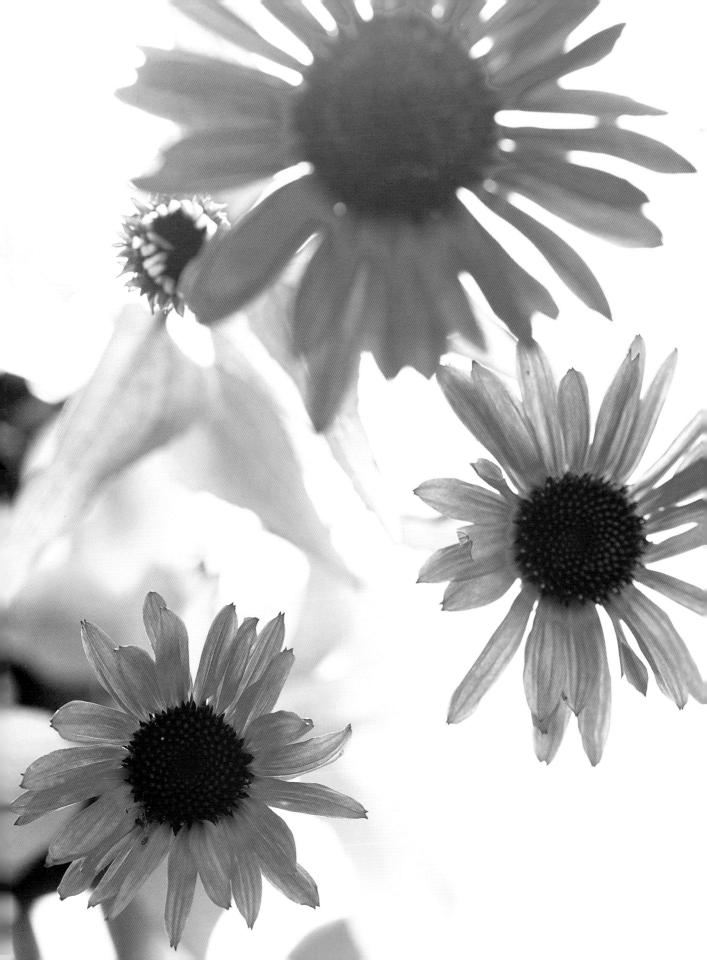

Global herbal traditions

Today's herbalists draw on a variety of healing traditions, from shamanic ritual to remedies proven by scientific trials. Many of the world's traditional systems of healing share a common thesis: that everything in the universe, including plants and human beings, is composed of energy and matter manifested as five elements, and keeping them in balance helps to ensure health and wellbeing. This is the basis of the humoral medicine of ancient Greek physicians, Indian Ayurveda, Traditional Chinese Medicine, Tibetan healing and Islamic Unani Tibb. Herbs play a central role in all these systems, preventing and treating instances of ill health.

Our medical roots

The use of herbs as medicines on both physical and more subtle levels is common to all cultures as far back as we know. We can trace the link between human life and healing herbs back to Neanderthal man 60,000 years ago, when herbs including Horsetail, Yarrow and Ephedra were used.

Ancient and modern medicine

With the vast network of communication that has developed in recent decades has come a wealth of information and wisdom from far and wide that has engendered a considerable merging of herbal traditions. This means that herbalists today have the advantage of drawing on a number of therapeutic systems and philosophies, as well as access to the herbs themselves from most corners of the globe.

Some therapeutic traditions – such as Chinese, Ayurvedic, Unani Tibb and Tibetan medicine – are based on systems of healing that have remained almost intact through thousands of years and still form the primary healthcare system for a significant proportion of the population in those countries. Many Western herbalists now study those traditions and incorporate their ancient practices into their own diagnosis and treatments.

Other age-old systems of herbal healing, particularly in the Western world, have been largely broken and replaced by modern drugs and allopathy, that is, conventional medicine. Currently, the popularity of herbal medicine has inspired a re-evaluation of global medical roots, with their rich sources of effective medicines that certainly have a place in modern medical practice. Herbs such as Garlic, Ginkgo, Ginseng, Echinacea and St John's wort have proved themselves to the world, almost becoming household names in the process, and are even recommended by some doctors.

In recent decades the scientific world has identified specific constituents of herbs and their properties and interactions. Modern studies into the efficacy of herbs and randomized controlled trials have proven that herbs can be effective medicines, and this research vindicates the ancient use of such plants that goes back thousands of years.

Traditional Chinese herbal treatment has been shown to be effective in treating eczema in a randomized controlled trial.

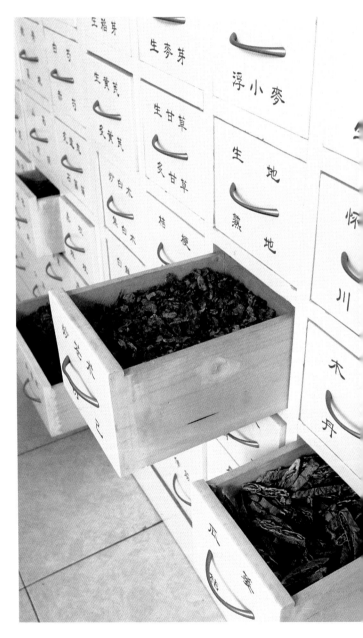

Shamanic healing

The earliest known herbalists of every culture were shamans – important men or women whose instincts were raised to a highly intuitive level through years of training to develop their inner eye. This deeper perception enabled them to communicate directly with the plant and spirit world, and to visit other realities through their spirit allies.

Origins

Shamanistic practices are said to predate all organized religions, dating back to the Paleolithic and Neolithic periods. Many shamanic traditions, including European, Tibetan, Mongolian, Korean, Japanese and Native American in both North and South America, originally came from Siberia and metamorphosed as they travelled to other parts of the world. African slaves took their shamanic traditions to America, where they merged divination and other rituals with Christian practices to produce, for example, Haitian voodoo (vodou), Cuban Santería and Brazilian Candomblé. Elsewhere, shamanism became absorbed into the religion of the area, as it clearly did in Tibetan Buddhism. In some cultures the early shamans were known as priest physicians. They were also sorcerers, magicians, diviners and intermediaries between the mortal and the spirit worlds.

Contemporary shamanism

Today, shamanism is still alive and well in a variety of forms, mainly among indigenous peoples in rural areas, especially in Siberia, where it is the main form of medical treatment available. Even in cities, shanty towns and areas with access to more modern medicine, shamanism forms an important part of the culture, particularly in Africa and Central and South America, where it is used alongside, or as an alternative to, modern medicine.

The belief in witchcraft and sorcery, known as *brujeria* in South America, is still prevalent in many shamanic cultures. Some societies, including several from Africa, distinguish shamans who cure from sorcerers who harm, while others believe that all shamans have the power both to cure and kill. Shamanism is also still practised in South Korea, Japan, Vietnam, Inuit and Eskimo cultures, Papua New Guinea, Australia and Tibet, and in each region the shaman will communicate with the local flora in order to be guided towards cures.

The shaman's journey

In some cultures the shaman's powers are believed to be inherited, while in others a shaman follows a 'calling', sometimes from his or her dreams, and endures rigorous training. Initiation occurs often through a transformational experience, which could be a serious illness or being struck by lightning. In North America Native Americans may seek communion with the world through a 'vision quest', while aspiring shamans in South America might apprentice themselves to a respected shaman.

Shamans enter altered states of consciousness, often ecstatic trance states, journeying to the beat of a drum or rattle, or using singing, music, sweat lodges, vision quests and fasting to communicate with other realms of reality – a teacher, a spirit guide from the animal or plant world or a totem – asking for wisdom and guidance. It is in this way that they gain their knowledge and power. The shaman's journey is intended to help the patient or community to rediscover their connection to nature and spirit. In the Ecuadorian and Peruvian rainforests shamans

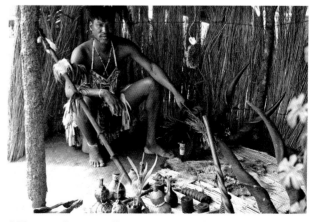

A Tongan shaman in Zambia sits among his remedies, which include gourds and animal horns.

are known as *curanderos*. Some base their healing work on the use of Ayahuasca, a hallucinogenic plant that can induce divine revelation and evoke mental and emotional as well as physical healing. Visiting an *ayahuasquero* has become popular among Western spiritual seekers, who can now go on tours into the jungle for just this purpose.

Other Native American shamans modify consciousness through the use of mind-altering plants, such as psychedelic mushrooms, cannabis, San Pedro cactus, Peyote, Datura, Fly agaric and *Salvia divinorum*. In so doing, shamans can put themselves at risk and therefore use rituals to protect them from enemies and rivals in the spirit and human world. Many of the plants employed are poisonous in large doses, and failing to return from out-of-body experiences can be fatal. These are best used under the guidance of an authentic shaman.

Healing approaches

There has been a surge of interest in shamanic healing in the past few years and many contemporary therapists are incorporating these traditional practices into their work. Some are attracted to healing practices from the East or Native American traditions, while others are accessing the roots of European shamanism and its mystical beliefs and practices that were suppressed by the Christian Church.

Illness in shamanism is generally attributed to spiritual causes, which could be the bad will of another towards the patient, the work of evil spirits, witchcraft or divine intervention. Both spiritual and physical methods are used to heal, depending on what is recommended in the spirit world. In the healing rituals the shaman will 'enter the body' of the patient to confront and banish the spirit responsible. Incense and aromatic plants are often burned as tools of transformation to help transport the minds of the participants to another dimension – the origins of modern aromatherapy (see pages 32–33). Spells, incantations, amulets and ritual dances are used or performed to dispel or placate the spirits thought to be responsible for the patient's ill health.

In his or her healing work a shaman can bring about transformation of the energy and experience of the patient. Loss of vital energy from stress, trauma, illness or accidents can cause what is known as 'soul loss', and this is remedied by 'soul retrieval', where the energy and part of the patient's life that has been traumatized is returned and healed. Loss of power caused by stress, pressure, abusive relationships and lack of love and support leading to low self-esteem can be remedied via the shaman's connection to the patient's power animal, and re-empowering the patient through their own relationship to their power animal to make changes in their lives. Plant

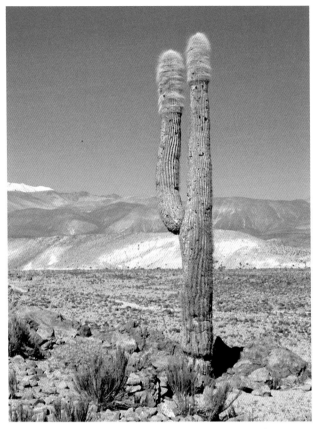

The San Pedro cactus is used by Native American shamans to free their minds from everyday consciousness.

spirit medicine, in which the shaman calls on the healing spirit of a plant to help the patient, often forms part of the healing approach. Plant spirits can be summoned by songs. Totem items such as rocks with special powers are also used.

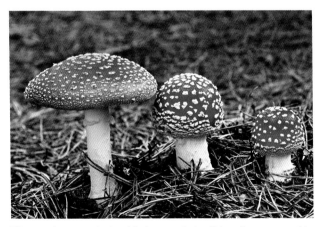

Fly agaric, a psychotrophic fungus, is traditionally consumed in shamanic rituals in Siberia to bring about a state of trance.

Humoral medicine

Around the time of the establishment of the ancient Greek empire, the transition from hunter-gatherer to nomadic tribes and then into farming communities meant the emergence of trade and agriculture. At this time, huge advances in the development of medicine were taking place.

Densely populated centres of trade that grew up incubated epidemics of diseases, including malaria, tuberculosis, measles and digestive and chest infections caused by insanitary living conditions. These presented challenges to shamans in their ritualistic approach to healing. Gradually shamanic practice and control gave way to more complex philosophical systems of medical theory and practice made possible by the increase in trade and travel, education and the exchange of ideas between the cultures of Egypt, Syria, Persia, China and India.

The father of medicine

The increasingly sophisticated and educated clientele of the physicians expected good results and a rationale behind their prescriptions, and stimulated the beginning of rational medicine in which theories were developed to explain patterns of illness. Physicians studied anatomy, physiology and surgery at the great medical schools such as those in Alexandria, Egypt. One of the greatest legacies of this period of learning was the development of holistic medicine, largely inspired by the great 5th-century BCE philosopher and physician Hippocrates. He observed that the body was subject to natural laws and that susceptibility to illness depended on a person's constitution and hereditary tendencies and the influence of environmental factors such as diet, water, hygiene, climate and society.

Hippocrates has been called 'the father of medicine', as he laid down many of the principles of medicine used today, and his work formed the basis of medical theory and practice that has been developed ever since. He emphasized the value of ethical medicine, working for the benefit of the sick and not the physician's pocket alone, and this is incorporated in the Hippocratic Oath, which is still used in modern medical schools today. He taught close observation of patients through the senses – touch, smell, taste and sound – as well as keeping written case histories and basing treatment on results. He also promoted addressing the whole person, not the suppression of symptoms, and enhancing the ability

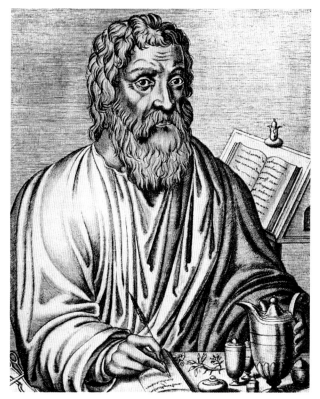

Hippocrates, the ancient Greek physician and philosopher, is widely regarded as the father of medicine.

of the body to heal itself through herbs, fresh air, exercise, bathing and diet. He is recorded as using around 400 herbs.

The five elements

Hippocrates' humoral system of medicine with its five-element theory, paralleled other great traditional systems which existed in India and China at the time. He believed that all matter could be explained by the five basic elements – ether, air, fire, water and earth – and the individuality of people explained by the four humours arising from these elements – blood, phlegm, choler or yellow bile, and melancholy. The proportions of these humours in each person would determine his or her personality and body type, and susceptibility to particular imbalances and illness. Hippocrates thus perceived that illness was not a punishment of the gods, as believed by his forefathers, but arose from imbalances of the four elements that composed everything in nature.

The element earth corresponded to the melancholic humour or temperament, black bile and the season of autumn. It had a cold and dry nature, giving rise to symptoms such as constipation, arthritis, depression or anxiety. Herbs like Ginger and Senna would be used to clear black bile and restore balance. Water corresponded to phlegm and a phlegmatic temperament. Phlegm had a cold and damp nature, epitomized by the season of winter, and gave rise to illnesses such as catarrh, respiratory infections, overweight and fluid retention. Warming and drying herbs like Thyme, Hyssop and Ginger were used to clear cold and damp symptoms and thereby restore the balance of the humours. Fire corresponded to choler or yellow bile, and related to summer. A choleric type would be hot-tempered and prone to liver and digestive problems. Cooling and

Senna is famous as a laxative to clear toxins and its medicinal use was first recorded by Arab physicians in the 9th century.

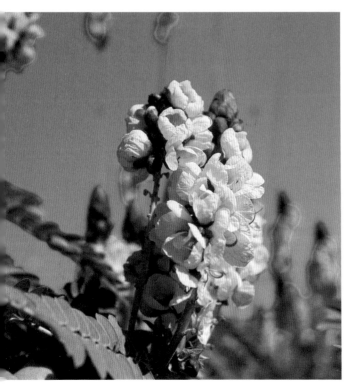

moistening herbs, for example Dandelion, Violet and Lettuce, would help to balance the excess heat and dryness of the choleric temperament. Air corresponded to blood and the sanguine temperament, characterized by spring. A sanguine type would be easy-going and good-humoured, but prone to excesses and overindulgence, giving rise to problems such as gout and diarrhoea. Cool, dry herbs like Burdock or Figwort were used to balance the humours.

Great Greek herbals

Another famous Greek physician was Theophrastus (372–286 BCE), a friend and pupil of Aristotle, who inherited Aristotle's garden and library and wrote the first important herbal, entitled *Enquiry into Plants*, to survive until the present day. He listed 500 healing plants and described the properties of oils and spices, basing much of his work on Aristotle's botanical writings, which expanded much of Hippocrates' work. The Alexandrian school was also a great source of herbal knowledge at this time that enabled Greek medicine to flourish, drawing on Egyptian, Sumerian and Assyrian healing traditions as well as Greek, and included knowledge brought back from campaigns in Asia. These strong traditions survived into medieval Europe through the writers and scholars of the Arab world.

Galen (c.131–200 CE), another notable Greek physician, studied at the school and later became renowned as surgeon to the gladiators in Rome, and personal physician to the Emperor Marcus Aurelius (121–180 CE). In his herbal *De Simplicibus* he expanded on Hippocrates' philosophy and classification of herbs into the four humours, and his works became the standard medical texts of Rome and later of the Arab physicians and medieval monks. His theories are still clearly to be found in Unani Tibb medicine today (see pages 16–19).

Pedanius Dioscorides was a Greek physician serving with the Roman army during the reign of Emperor Nero, which allowed him to travel extensively in Asia Minor. Around 60 CE he set himself the enormous task of collating all the current knowledge on medicinal plants and healing substances in one work: *De Materia Medica*. It included discussion of the components of perfumes and their medicinal properties, and aromatic herbs used for these included Lemon balm, Basil, Coriander, Fennel, Garlic, Hyssop, Marjoram, Mint, Myrtle, Rosemary and Violet. His famous herbal provided the major source of herbal knowledge for all the herbals that followed for the next 1,500 years, and has been copied and quoted to the present day.

Continuing legacy

Under the Romans, the Catholic papacy grew more powerful and the early Christians, feeling that the Church rather than the physicians should be responsible for the health of mind and soul, started to repress the use of many 'pagan' herbs. In 529 CE Pope Gregory the Great ruled that learning that was not in accordance with the political ambitions of the papacy should be forbidden. Thus, during the Dark Ages (c.200–800 CE), knowledge of herbs and the use of the great herbals was pushed underground and scientific research and writing across Europe came to a halt.

However, the highly sophisticated Arab culture of the time maintained and developed the healing legacy of the Greeks, merging it with their ancient folk medicine and surviving Egyptian tradition. By 900 CE all the Greek herbal and botanical texts that had survived had been translated into Arabic in the cultural centres of Cairo, Damascus and Baghdad. When Arab armies invaded North Africa and Spain, they took with them their knowledge of healing plants and medicine. In Spain, particularly in Cordoba, schools of medicine were established that kept alive the Greek and Arabic medical traditions in the medieval period, spreading the teachings throughout the continent of Europe. Indeed, as late as the 18th century, the standard textbook in use in medical schools across Europe – *Avicenna Canon Medicinae*, or *The Canon of Medicine* – was a fusion of ancient Greek, Arabic and Indian systems of medicine and herbal healing.

The knowledge preserved by the Arabic schools continues into today's practice of healing. One can see the influence of humoral theory, for example, in various different modern philosophies. The Austrian philosopher Rudolf Steiner (1861–1925) derived many of his ideas of Anthroposophical medicine from Graeco-Arabic healing traditions. He introduced the notion of four temperaments related to the dominance of one or other of the four levels of the self: choleric with the ego; sanguine with the astral body; phlegmatic with the etheric body; and melancholic with the physical body. The personality types described by psychologist Hans Eysenck (1916–1997) – basically extrovert and introvert – are also divided into four different types resembling the influence of the humours. According to Eysenck's theory, introverted types tend to be melancholic and phlegmatic; extroverts choleric and sanguine. Modern professional herbalists might call on the four temperaments or a type of personality analysis when assessing a patient and choosing a course of treatment.

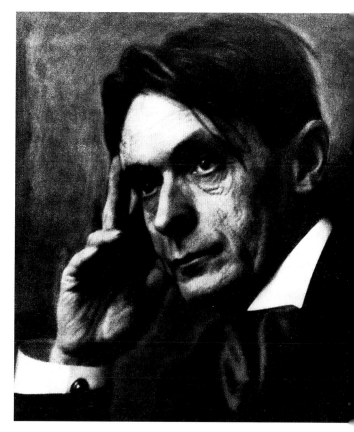

Rudolf Steiner drew on the notion of humours when developing his philosophy known as Anthroposophy.

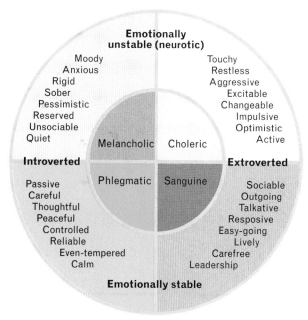

Emotionally unstable (neurotic)

Moody
Anxious
Rigid
Sober
Pessimistic
Reserved
Unsociable
Quiet

Touchy
Restless
Aggressive
Excitable
Changeable
Impulsive
Optimistic
Active

Introverted

Melancholic   Choleric

Extroverted

Passive
Careful
Thoughtful
Peaceful
Controlled
Reliable
Even-tempered
Calm

Phlegmatic   Sanguine

Sociable
Outgoing
Talkative
Resposive
Easy-going
Lively
Carefree
Leadership

Emotionally stable

Steiner's theory of temperaments divides personalities into four types and explains how each relates to others and the world.

Unani Tibb

Between the 9th and 13th centuries, Graeco-Roman medicine from Hippocrates and Galen was assimilated by the Arabs and an Arabic tradition of medicine known as Unani Tibb developed. The word *Unani*, meaning 'Ionian', reflects the strong Greek influence in this tradition, while *tibb* means 'knowledge of the states of the human body in health and disease' – medicine.

A succession of renowned Arab physicians, including Albucasis, Razis and Ibn Sina (known as Avicenna), were particularly responsible for the development of medicine at this time, adding their own inventions and discoveries to the sum of herbal and botanical knowledge. Avicenna (980–1037 CE) brought together all the information that was available on the nature of disease, plant medicines, aromatics and medical theories, including the teachings of Susruta and Charaka from the Ayurvedic tradition (see pages 22–25), in his *Canon Medicinae*. He developed the process of distillation, originated in the Alexandrian school around the 3rd century CE, inventing the apparatus and method of alembic distillation to extract essential oils from aromatic plants – a great landmark in the history of aromatherapy (see pages 32–33). Fragrant oils were used particularly for their purifying and restorative properties at this time and were thought to reduce the impact of destructive emotions such as grief and fear on the health of the body.

Practice in India and beyond

When the Mongols invaded Persia and Central Asia, many scholars and physicians of Unani fled to India. Once established in India, Unani suffered setbacks under British rule, although it continued to flourish unofficially. In the ensuing struggle against British colonialism, a friend of Mahatma Gandhi, Muhammad Ajmal Khan, founded the Unani Tibb and Ayurvedic College in Delhi in 1916. Unani is currently practised in Bangladesh, Pakistan, Sri Lanka, Iran, China, Afghanistan and other parts of the Middle East. In India there are many Unani medical colleges, where, after a five and a half year course, graduates are awarded a BUMS (Bachelor of Unani Medicine and Surgery) degree and can practise as government-approved doctors. Some ten Unani medical colleges award postgraduate degrees, and there are schools in Australia and the USA. The American Institute of Unani Medicine was founded in 1986.

The seven components

According to Unani, the human body is composed of seven components called Umoor e Tabaiyah, which are responsible for the maintenance of health. Changes to any of these can predispose to imbalance and disease, and each needs to be taken into consideration in diagnosis and assessment of the correct treatment. These are:
- arkan (elements)
- mizaj (temperament)
- akhlaat (humours)
- aaza (organs)
- arwah (vital forces)
- quwa (faculties)
- afaal (functions)

The balance of a person's constitution can be impaired by emotional, psychological, social, environmental or spiritual factors, or by diet. The environmental and lifestyle factors that are vital to good health in Unani Tibb are divided into five categories: fresh air, food and drink, movement and rest, sleep, and emotions. An imbalance in any of these five categories leads to disturbance of the humours, causing ill health.

The four humours

The four elements, known as Anasir-e-Arba, are earth (hava), water (pani), fire (mitti) and air (dhup). In varying combinations, these four elements constitute the four bodily humours (akhlaat):
- blood (dam)
- phlegm (kafa)
- bile (safra)
- black bile (souda)

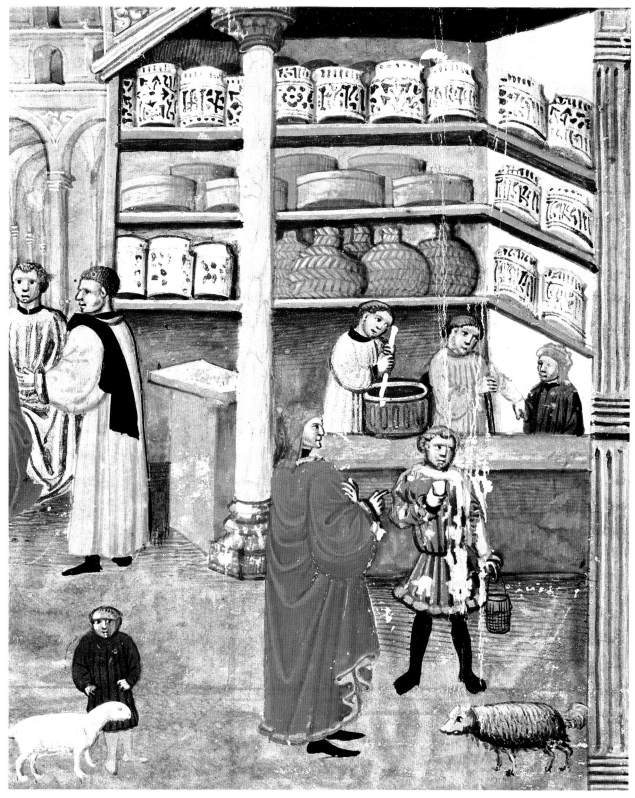

A pharmacy from the pages of *Canon Medicinae*. Finished in
1025, the 14 volumes were published in Latin, Hebrew and Arabic.

The humours originate in the liver from digested nutrients and are carried around the body in the blood. Each person's unique balance of these substances determines his or her temperament or mizaj (individual metabolic constitution): a predominance of blood gives a sanguine temperament; a predominance of phlegm makes one phlegmatic; yellow bile, bilious (or choleric); and black bile, melancholic. As long as these humours are in balance, the human system is healthy; it is imbalance in the humours that leads to ill health and disease. Each individual has his or own innate healing mechanisms, akin to ojas in Ayurveda and known in Unani as the Tabiyat-e-Muddabare Badan, which is considered the best physician, and it is this that maintains the equilibrium of the four humours, or akhlaat, and helps ensure health and a happy state of mind, which is our birthright.

Disciplines and diagnosis

There are ten branches of Unani medicine, resembling those in the Ayurvedic system:

- internal medicine (moalijat)
- gynaecology, including obstetrics and paediatrics
- diseases of the head and neck
- toxicology
- psychiatry
- rejuvenation therapy, including geriatrics
- sexology
- regimental therapy
- dietotherapy
- hydrotherapy

The diagnostic skills of practitioners of Unani, known as hakims, include observation, pulse taking, questioning, palpation and urine analysis. Pulse diagnosis requires the hakims to be in a clear state of spiritual awareness to enable them to analyse the subtle qualities of the pulse. Practices including breathing and voice exercises and visualizations are recommended to help to calm and clear the mind. In the initial consultation, the practitioner will take a detailed case history from the patient and make observations of the patient's skin, tongue, eyes, hands and nails. The practitioner will also take the patient's pulse, as an enormous amount of information can be gleaned from this in just minutes. Unani classifies health in three different stages: health, disease and neutral. Neutral exists between health and disease when symptoms have not yet manifested. Disease occurs when the functions associated with the vital, natural and psychic forces of the body are obstructed or unbalanced due to some form of deviation.

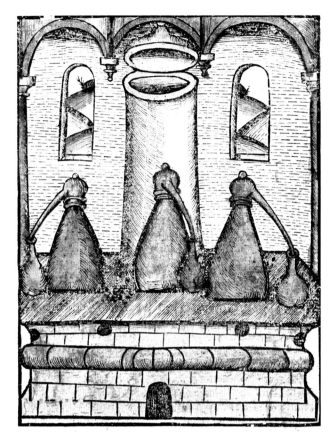

Alembic distillation was perfected by Arab physicians to extract oil from plants.

Symptoms of illness are seen in a positive light as an opportunity to cleanse and balance us on a physical, emotional and mental as well as spiritual level. Experiencing pain, for example, is viewed as a message that something is wrong, the underlying causes of which need to be addressed so that a person's health can be better in the future. A 'healing crisis' is simply 'tabiyat', or the homeostatic mechanisms of the body attempting to eliminate toxins through vomiting, diarrhoea, fevers, sweating and increased urination in order to re-establish equilibrium of the humours, and thus restore health and general wellbeing.

Treatment

Healers in the Unani Tibb tradition follow strict ethical codes of conduct and practice based on Islam. This includes earning the respect of their patients, proper cleansing routines, moderation in their intake of food and drink and spiritual purification techniques. As in Ayurvedic and Tibetan medicine, prevention and treatment of health problems is based on each person's body type, personality and mizaj or individual metabolic

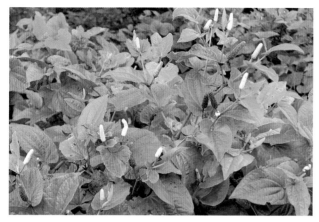

Long pepper might be included by Unani healers in herbal remedies to treat gastric problems and strengthen digestion.

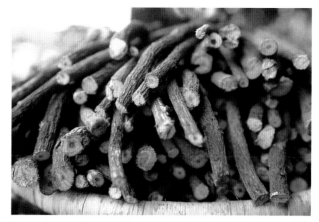

Liquorice root is classified as dry in the first degree (very mild) and hot in the second degree (relatively mild).

constitution. It is aimed at rebalancing the patient physically, emotionally, mentally and spiritually, and is largely based on lifestyle advice, including advocating bathing, fresh air, fresh food and codes of conduct to promote and maintain health. Hakims also prescribe herbs, precious metals and stones (gold, silver, gems and pearls), detoxification and dietary regimes, minerals and aromatherapy. Oils or attars extracted from herbs are given singly or in combinations, according to the needs of the patient, to affect body, mind and emotions. Some of the herbs, such as Saffron, Fennel, Caraway, *Terminalia chebula*, *Terminalia bellerica* and Amalaki/Indian gooseberry, are also used in the Ayurvedic and Tibetan medical traditions. Other herbs used in the Unani tradition include Guggulu, Ashwagandha, Coriander, Bacopa, Sweet violet, Liquorice, Long pepper and Guduchi. Massage or cold/heat suction cups might be used, as well as puncturing certain reflex points to release a few drops of blood in acute disease.

Food and taste

Foods and herbs are categorized according to their own miza, or balance of the humours and elements. Appropriate treatments are prescribed to suit imbalances of a patient's constitution, and these vary from one person to another. Substances in foods and herbs are also classified according to whether their therapeutic effects are mild (which can be used by anyone), moderate or powerful (including potential poisons and for use only by hakims). Qualities of hot and cold, wet and dry are also attributed to physical conditions, foods and herbs. In common with Chinese, Tibetan and Ayurvedic medical systems, Unani Tibb emphasizes the importance of tastes as well as the manner in which food is prepared to adjust the imbalances that contribute to ill health. There are five

tastes: salty, sweet, bitter, pungent and sour, each of which affect the humours in its own way. In addition, appropriate warming and cooling spices and herbs are added to cooking to help address underlying imbalances of the humours. Even the aromas from preparing, cooking, eating and digesting food contribute to the healing benefit and are taken into consideration in planning meals. Cooking and eating are seen as rituals that, if containing the right foods and herbs and practised with a pure heart, good intent and clear focus, can help transform the energy of the meal and contribute to the healing process.

HERBS COMMONLY USED IN UNANI TIBB

Marshmallow *(see page 105)*
Senna *(see page 118)*
Cinnamon *(see page 120)*
Coriander *(see page 123)*
Cardamom *(see page 127)*
Amalaki *(see page 128)*
Fennel *(see page 131)*
Liquorice *(see page 135)*
Peppermint *(see page 144)*
Long pepper *(see page 150)*
Sweet violet *(see page 171)*
Ginger *(see page 175)*

Tibetan medicine

Tibetan medicine is a highly evolved system that developed as a synthesis of medical knowledge and wisdom from Indian Ayurveda, Traditional Chinese Medicine, Greek medicine and Unani Tibb, the origins of which can be traced back to at least the 7th century. It is deeply rooted in Buddhist philosophy, which was also introduced over 2,000 years ago, and views physical illness as being inextricably bound up with mental, social and spiritual illness.

Sangye Menla, the 'Medicine Buddha', is respected as the source of medical teachings and the inspiration for correct practice as a physician. Tibetan medicine has developed into a sophisticated and complex medical science with intricate theories about causes of disease, diagnosis and therapeutics, and has existed in its present form for over a thousand years. The essential aspects of this teaching are summarized in the *rGyud-Bzhi* (pronounced *giu shi*) or the *Four Medical Tantras*, the 12th-century text in four volumes, which is still taught today. The Tibetan system of healing, known as Sowa Rigpa or the Knowledge of Healing, is practised in Tibet, India, Nepal, Bhutan, Sikkim, Ladakh, Siberia, China, Russia and Mongolia, and in Europe and the USA.

The three humours

Like other Asian systems of medicine, Tibetan medicine is based on the principle that everything in the cosmos, including human beings, is composed of five elements: earth, water, fire, wind and space. These are symbols for matter, energy, cohesion, movement and space, which affect the mind as well as the body. The universe and the body are a result of the interplay of these five elements, which manifest themselves in the form of energy into three different humours or energies, each of which is further divided into five sub-categories, with different locations and functions:

Wind (rLung, pronounced *long*) is vital for movement, responsible for breathing, circulation of bodily fluids including blood and lymph, and mental activity such as thinking, speech, energy and transfer of nerve impulses.

Bile (mKhrispa, pronounced *tripa*) is heating energy that regulates digestion, metabolism and liver function, and maintains body temperature and the discriminating mind.

Phlegm (Badkan, pronounced *beken*) governs the structure of the physical body, such as bone, muscle and mucous membranes. It is responsible for some aspects of digestion, the maintenance of our physical structure, joint health and mental stability.

Health depends on the equilibrium of the humours, so disease is likely to develop when they are out of balance. The three energies are present in different proportions in each person and determine his or her constitution, including his or her body shape, temperament and susceptibility to specific health problems.

Balancing the humours

Another important concept in Tibetan medicine is the dichotomy between warm and cold. Diseases as well as remedies and food are distinguished as warm and cold or as warming and cooling respectively; mKhrispa is warm and Badkan is cool. rLung is a special case and is basically neutral; it can aggravate warm and cold, much like wind is able to boost a fire as well as cool down the body. A rLung imbalance is at the root of most diseases.

An understanding of physiology is governed by the dynamic interaction of the three humours (rLung, mKhrispa and Badkan). Health is a dynamic equilibrium and is therefore relative because all three humours must be in a corresponding balance for each individual.

Diagnosis and treatment

As in Ayurveda and Unani medicine, the balance of the humours determines the constitution of each individual, and this is influenced by a person's external and internal environment, including diet, lifestyle, relationships and his or her internal emotional, mental and spiritual state. The dynamic equilibrium of the humours also changes with the climate, seasons and age. In Buddhist thought,

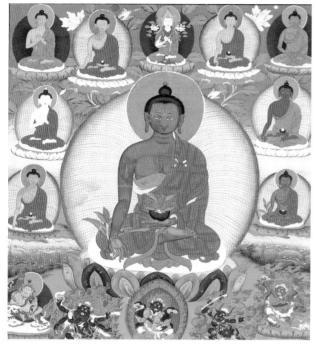

This thangka painting (c.1780–1880) depicts Sangye Menla with nine other Medicine Buddhas.

all physical and mental suffering, and hence all illness, is caused by the three mental poisons: attachment, anger and ignorance, as well as the effect of past karma. The importance of compassion in healing is stressed.

Diagnosis of imbalance and disease involves observation and an in-depth interview with the patient, taking the pulse and examining the tongue as well as urine and faeces. Once the imbalance of the humours has been ascertained, treatment specific to the individual is designed to re-establish mental harmony and equilibrium of the three humours. This can include advice on lifestyle, exercise, conduct and behaviour, healing of the mind through mantras and meditation, yoga, moxibustion (burning Mugwort), herbs, vegetable and mineral supplements, massage and inhalations with specially formulated herbal oils, bathing, cupping and occasionally acupuncture. Foods and herbs all comprise their own individual balance of the five elements and three humours, so diets appropriate to each patient and the balance of the humours are suggested.

Herbal medicines

If dietary and behavioural changes are not sufficient to remedy the condition, herbs are prescribed. The Tibetan materia medica consists largely of medicinal herbs and includes minerals and, to a lesser extent, animal substances. As in Ayurveda, medicinal substances are grouped according to their properties, their taste (sweet, sour, salty, bitter, pungent and astringent) and potency (heavy/light, oily/rough, hot/cold and blunt/sharp), and the effect of these on the humours. Tibetan medicines are generally composed of 20 or more different ingredients, including one major group of ingredients and two minor ones aimed at supporting the major group and preventing unwanted side effects. Herbs that are used in the Tibetan tradition include Amalaki/Indian gooseberry, Rose, Marigold, Nettle, Coriander, Cinnamon, Cardamom, Ginger, Garlic, Rhodiola, Gentian, Liquorice and Nutmeg. Medicines are considered to be offerings to the Medicine Buddha and other medicine deities, and are prepared with spiritual rituals by traditional methods of drying, grinding, mixing and pressing the plants to make pills, powders or decoctions.

The annexation of Tibet by the People's Republic of China in the 1950s had a great impact on Tibetan medicine. Despite the fact that practitioners have suffered great persecution and clinical practice, study and research has been largely censored by the Chinese, particularly during the Cultural Revolution, Tibetan medicine has survived almost intact. His Holiness the 14th Dalai Lama, living in exile in Dharamsala, has been a powerful influence in Tibetan medicine. In 1961 he founded the Men-Tsee-Khang, the Tibetan Medical and Astrological Institute (TMAI), which has a college of Tibetan medicine, a clinic and a pharmacy that produces and dispenses medicines, and carries out research and the publication of medical and astrological texts.

HERBS COMMONLY USED IN TIBETAN MEDICINE

Garlic (see page 104)
Marigold (see page 116)
Cinnamon (see page 120)
Coriander (see page 123)
Cardamom (see page 127)
Amalaki (see page 128)
Gentian (see page 134)
Liquorice (see page 135)
Nutmeg (see page 145)
Rhodiola (see page 152)
Rose (see page 153)
Nettle (see page 167)
Ginger (see page 175)

Ayurvedic medicine

The name 'Ayurveda' derives from two Sanskrit words: *ayur*, meaning 'life', and *veda*, meaning 'knowledge' or 'science'. Ayurveda is more than just a system of medicine; it is a way of life encompassing science, religion and philosophy that enhances wellbeing, increases longevity and ultimately enables self-realization. It aims to bring about a union of physical, emotional and spiritual health, or swasthya, which is a prerequisite for attaining moksha, or liberation.

Ayurveda is thought to be the oldest healthcare system in the world, with its roots stretching back over 5,000 years into the Vedic Age. It evolved on the far reaches of the Himalayas out of the deep wisdom of spiritually enlightened prophets, or rishis. Their wisdom was transmitted orally from teacher to disciple and eventually set down in the books of Sanskrit poetry known as the Vedas. These writings, dating from c.1500 BCE, distilled the prevailing historical, religious, philosophical and medical knowledge, and form the basis of Indian culture. The most important of these texts

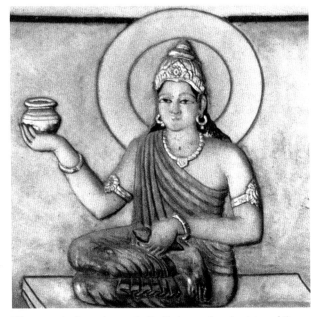

Dhanwantari was known in the Vedas as the physician of the gods and the patron saint of Ayurveda.

are the *Rig Veda* and the *Atharva Veda*. Ayurveda has survived largely as an oral tradition until the present day, one of its greatest values being its timelessness. It has as much to teach us now about every facet of contemporary everyday life as it had in its beginnings, all those centuries ago.

Ayurveda has had a strong influence on many systems of medicine, from ancient Greek medicine in the West to Traditional Chinese Medicine in the East. The Chinese, Tibetan and Islamic (Unani Tibb) systems of medicine are thought to have their roots in Ayurveda. The Buddha, who was born c.550 BCE, was a follower of Ayurveda, and the spread of Buddhism into Tibet during the following centuries was accompanied by the increased practice of Ayurveda. The ancient civilizations were linked to one another by trade routes, campaigns and wars. Arab traders spread knowledge of Indian plants in their materia medicas, and this knowledge was passed on to the ancient Greeks and Romans, whose practices were eventually to form the basis of European medicine, as taught in the medical schools of medieval Europe.

The first Ayurvedic medical school was founded c.800 BCE by Punarvasu Atreya. He and his pupils recorded medical knowledge in treatises that would in turn influence Charaka, a scholar who lived and taught c.700 BCE. His writings in the *Charaka Samhita* describe 1,500 plants, identifying 350 as valuable medicines. This major work is considered the main authority of Ayurveda to this day and the text is referred to constantly in both the teaching and practice of contemporary Ayurveda. The second major work of Charaka was the *Susruta Samhita*, written a century later, which forms the basis of modern surgery and is still consulted today. It sets out the medicinal properties of 700 healing plants.

The five elements

According to Ayurveda, the origin of all aspects of existence is the field of pure intellect or consciousness, known as purusha, and this appeals to those influenced by the theories of modern quantum physics that locate the basis of the physical universe in a single unified field that directs and orchestrates the continuous flow of matter. Energy and matter are one. Ayurveda does not separate the external world from the inner world. Everything that exists in the macrocosm has its counterpart in the microcosm of the inner universe of the human being. Cosmic energy manifests in the five elements, which are the basis of all matter: ether, air, fire, water and earth. In the body, ether is present in the spaces such as the mouth, abdomen, thorax, capillaries and cells. The movement of space is air, manifest in movements of, for example, the muscles, pulsations of the heart, peristalsis of the digestive tract and nervous impulses. Fire is present in the digestive system, governing enzyme systems and metabolism, as well as body temperature, vision and the light of the mind – intelligence. Water is present in secretions like the digestive juices, saliva, mucus, plasma and cytoplasm. Earth is responsible for the solid structures holding the body together: bones, cartilage, muscles and tendons, as well as skin, hair and nails.

The five elements manifest in the functioning of the five senses, and these in turn enable us to perceive and interact with the environment in which we live. Ether, air, fire, water and earth correspond to hearing, touch, vision, taste and smell respectively.

The three doshas

From the five elements derive three basic forces, the tridoshas, which exist in everything and influence all mental and physical processes. Vata, the air principle, is created from ether and air; pitta, the fire principle, from fire and water; and kapha, the water principle, from earth and water. The balance of the doshas in each person is believed to promote health and wellbeing, while imbalance leads to ill health and disease. According to Ayurveda, everyone is born with a certain balance of doshas brought about mainly by the dosha balance in their parents at the time of conception. This constitutes a person's basic constitution (prakruti), which remains unchanged throughout their lives. The dominant dosha largely determines body type, temperament and illness to which an individual may be susceptible. A person's vikruti, or present dosha balance, reflects the effect that lifestyle has on prakruti to cause imbalances that predispose them to ill health.

Diagnosis and treatment

The first requirement for health in Ayurveda is proper balance of the doshas according to the person's prakruti. If the balance is disturbed by diet, lifestyle or state of mind, for example, illness (vyadhi) of one kind or another eventually results. The disruption may be felt in physical discomfort and pain, or in mental and emotional suffering such as fear, anxiety, anger or jealousy. The current state of imbalance causing such symptoms to manifest is known as vikruti.

Both prakruti and vikruti can be ascertained by careful diagnosis, which involves taking a detailed case history and examining the body, paying attention to build, skin and hair type, temperature of the body, digestion and bowel function, all of which point to more profound aspects of the patient's condition. Pulse and tongue diagnoses are exceptionally valuable tools for confirming analysis of health and constitution. In these respects Ayurveda has much in common with Chinese and Tibetan medicine, in which these two indicators of the state of health are also of the greatest importance. A highly complex technique for taking the patient's pulse has been developed by Ayurvedic practitioners, which requires many years of practice to perfect.

Once the dosha balance has been diagnosed and the causes of imbalance have been established, treatment and lifestyle advice are given. The first step back to health is the elimination of toxins and enhancing digestion or raising digestive fire, or agni. Treatments fall into three

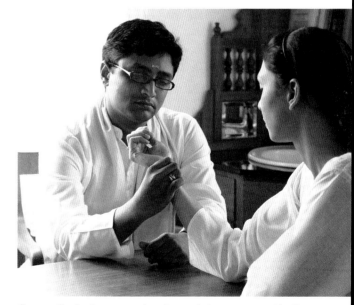

Ayurvedic doctors use pulse diagnosis to assess a patient's constitution and his or her present state of health.

main categories: natural medicines, dietary regimes and lifestyle changes. These are all classified according to their effect on the three doshas. To illustrate, a health problem associated with excess kapha could be characterized by catarrh, lethargy, overweight and fluid retention. A diet consisting of warm, dry, light food would be advised, since kapha is cool and damp. Avoidance of foods with a cold, damp quality, such as wheat and milk products and sugar, which tend to increase kapha, would also be recommended. Herbal remedies would include warming spices such as Ginger, Cinnamon, Cloves and Pepper to raise digestive fire and cleanse toxins from the body. Bitters such as Turmeric and Aloe vera may also be prescribed. The specific choice of herbal remedy depends on its 'quality' or 'energy', which Ayurveda determines according to 20 attributes, or vimshati gunas, such as hot, cold, wet, dry, heavy or light. Ayurveda also classifies remedies according to six tastes: sweet, sour, salty, pungent, bitter and astringent. Sweet, sour and salty substances increase kapha and decrease vata; pungent, bitter and astringent tastes decrease kapha and increase vata; sweet, bitter and astringent tastes decrease pitta; and pungent, salty and sour tastes increase pitta. Herbs from the Ayurvedic tradition include Amalaki, Shatavari, Ashwagandha, Bacopa, Guduchi, Brahmi, Long pepper, Holy basil, Ginger, Cumin, Fenugreek, Gymnema, Bhringaraj, Guggulu, Cinnamon, Coriander, Andrographis, Aloe vera, Neem, Frankincense and Turmeric.

Herbal remedies are prepared in varying mediums according to the predominant dosha being treated. Herbs used to balance vata are often given in warm milk, those for reducing pitta in ghee and those to reduce kapha are prepared in honey or hot water.

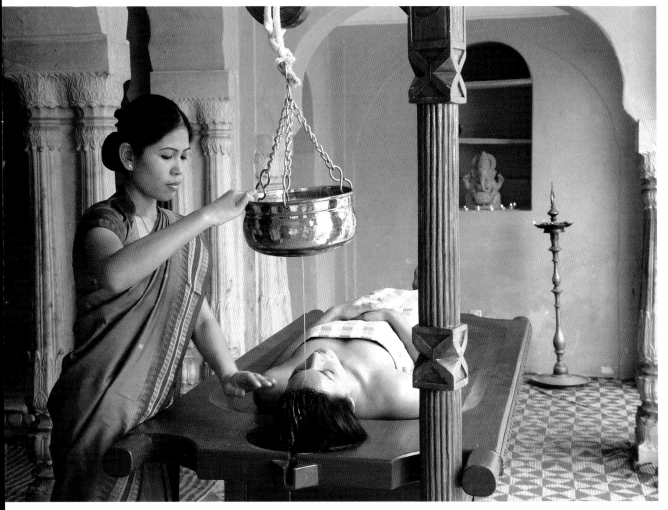

Panchakarma treatment includes *shirodhara*, the continual pouring of warm herb-infused oil onto the forehead.

Sometimes minute doses of minerals such as salt are also mixed with the herbs. Other formulae take the form of pills, powders, decoctions and alcohol extracts, and most contain several ingredients, all carefully tailored to individual needs.

Panchakarma, a thorough cleansing and rejuvenation programme, is available in treatment centres particularly in southern India and Sri Lanka, as well as in Europe and the USA. It includes the use of oil massage, sweating, therapeutic vomiting, purging, enemas, nasal administration of medicine and purification of blood.

Ayurveda today

The value of Ayurveda is proved partly by its timelessness, since it has existed as an unbroken tradition for thousands of years, despite a number of setbacks. Following the rise of the Mogul Empire in the 16th century, the dominance of Unani Tibb medicine led to the partial repression of Ayurveda in India. In the 19th century, the British dismissed it as nothing more than native superstition and in 1833 they closed all Ayurvedic schools and banned the practice of Ayurveda altogether. Great centres of Indian learning thus fell apart and Ayurvedic knowledge retreated into the villages and temples. At the turn of the century, however, some Indian physicians and enlightened Englishmen began to re-evaluate Ayurveda, and by the time India became independent in 1947 it had regained its reputation as a valid healing system. Today in India, Ayurveda flourishes alongside Unani Tibb and Western allopathic medicine, and is actively encouraged by the Indian government as an inexpensive alternative to Western drugs.

In recent years Ayurveda has increasingly attracted attention from medical scientists in Japan and the West, and the World Health Organization has resolved to promote its practice in developing countries. In the West the popularity of Ayurveda is growing daily as more and more people recognize its value. Westerners are not drawn to Ayurveda simply as a form of treatment for a specific health condition. Many people first encounter this system of healing in one of the many spas around the world that have embraced Ayurvedic detoxification or rejuvenation techniques. Others may start to investigate its principles following a period of yoga practice or spiritual study. Practitioners and patients worldwide understand that Ayurveda provides immense value not only in the prevention and treatment of disease but also in its comprehensive recipe for a better, healthier way of life that addresses all facets of our existence – mind, body and spirit.

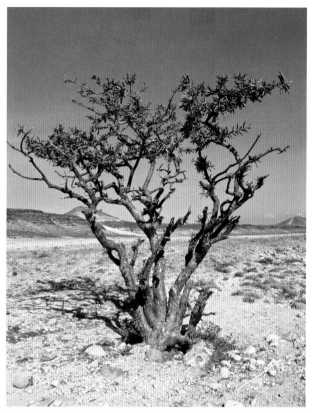

Frankincense The gum resin of this tree is used in Ayurveda to cleanse the heart and blood, and nourish the nerves.

HERBS COMMONLY USED IN AYURVEDA

Andrographis *(see page 105)*
Dill *(see page 106)*
Shatavari *(see page 111)*
Neem *(see page 113)*
Brahmi *(see page 113)*
Frankincense *(see page 116)*
Forskohlii *(see page 121)*
Myrrh *(see page 122)*
Guggulu *(see page 122)*
Bhringaraj *(see page 126)*
Amalaki *(see page 128)*
Gymnema *(see page 136)*
Holy basil *(see page 146)*
Long pepper *(see page 150)*
Fenugreek *(see page 164)*
Ashwagandha *(see page 174)*

Traditional Chinese Medicine

Traditional Chinese Medicine is a system of healing as ancient as Ayurveda that can be traced back to *c*.2500 BCE and includes oriental traditions of South East Asia that originally came from China. The first, perhaps mythical Chinese herbalist was Shennong, who imparted his knowledge of hundreds of medicinal and poisonous plants to farmers.

The first major text, the *Shen Nong Bencao Jing* (*The Yellow Emperor's Classic of Materia Medica*), dating from *c*.1000 BCE in the Han dynasty, describes 365 medicines, over 250 of which are herbs, their physical actions and applications. Later additions to herbal knowledge followed the style and format of the *Shen Nong*, placing emphasis on the herb's taste, its heating or cooling nature, which organs and meridians it primarily affects, dosage ranges, degree of toxicity and overall effects of the herb on specific patterns of symptoms. The *Shen Nong* divided medicines into three categories: superior herbs that are the main remedies for returning the body and mind to health; middle-level tonic herbs that boost energy and immunity; and low-level, more powerful herbs that should be taken only in small doses for specific symptoms. The *Bencao Gangmu* (*Compendium of Materia Medica*) was compiled in the 16th century during the Ming dynasty by Li Shizhen, and lists all the plants,

animals and minerals used in Chinese medicine at the time. It includes herbs that are still used, including Opium, Ephedrine, Rhubarb and Iron, and is still a major reference book today.

Traditional Chinese Medicine today

As in Ayurvedic medicine, these early texts are still studied and their precepts adhered to by modern practitioners of Traditional Chinese Medicine. At the same time, Traditional Chinese Medicine has continually been developed and refined in response to cultural and clinical advances and ongoing research. It has survived through the rise and fall of several dynasties, and still exists happily in China alongside Western allopathic medicine, providing healthcare for the majority of the Chinese population. It continues to grow in popularity in the West, despite occasional bad press concerning the adverse effects of certain Chinese herbs.

The life force

The Chinese, like the Indians, regard the human body and all its functions as a microcosm of the macrocosm. All forms of life are seen to be animated by the same essential life force, called 'qi' or 'chi'. By breathing we take in qi from the air and pass it into the lungs, and by digesting we extract qi from food and drink and pass it into the body. When these qi meet in the bloodstream, they become known as human qi, which circulates around the body as vital energy. The quality, quantity and balance of qi in each person influences their state of health and lifespan, and this in turn is affected by factors such as the season, climate, lifestyle, diet and air breathed. Wind, dampness, dryness, heat and cold can derange the internal balance of the body, obstructing the movement of qi in the organs. Disturbance of internal wind causes vertigo, unsteady movement and trembling;

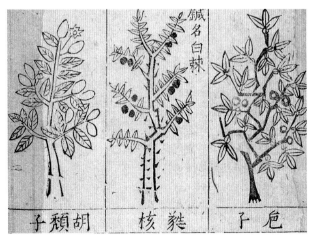

Bencao Gangmu This 16th-century pharmaceutical encyclopedia features 1,892 medicinal substances.

dampness causes increased phlegm and oedema; dryness causes drying of the mucous membranes; cold decreases circulation and slows metabolism; and excess heat leads to inflammation.

Qi flows through a network of channels, or meridians, throughout the body and can be stimulated and balanced using acupuncture, acupressure, diet and herbal medicine. The body is also composed of moisture, which is the fluid in the body that protects, nurtures and lubricates the tissues and blood – the basic material from which bone, muscle, nerves, organs and skin are made. For the body to be healthy, adequate qi, moisture and blood need to circulate within a network of channels that connects all parts of the body. Forms of illness are regarded as a result of either depletion or congestion of qi, moisture and blood. This may be caused by an unhealthy diet and lifestyle, stress, tension, overwork, lack of exercise and so on, all of which impair the ability of the organ networks to function properly.

Yin and yang

The principles of Traditional Chinese Medicine originate in traditional Taoist philosophy, China's most ancient school of thought. Central to this philosophy is the idea of fluctuation and mutability, explaining natural phenomena in terms of the constant ebb and flow of cosmic forces. Yin and yang, the two primordial cosmic forces, are concepts that are familiar to many. Yin symbolizes a passive yielding force that is cold, dark, negative, contractive and female, represented by water. Yang is active, positive, hot, light, expansive and male, symbolized by fire. The constant interplay between these opposite and mutually dependent forces produces all the change and movement in the universe. Different parts of the body are described as predominantly yin or yang. Yin is found in the internal, lower and front part of the body, body fluids and blood, and governs innate instincts, while yang governs qi, vital energy and learned skills, and presides in the upper, external and back parts of the body. To maintain health, yin and yang need to be in balance.

The five elements

As in Ayurveda, the theory of the five elements is vital to the Traditional Chinese Medicine understanding of life in all its variety. Wood, fire, earth, metal and water are the elements that compose and relate to all aspects of life, including parts of the body, vital organs, emotions, seasons, colours and tastes. For example, wood relates to spring, the colour green, the liver and gall bladder, anger and the sour taste, while fire corresponds to summer, the heart and small intestine, joy and bitter taste.

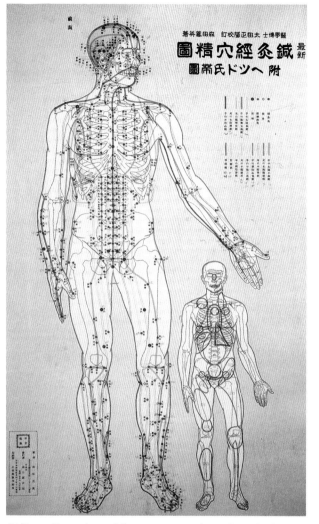

Qi flows through meridians, or energy channels, in the body; stimulating acupoints along them rebalances energy flow.

The constant interplay of the five elements along with that of yin and yang spark off all change and activity in nature. The fundamental relationships among the five elements are the key to understanding how our bodies and the environment interact and influence each other. To maintain good health the elements need to be in harmony, and if one element becomes over-dominant, imbalance and illness can result. Although the emphasis is on the internal causation of a disease, Traditional Chinese Medicine recognizes that outside factors play a role. A 2nd-century CE physician called Zhang Zhongjing wrote the *Treatise of Cold-Damage Disorders*, which described the diagnosis and treatment of diseases caused by external cold factors; in effect, this referred to infectious diseases.

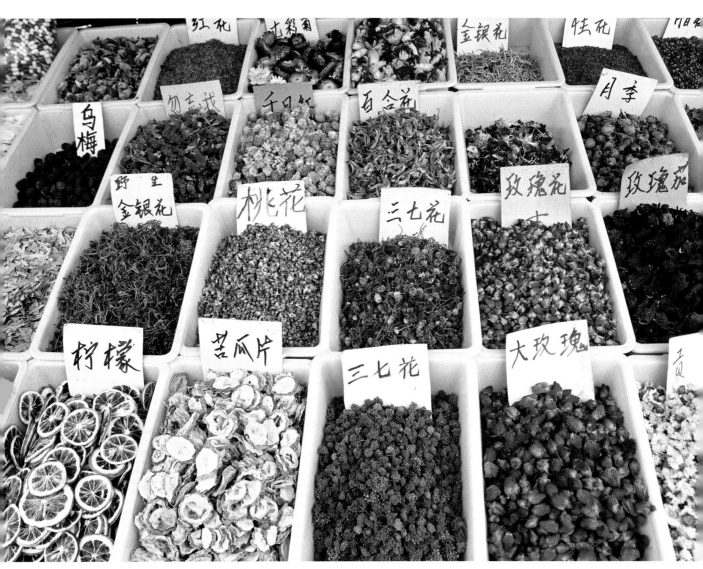

Chinese herbs are often used combined in formulae; synergy increases their therapeutic benefits.

The organ networks

The body is also divided into five functional systems called organ networks, which govern certain tissues and mental and physical activities by regulating and preserving qi, moisture, blood, spirit, or shen, and essence, or jing. The kidney network is responsible for fluid balance in the body and also stores the essence, or jing, which is responsible for fertility, growth and regeneration. Its province is the teeth, bones, marrow, brain, inner ear, pupil of the eye and the lower back; the emotion of fear; the will; and the ability to think and see things clearly. The heart network circulates blood; it is the home of the spirit, or shen, and governs the mind. The spleen network governs the digestion and assimilation of food and fluids, as well as the digestion of information and ideas. The liver network controls the storage of blood, the flow of qi and the stability of mood and temperament. The lung network governs breathing, circulation and the distribution of moisture.

Diagnosis and treatment

This involves taking a case history, including the patient's present and past complaints, lifestyle, physical environment, family health history, work, home and emotional life. It includes reading of the basic indicators of health and disease such as the complexion, lustre of the eyes and hair, and colour and texture of the tongue and its coating. Pulse and tongue diagnoses are the principal diagnostic tools of the practitioner of Traditional Chinese

Medicine and enable him or her to detect imbalances and ill health before they may show up on other modern diagnostic apparatus such as blood tests and x-rays

Treatment is aimed at harmonizing yin and yang, wet and dry, cold and heat, inner and outer and body and mind by regulating the qi, moisture and blood in the organ networks. It may combine herbs, diet, exercise and massage. Chinese herbs have been classified according to the four natures, the five tastes and the meridians. The four natures relate to the degrees of yin and yang: cold (extreme yin), cool, warm and hot (extreme yang). As in Tibetan and Unani medicine, herbs and foods are all composed of five tastes: pungent, sweet, sour, bitter and salty, each of which has different qualities and actions in the body. Pungent herbs increase the production of sweat and direct and increase qi and blood. Sweet herbs are nourishing and tonify, some acting as diuretics to drain dampness. Sour herbs are astringent, while bitter herbs clear heat and dampness, and salty herbs are used to stimulate the bowels and reduce hard masses. Herbs that nourish qi have an energizing effect, herbs to enrich the blood help sleep, vision and mood, while herbs to replenish moisture soften the skin and relieve thirst. The meridians relate to the organ networks that can be supported by herbs to do their work.

Herbs are usually combined in formulae to enhance their action either in the form of dried herbs for decoctions, ground and produced as pills and powders or used in liquid extracts. Some practitioners use patent formulae in the form of pills, which are certainly easier and more convenient for the patient than boiling up herbs in decoctions, but do not allow for individualized remedies that practitioners can formulate themselves in response to the specific needs of each patient. Herbs used in Traditional Chinese Medicine include Codonopsis, Astragalus, Liquorice, Ginger, Chinese angelica, Sweet Annie, Coriander, Honeysuckle, Peony, Polygonum, Rehmannia, Schisandra, Baikal skullcap and Selfheal.

Research into the medicinal properties of Chinese herbal remedies has led to some being adopted into Western medicine. For example, the drug artemisinin, used to treat drug-resistant malaria, has been derived from Chinese wormwood (Qing-hao). In China, traditional herbs have also been fused successfully with Western drugs – for instance, aspirin has been combined with *Gypsum fibrosum* to treat a form of arthritis.

HERBS COMMONLY USED IN TRADITIONAL CHINESE MEDICINE

Chinese angelica *(see page 107)*
Sweet Annie *(see page 110)*
Astragalus *(see page 112)*
Codonopsis *(see page 121)*
Honeysuckle *(see page 143)*
Peony *(see page 148)*
Polygonum *(see page 151)*
Selfheal *(see page 151)*
Rehmannia *(see page 152)*
Schisandra *(see page 156)*
Baikal skullcap *(see page 157)*

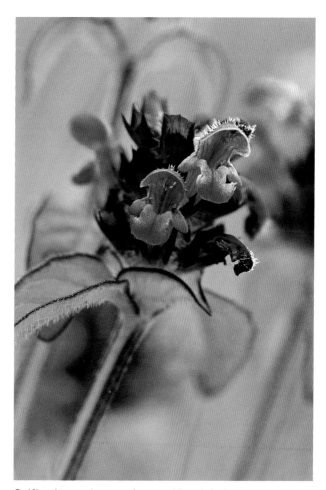

Selfheal is used to treat fever and liver imbalance and is also valued for accelerating wound-repair.

The healing tradition of North America

Native North American herbalism, like South American herbalism, was a shamanic tradition (see pages 11–12) – ritualistic dances, the playing of drums and rattles and the use of mind-altering plants such as Peyote and Datura enabled the shaman or medicine man or woman to enter a trance-like visionary state in order for him or her to communicate with the spirit world – including the Great Spirit (called Wakan Tanka in the language of the Lakota Sioux), which permeates everything like the notion of God – and the soul of the ill person to bring about healing.

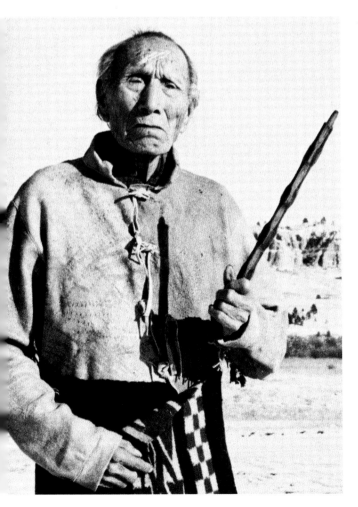

The medicine man or woman sought help from the Great Spirit for healing physical ills and troubles of the psyche, and to engender harmony within communities or between individuals. Plants were revered for their ability to cure not only diseases of the body but also imbalances in the mind, emotions and spirit. They were a vital part of the shamans' tradition and were used in ceremonies and rituals. Disease was considered to be caused by human, supernatural or natural causes and the medicine man or woman was called upon to administer herbs for anything from wounds and broken bones to unfulfilled dreams, spiritual intrusion and soul loss. The circle was an important part of ceremony for the Native North Americans, and according to Black Elk of the Teton Dakato, the 'Power of the World' always worked in circles. 'All our power came to us from the sacred loop of the nation', he reported, and his people flourished as long as the circle was unbroken. 'The flowering circle of the four quarters nourished it. The east gave peace and light, the south gave warmth, the west gave rain and the north with its cold and mighty wind gave strength and endurance.'

Physiomedicalism

A group of herbalists in 19th-century North America known as Physiomedicalists blended together the traditions of European herbalism brought to America by the Pilgrim Fathers with the herbal wisdom of the Native

Black Elk of the Teton Dakato is one of the most respected visionaries of Native American spiritual healing.

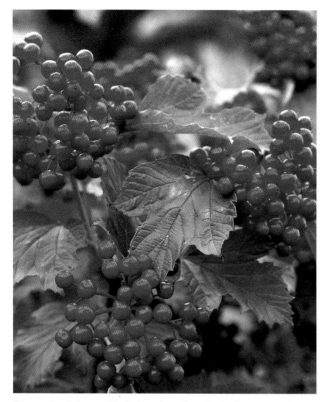

Cramp bark is used in Native American herbalism to treat nervous problems and cramp.

stomach of infection and diarrhoea to remove toxins from the bowel. This self-healing mechanism is called homeostasis in modern science.

Thomson also held that all bodies were composed of the four elements – earth, air, fire and water – and that good health derived from their harmonious interplay. Herbs were used primarily to maintain or correct this balance, and prescriptions were designed to do one of four things: astringe (tone) or relax; stimulate or sedate. Toning herbs include Shepherd's purse, Agrimony and Beth root; relaxing herbs include Cramp bark and Lemon balm; Ginger and Cayenne are stimulating; and Chamomile and Yellow jasmine are sedating.

Thomson's model of Physiomedicalism was followed in the USA by other botanic schools, notably the Eclectics founded by Dr Wooster Beech in the 1830s, who also combined Native American traditions with European knowledge as well as orthodox practices. Physiomedicalism was brought to England in 1838 by Dr Albert Coffin and Wooster Beech arrived in the 1850s to bring Eclectic medicine to Europe. Although Thomson's ideas met with enormous opposition from allopathic doctors in the USA, as the same ideas have in Europe until more recently, they are the same ideas that formed the basis of Hippocrates' Humoral medicine, and the vast systems of Chinese, Indian and Tibetan medicine.

North Americans. The herbs they used included Pleurisy root, Barberry, Black cohosh, Gravel root/Joe Pye weed, Boneset, Golden seal, Witch hazel, Poke root, Cramp bark and Black haw. The renowned founder of Physiomedicalism was Dr Samuel Thomson (1769–1843), who was the first to bring the Native American remedy Lobelia to the attention of the medical world. He kept alive traditional ideas of allowing the body to heal itself and helping to create the ideal conditions for this with the use of herbs. He mixed it with the knowledge he had gained by observation of the Native American medicine men, such as the value of sweating in clearing toxins from the body.

Thomson, like ancient as well as modern herbalists, recognized the presence of the vital force – the energy that flows throughout nature and animates all in existence. The same wisdom described as the spirits in plants by the ancient Greeks and American cultures, the 'qi' of Traditional Chinese Medicine and philosophy, and 'prana' of Ayurveda is our innate healing energy that manifests itself daily in the amazing feats of the body – the cough to clear the airways of phlegm, the sneeze to shift irritants from the nose, vomiting to clear the

HERBS COMMONLY USED IN NATIVE AMERICAN MEDICINE

Pleurisy root *(see page 111)*
Wild indigo *(see page 114)*
Oregon grape root *(see page 114)*
Barberry *(see page 115)*
Globe artichoke *(see page 124)*
Wild yam *(see page 125)*
Echinacea *(see page 126)*
Boneset *(see page 129)*
Gravel root *(see page 130)*
Witch hazel *(see page 136)*
Golden seal *(see page 138)*
Bayberry *(see page 145)*
Poke root *(see page 149)*
Sarsaparilla *(see page 158)*
Beth root *(see page 165)*
Slippery elm *(see page 166)*
Cramp bark *(see page 170)*
Black haw *(see page 170)*
Prickly ash *(see page 174)*

Aromatherapy

The use of essential oils distilled from highly scented plants is enormously popular – a natural enough fact given that people have enjoyed the perfumes of plants as far back as we can remember. Most ancient civilizations have used fragrant oils and plants. Herbs, flowers and aromatic woods were burned in temples to purify the atmosphere and to please the gods. Their perfumes were believed to rise higher than the temple ceilings to the heavens, where they scented the realms of paradise.

In Biblical times aromatic oils were used for anointing and as temple incense, and mention is made in the Bible of the smell of Spikenard, smoke perfumed with Myrrh and Frankincense, and Camphor and Cinnamon to perfume rooms. Myrrh and Frankincense were obviously so highly valued that the Magi considered them worthy gifts for the infant Jesus. The ancient Egyptians skilfully employed aromatic oils in their healing ointments and in the mummification process, and used perfumes just as we do today in courtship. Queen Cleopatra's royal barge apparently emitted the most exotic perfumes as it sailed down the Nile to meet Mark Anthony. Cleopatra is said to have bathed several times daily with essence of Rose and Orange blossom. The Romans loved aromatic oils, favouring Rose above all for wine-making, perfumes and their famous baths.

When the fashion for bathing died out or when water was short, aromatic oils would be applied to skin and clothes to mask more unpleasant smells; they were particularly popular in Tudor and Elizabethan times. In Queen Elizabeth I's reign, perfumed gloves were the height of fashion, and in fact Queen Elizabeth herself possessed her own still room for distilling oils for the making of the royal floral perfumes. So powerful was the effect of scent, with its sensual, often mind-altering properties, that when the Crusaders returned to England from the Holy Land laden with perfumes of the Orient, the medieval clergy were greatly alarmed and associated it with the forces of evil. Later, in the 18th century, the House of Commons considered applying the laws of witchcraft against women who tried to seduce any of His Majesty's subjects into marriage with the aid of scent! Certainly, the fragrances of plants have always been

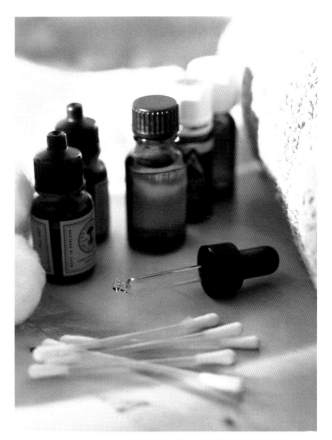

Essential oils are stored in dark glass bottles to preserve active ingredients that are destroyed by light and heat.

associated with the supernatural, used in magical or religious ceremonies to heighten perception and for divination and love potions.

Healing heritage

Fragrant oils have also long been associated with healing. From Hippocrates onwards we know that aromatic baths, massages and inhalations were employed to remedy all kinds of health problems. Herbs such as Rosemary, Pine and Juniper were burned and pomanders were worn to keep contagion away during epidemics. With the development of scientific analysis of plants and their constituents, more has become known about the amazing range of biochemical constituents that make up volatile oils. In the 1920s a French chemist, René Gattefossé, brought the healing benefits of oils to the attention of the orthodox scientific world, which was by now disregarding much of the benefit to be derived from the plant world, preferring to develop the synthesis of more powerful drugs in the laboratory. Gattefossé had a family perfume business, and while experimenting in his laboratory, he burned his arm badly and plunged it into the nearby vat of Lavender oil. To his great delight his arm healed quickly with no scarring. Consequently, Gattefossé was inspired to devote much time researching essential oils and their medical application, particularly in relation to their benefit on the skin. In 1937 he published his book *Aromatherapy*, the name he coined for describing the healing benefits of essential oils used to this day.

Gattefossé's research papers were read by a French army doctor, Jean Valnet, who was so interested in the subject that he began his own clinical research using oils on soldiers as antiseptics and wound healers, and was greatly impressed by their efficacy. He then began to experiment with treating the emotional or psychological problems experienced by war veterans, and to write extensively about aromatherapy. His *Practice of Aromatherapy*, published in 1964, is a standard text for all present-day professional aromatherapists.

Modern aromatherapy

The modern practice of aromatherapy, using essential oils with massage for health and wellbeing, was popularized by an Austrian biochemist, Marguerite Maury (1895–1968), who was particularly interested in the healing and rejuvenating properties of essential oils and carried out an extensive research programme on the effectiveness of oils when absorbed through the skin. She went on to write about essential oils, publishing *La Capital 'Jeunesse'* in 1961, which has been reprinted and translated into English as *The Secret of Life and Youth*. Dr Maury opened several clinics for aromatherapy, as have many practitioners since, offering massage using essential oils to treat a wide range of physical problems

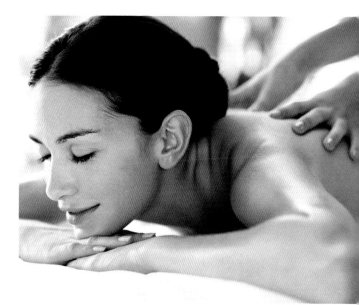

For massage, essential oils are diluted in a carrier oil, such as sweet almond or sesame, ensuring safe application to the skin.

and to address underlying emotional and mental problems. As well as the great versatility of the effects of the essential oils, massage gives the opportunity of benefiting from the comfort of touch and the great therapeutic value that brings.

Volatile oils can be taken into the body in a variety of different ways: through aromatic herbs used in foods, drinks and medicines; diluted oils inhaled through the nose; and rubbed on to the skin. When oils are inhaled, olfactory receptor cells are stimulated and carry nerve impulses to the brain, especially the limbic system, thereby potentially affecting instinctual responses, emotions and memory. As the oils are inhaled, molecules are also taken via the lungs to the bloodstream and the systemic circulation. Their actions are felt throughout the digestive tract, the urinary tract and the respiratory system, as well as affecting sweat and salivary, vaginal and lacrimal secretions. It is probable that the oils are passed in some amount through breast milk. Fennel, Dill and Chamomile tea have been drunk for centuries by lactating women to soothe babies' colic and help induce sleep.

When oils are absorbed via the skin through massage or baths, they stimulate nerve endings in the skin and messages are relayed to underlying tissues, muscles, blood and lymphatic vessels, and also via the nervous system to the pituitary gland, thereby having the ability to regulate the action of other endocrine glands, including the adrenals. This can be helpful in balancing hormonal problems and stress-related symptoms.

Flower remedies

Flower remedies were described as early as the 1500s by Paracelsus, who prepared remedies from dew he had collected from flowers to treat his patients' emotional problems. Today flower remedies are most strongly associated with **Dr Edward Bach (1886–1936)**, whose deep compassion for those suffering pain or distress led him to train in medicine and become a respected immunologist, pathologist and bacteriologist.

It was, however, Dr Bach's dissatisfaction with medicine's palliative rather than curative effect on illness that drove him to continue studying, in the belief that true health and wellbeing come from within and depend on harmony of body, mind, emotions and spirit. His research as a bacteriologist led to his discovery of the relationship between bacteria in the gut and chronic illness, and the use of vaccines derived from these bacteria.

In 1919, when working in the London Homeopathic Hospital, Dr Bach realized that the work and philosophy of Dr Samuel Hahnemann (1755–1843) echoed much of his own approach to medicine – focusing on the treatment of the person, not the disease. He began to prepare vaccines homeopathically and used them with great success. However, he still felt that he was working with physical disease rather than addressing its underlying causes. His understanding was that disease resulted from inner disharmony and negative thoughts and feelings, which frequently manifested on a physical level. He saw that stress – fear, anxiety, panic, anger, intolerance, impatience – put a strain on an individual, depleting vitality and resistance to disease.

Dr Bach's discoveries

Dr Bach had a great love of nature and intuitively understood that remedies for emotional pain and suffering could be found among flowers, herbs and trees. At the height of his medical career, he left to spend the rest of his life travelling in Wales and southern England in search of such remedies to restore peace of mind and happiness, which he believed to be the essential nature of our being. During this time he discovered 38 plants that provided answers to the many sufferings of people, derived (with the exception of one) from flowering trees and plants. He discovered that the early morning dew on plants exposed to sunlight absorbed the properties of that plant far better than on those growing in the shade. So he devised the sun method of extracting the properties of the plants, which involves floating the picked flower heads in a glass bowl of spring water. The bowl is placed on the ground near the parent plants and exposed to sunlight for a few hours, after which time the flowers are carefully removed with a twig or leaf. The essence is then poured into bottles half full of brandy to preserve it. The boiling method involves placing the plant in an enamel pan of spring water and simmering it for 30 minutes. Once cool, the essence is filtered and preserved in equal parts of brandy. Dr Bach published his discoveries in the main homeopathic journals of the day and produced several

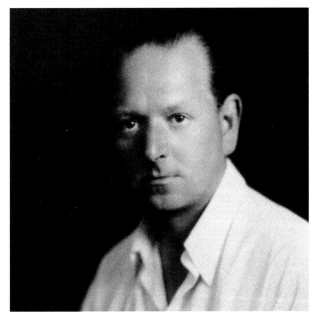

Dr Edward Bach wrote that flower essences could 'bring us peace and relieve our suffering'.

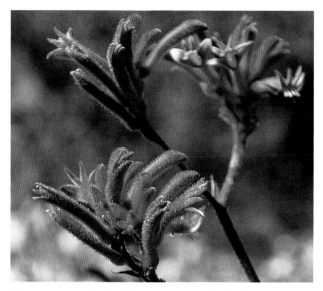

Kangaroo paw is a Bush Flower Essence derived from the native Australian plant; it helps to encourage social interaction.

booklets for lay people so that his remedies would be accessible to everyone. These included *Heal Thyself, Free Thyself* and *The Twelve healers.*

The Flower Essence Society

In the early 1970s, 'flower power' was the message on many people's lips, particularly in California, as were 'good vibrations', the wisdom of the East and the power of love and meditation. Flowers were in vogue and a variety of people in the healing and psychic world began intuitively to discover a whole host of new flower essences. Within the context of mind-altering substances and popular New Age concepts, the profusion of flower remedies was causing some confusion, with some doubt as to whether claims for their remarkable healing abilities were actually valid or not.

Richard Katz and Patricia Kaminski were among those who were developing flower essences, having worked with the Bach flower remedies for many years, but were concerned that charlatans in the area would bring flower healing into disrepute. In 1979 they set up the Flower Essence Society to separate the chaff from the wheat, to gather case studies from practitioners worldwide, to confirm the genuine effects of flower essences and to run training courses for students and seminars for practitioners. After extensive testing of their remedies on health practitioners, the Flower Essence Society (FES) produced a range of flower essences called Quintessentials, made from organically grown flowers cultivated around the Californian Sierra Nevada.

While Dr Bach's remedies reflected the spirit of his era during the Depression, with flowers for negative emotions such as fear, anger, resentment, depression and discouragement, the Californian flower essences were influenced by the backdrop of 1970s California. Their remedies included those for enhancing spiritual development and for dealing with sexual inhibitions, blocks to creativity and problems in relationships. From that period onwards the world of flower essences has continued to blossom, with ranges of flower essences originating from all corners of the world, including New Zealand, Hawaii, Alaska, Scotland, the Himalayas, Africa, the Amazon and Australia.

Australian Bush Flower Essences

These were evolved by naturopath Ian White, who had used the Bach flower remedies and wanted to explore the healing potential of flowers closer to home. As a boy he had grown up in the Australian bush, and there his appreciation and respect for nature developed as he accompanied his herbalist grandmother on walks searching for medicinal herbs. As an adult, information about bush essences, a picture of the flower, where it could be found and often its name were channelled to Ian White during meditation. Working with other practitioners who were excited by this new discovery, he set about verifying the effects of the bush remedies, not only by working with patients but also by testing them with Kirlian photography, kinesiology and vega machines, and with other mediums. His book *Bush Flower Essences* describes 50 of these Australian essences and their applications, and since then 12 more remedies have been discovered and researched.

Healing nature

Flower remedies are highly diluted from a physical or chemical perspective. They are effective not because of their chemical constituents but for the life force derived from the flower contained within the water-based fluid. Like homeopathic remedies, their presence is more subtle than physical. They address profound issues of spiritual wellbeing, emotional and mental harmony, and help to heal emotional and mental difficulties that create blocks to spiritual development and the realization of an individual's full potential. They can act as catalysts, helping people to heal themselves, understand their purpose and direction in life, and free themselves from the mental or emotional suffering that hinders them on their life path. Dr Bach said that flower essences, '…raise our vibrations and open up our channels for the reception of our spiritual self'.

The chemistry of herbs

How do herbs work on the human organism? Much of their medicinal action can be classified according to a plant's therapeutic constituents, measured using the tools of biochemistry and pharmacology. However, plants work synergistically – the whole being more than the sum of the parts – and this has been less well studied. As a result, many herbalists are happy to evaluate the healing potential of plants according to both modern scientific findings and more holistic philosophies of energy medicine.

Re-evaluating herbal medicines

Modern evaluation of herbal medicines is divided between 'rationalistic/scientific' and 'energetic' viewpoints. With the emergence of modern Western scientific medicine, herbs have been seen either as old-fashioned and obsolete or as sources of pharmacological constituents for using as building blocks to make drugs.

For thousands of years, until the last 200 years or so, plants provided the sole source of medicines, and many familiar and potent medicines of the 21st century have been derived directly or indirectly from herbs. Despite this, there are still those who persist in the view that the value of herbs is unproven scientifically. Cinchona bark, for example, is the source of quinine, the antimalarial drug, Periwinkle is the source of vincristine, the

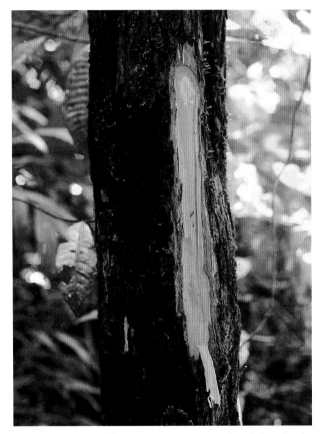

The bark from the Cinchona tree, native to South America, is the source of quinine in antimalarial drugs.

antitumour drug, and the Opium poppy is the source of morphine and codeine. Atropine, aspirin, digoxin and ephedrine are all plant-derived drugs found in modern pharmacological textbooks and dispensaries. At the same time, however, the unquestionable value and popularity of herbs as medicines in the last 20–30 years has prompted an increasing amount of research into the action of plant components, which is not only fascinating but also greatly helpful to the modern practitioner.

Alongside this enquiry into the world of herbs has come a re-emergence in popularity of more ancient systems of medicine, with their 'energetic' or 'holistic' philosophies, as well as more modern systems of healing using plants, such as aromatherapy and flower essences. This has occurred amid a milieu of natural healing that has challenged modern allopathic medicine to the point that now many people are conscious that valid choices exist for the patient before embarking on a course of treatment, particularly for chronic problems.

Whole-plant medicines

To stand up to scrutiny in a modern scientific world, herbalists now have to provide evidence of the efficacy and safety of therapeutic herbs they use and apply the tools of the scientific world – biochemistry and pharmacology – to their task. While herbalists advocate the use of whole-plant medicines, their enquiry necessitates that, for study and evaluation purposes, ingredients are singled out and their actions are ascertained. Such research enables quality testing and efficient extraction methods, and provides pointers to potential side effects and herb–drug interactions. Once this is accomplished, it does not, however, tell the whole story, and the knowledge gained from such study still needs to be incorporated into a more overall view of the whole plant. It has long been held that a herb is more than the sum of its parts, and despite investigations into

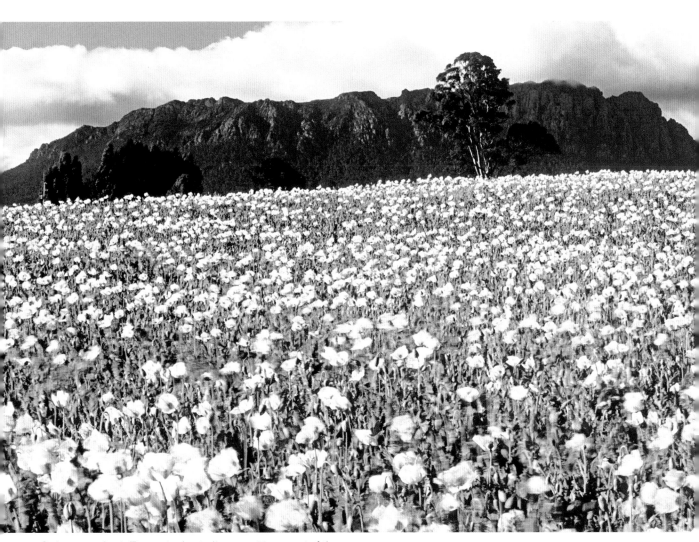

Opium poppies in Tasmania, Australia; some 50 per cent of the world's crop used in medicine is grown here.

what are seen as the active ingredients in a given plant, there are other 'lesser' constituents that have an equally important role to play therapeutically. They are essential in determining how effective the primary healing agents will be by rendering the body more or less receptive to their powers. Some of these 'synergistic' substances will make the active constituents more easily assimilated and readily available in the body, while others will buffer the action of other potent plant chemicals, thus preventing the risk of side effects. It is the natural combination of both types of substance that determines the healing power and safety of any herbal medicine.

Before the development of modern scientific methods for isolating active constituents, whole-plant medicines were used. Then, as science progressed, many of these constituents were able to be synthesized in the laboratory, perhaps in the assumption that synthetic compounds were similar to those derived from the plant world and, as such, would be assimilated just as easily by the body, and so herbs became more or less redundant. However, chemical analysis of medicinal plants has demonstrated that there is a similarity in the molecular structure of components of plants and the human body that makes the foods we eat and herbs used as medicines easily assimilated. The isolation and synthesis of potent active ingredients can produce an array of side effects. Plant-derived drugs such as morphine, digoxin, ephedrine and atropine clearly need to be used with great caution. Even aspirin carries its risks, and since 1986 all children's aspirin-based drugs have been withdrawn from the market due to their implication in association with Reye's syndrome as a sequel to other children's diseases, which can cause damage to the kidneys and brain.

Constituents of herbal medicines

Through photosynthesis, plants manufacture carbohydrates and give off oxygen, and in this process they create metabolic pathways that provide building blocks for the production of a vast array of compounds. In medicinal plants these include minerals, vitamins and trace elements, and a vast assortment of substances known to have specific therapeutic actions in the body. The more widely known of these are detailed below.

Phenols

Phenols, sometimes called phenolic compounds, are a large class of secondary plant compounds. They are aromatic alcohols and the building blocks of many plant components, and generally have antiseptic, antibacterial and anthelmintic actions.

The simplest of the class is the antimicrobial phenol (CHOH65). Another simple phenolic compound is salicylic acid, which forms glycosides found in Willow, Cramp bark and Meadowsweet. It has antiseptic, painkilling and anti-inflammatory properties and forms the basis of aspirin. Among other compounds are the hydroxycinnamic acids including caffeic, ferulic and sinapic acids. These form the basis of phenolic esters, coumarins, glycosides and lignans, as well as cynarin, the main constituent of Globe artichoke, which has liver-protective and cholesterol-lowering actions, and curcumin, the main component of Turmeric, famous as an anti-inflammatory agent which also lowers blood pressure and protects the liver[1].

Other phenolic compounds include stilbenes, which occur in grape skins and red wine, with antioxidant, anti-inflammatory, anticlotting and antiallergy actions, and quinones, including anthraquinones (see below) and naphthaquinones. The latter have antimicrobial and antitumour properties, such as juglone in Walnut bark and lapachol in Pau d'arco.

Coumarins

These occur widely in plants, including Black cohosh, Wild oats, Angelica and Horse chestnut, and are generally antimicrobial and antifungal. The evocative smell of hay is due to the coumarins that are lactones of hydroxycinnamic acids. They generally occur as glycosides, for example aescin in Horse chestnut. Dicoumarol, originally derived from Sweet clover (*Melilotus officinalis*), is used as a strong anticlotting agent in the form of warfarin in allopathic medicine.

Furanocoumarins include angelican and archangelican from Angelica root, which are antispasmodic. These need to be used cautiously, as they can cause photosensitivity, increasing the effect of sunlight on the skin, but could be used therapeutically for vitiligo and psoriasis[2].

Anthraquinones

These occur as glycosides and have a yellow-brown colour that has often been used for producing commercial dyes. They are found in Senna, Aloe vera skin, Yellow dock and Cascara, and pass unaltered through the stomach and small intestine and are

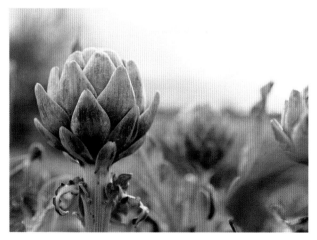

Globe artichoke is a rich source of cynarin, a phenolic compound that supports the liver and can lower cholesterol.

converted to their active form by micro-organisms. 8–12 hours after ingestion they stimulate peristalsis and inhibit water reabsorption in the large intestine, producing a laxative effect. Their peristaltic action can sometimes cause griping in the bowel, so they are best combined with herbs such as Peppermint, Ginger or Fennel, and are contraindicated in spastic bowel and pregnancy. They should not be used over a long period, as they can reduce normal bowel reflexes and cause habituation.

Tannins

These occur widely in nature, often as glycosides, and represent the largest group of polyphenols. Tannins are the main therapeutic constituents in Witch hazel, Agrimony, Raspberry leaf and Meadowsweet. Their main therapeutic action is astringent, brought about by their ability to bind albumin, a protein in the skin and mucous membranes, to form a tight, insoluble protective layer that is resistant to infection. On the skin or in the delicate linings of the mouth and respiratory, digestive, urinary and reproductive systems, tannins can separate bacteria that threaten to invade from their source of nutrition.

They occur either as hydrolysable or condensed tannins. Hydrolysable tannins protect the skin and mucosa from irritation and reduce swelling and inflammation. They have a drying effect, useful for over-secretion of mucus, bleeding and diarrhoea. Herbs rich in tannins make useful mouthwashes for infected and bleeding gums, gargles for sore throats, eyewashes, remedies for catarrh, inflammation of the gastrointestinal tract, diarrhoea and heavy menstrual bleeding. They can be used as compresses to heal burns, abrasions and cuts, and lotions to bathe haemorrhoids and soothe inflamed skin.

Condensed tannins include oligomeric procyanidins, widely known for their antioxidant and cardiovascular properties. They are found in green and black tea, red wine and grape seeds. Grape seed extract has been shown to have strong antioxidant activity, protecting against free radical damage and cardiovascular disease, and preventing degeneration of connective tissue.

Flavonoids

Flavonoids and flavonoid glycosides occur widely in nature and impart a yellow, orange and red colour to fruits and flowers. Their antioxidant action makes them an important part of our diet, having a beneficial effect on the heart and circulation, strengthening and healing blood vessel walls and enhancing resilience to stress. They act synergistically with ascorbic acid to enhance the body's ability to metabolize it. They are anti-inflammatory (as in quercetin), hepatoprotective (silymarin and quercetrin), antitumour,

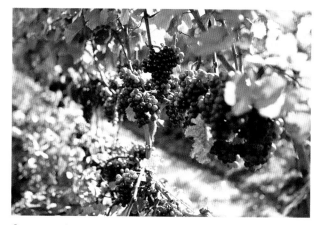

Grape seeds are good for cardiovascular health and the red skin includes phenols and flavonoids.

antiviral and hypotensive. Herbs rich in flavonoids, such as kaempferol, myricitin and quercitrin, protect against cardiovascular disease and treat vascular problems like venous insufficiency, bruising, piles and nosebleeds.

Isoflavones, such as genistein from soya, have a similar structure to oestrogen. Such phytoestrogens in Wild asparagus/Shatavari, Wild indigo, Liquorice, Red clover and Black cohosh bind to oestrogen receptors, and have been found to help prevent tumours and breast cancer and ease menopausal symptoms.

Anthocyanins and anthocyanidins are found in red, blue and black fruits and are high in Red grape skins, Elderberries and Blueberries/Bilberries. They also occur in Ginkgo, Cat's claw and Corn silk. They are antioxidant, and protect the eyes and connective tissue.

Terpenes

Terpenes or terpenoids occur widely in a variety of forms, including monoterpenes, sesquiterpenes and triterpenes.

Monoterpenes

These are the main components of volatile oils (see page 42), and include bitter iridoids as in the sedative valepotriates in Valerian, hypotensive asperulsides in Cleavers and paeoniflorin in Peony, which has anti-inflammatory, febrifuge and sedative actions[3].

Sesquiterpenes

These are also found in volatile oils or as lactones, and have a bitter taste, anti-inflammatory and antimicrobial actions. Sesquiterpenes are found in Myrrh, Hops, Chamomile and Chaste tree, and sesquiterpene lactones occur in Boneset, Feverfew, Yarrow, Wormwood, Globe artichoke and Elecampane.

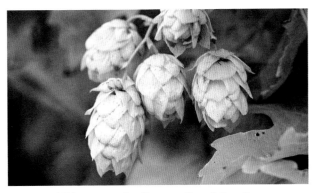

Hops are bitter, promoting the secretion of digestive enzymes, bile and certain hormones; they also have sedative properties.

Triterpenes

These have a similar structure to steroids (see below).

Bitters

'Bitter principles' is a term for a group of chemicals that have a very bitter taste and a cooling effect. They are diverse in structure, but have certain therapeutic actions in common and include mostly terpenes, flavonoids and some alkaloids. Through their effect on the bitter receptors on the tongue they promote the secretion of digestive enzymes from the stomach and intestines, the flow of bile from the liver and the release of hormones. Bitters are prescribed for poor appetite and digestion, gastritis, heartburn, to regulate blood sugar, relieve allergies and inflammation and to aid convalescence. Many bitter herbs have other actions: some are relaxant or sedative, like Hops and Valerian, others are anti-inflammatory, such as Devil's claw, and some, like Marigold, exert a beneficial action on the immune system, acting as natural antibiotics and antineoplastics. Well-known 'bitter tonics' include Dandelion, Cleavers, Holy thistle, Wormwood, Yellow dock and Gentian.

Triterpenoids and saponins

Triterpenoids represent a large and diverse group that includes phytosterols, triterpenoid saponins, steroidal saponins and cardiac glycosides.

Phytosterols

Those such as sitosterol and stigmasterol are vital to the formation of cell membranes and help regulate cholesterol. Guggulsterones in Guggulu lower harmful cholesterol and triglycerides by their regulatory effect on the thyroid. Phytosterols have been used as building blocks for making steroid drugs and may have the ability to inhibit tumour formation. For instance, withanolides in Ashwagandha have antitumour and hepatoprotective properties[4].

Saponins

These are glycosides that form a soap-like lather when they are mixed with water and precipitate cholesterol. Herbs containing saponins have a bitter taste and haemolytic activity[5]. They can dissolve red blood cell walls, so should never be injected into the bloodstream. Taken orally, however, they are hardly absorbed through an intact intestine and help to promote digestion and absorption of nutrients such as calcium and silicon. Some have beneficial action on blood vessel walls, such as Horse chestnut, while others decrease blood coagulation, blood sugar and harmful cholesterol levels[6]. Some are diuretic, including Goldenrod and Horsetail. Others are expectorant, such as Mullein, and several have hepatoprotective and immunomodulating effects, for example Korean ginseng and Liquorice.

Triterpenoid saponins

These help regulate steroidal hormonal activity and counter the effects of stress, and often have antifungal properties. Herbs containing these hormone-regulating properties are known as adaptogens, the most famous of which is Korean ginseng. Others include Liquorice, Wild yam and Fenugreek. Some, such as Wild yam and Liquorice, act as anti-inflammatories.

Steroidal saponins

These, such as diosgenin in Wild yam, are used in the body as building blocks for the production of hormones secreted by the testes, ovaries and adrenal glands, and vitamin D.

Cardiac glycosides

Discovered in 1785 in Foxglove, these have been widely researched for their ability to increase cardiac output by affecting the force and speed of heart contractions, which is beneficial in heart failure. Herbs containing these are generally for use by practitioners only.

Volatile oils

The exotic perfumes and delicious tastes of aromatic herbs are derived from volatile oils, which are complex combinations of compounds. Their varying compositions produce a wide variation in scent and therapeutic effects; up to 60 different chemical constituents have been identified in some oils. Categories of volatile oils include terpenoids and phenylpropanoids.

All volatile oils are antiseptic, stimulating the production of white blood cells and enhancing immunity. Many oils have antibacterial, antifungal and antiviral actions, and also anti-inflammatory and antispasmodic properties, particularly those containing sesquiterpenes such as azulene in Chamomile which are particularly applicable for relieving an inflamed and irritated digestive tract, while those in Dill relax spasm and colic in the gut. Some oils have an expectorant action, such as in Thyme and Hyssop; others are diuretic, useful for fluid retention and urinary infections. While they exert beneficial effects on the body, oils also reach the brain and nervous system and have a wide range of mento-emotional applications.

Fixed oils

These are lipids found in all plants, especially the seeds, and contain fatty acids that are either saturated, monounsaturated or polyunsaturated. They are vital for growth and health, the formation of cell membranes and healthy functioning of the immune and cardiovascular systems. Two that exist in every cell, particularly in the nervous system, known as essential fatty acids, are linoleic acid (found in Evening primrose and Borage seed oil and Saw palmetto berries) and linolenic acid (found in Flax seed), which are not able to be synthesized in the body and need to be taken in the diet. In the body, linoleic acid is converted into gamma-linolenic acid (GLA). Atopic allergies such as eczema and asthma and other immune problems are related to the lack of the enzyme responsible for this conversion in some individuals. Borage seed oil and Evening primrose oil contain GLA and are very useful for treating such problems.

Polysaccharides

These large sugar molecules are found widely in the plant world, for example in fructose, glucose and cellulose, and consist of chains of sugars linked to other molecules. They include mucilage, gums and fructans. Some polysaccharides, particularly beta-glucans found in, for instance, Reishi and Shiitake mushrooms, have immunostimulating properties. They activate cytokines that enhance the production of white blood cells and antibodies, and also have anti-inflammatory and antitumour actions. Liquorice, Rehmannia and Cinnamon also contain immunostimulating polysaccharides.

Mucilage

This sugary, gel-like substance draws water to it to form a viscous fluid. When taken orally, mucilage coats the mucous membranes of the digestive, respiratory and genitourinary tracts, protecting them from irritation and inflammation. Herbs rich in mucilage such as Slippery elm, Marshmallow, Plantain and Coltsfoot are prescribed for their cooling and soothing properties. They relieve diarrhoea by reducing peristalsis caused by irritation of the gut lining, but can be used as laxatives, absorbing water into the bowel and bulking out the stool, as in Psyllium seeds.

Gums

These are protective and healing exudates of monosaccharides which are released when a plant is damaged. Those in Guggulu enhance the liver's metabolism of cholesterol, promoting the uptake of harmful low-density lipoprotein (LDL) cholesterol. Marigold is high in gums with antimicrobial, antifungal and anti-inflammatory effects.

Fructans

These are composed of fructose and occur especially in herbs in the Compositae family as inulin, such as Elecampane, Globe artichoke, Goldenrod, Gentian, Codonopsis and Burdock. Inulin helps regulate blood sugar and enhances the immune system.

Alkaloids

The chemicals in this diverse group contain a nitrogen-bearing molecule and are pharmacologically very potent. Many of the more toxic plants contain alkaloids, such as atropine in Belladonna and morphine in the Opium poppy, the first alkaloid to be isolated in 1806[7]. Caffeine, ephedrine, quinine, strychnine, piperine, nicotine and codeine are all alkaloids with diverse actions ranging from stimulants, bronchodilators, antimicrobials and anti-inflammatories to narcotics and painkillers.

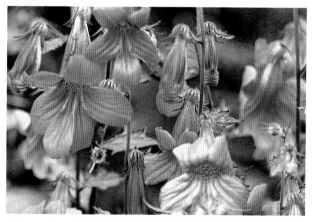

Chinese foxglove is prescribed by herbalists for its cardiac glycosides, a type of saponin that increases cardiac output.

Medicinal actions of herbs

The following guide classifies herbs according to their medicinal action (see The Herb Directory, pages 100–175).

Alteratives
Barberry, Bearberry, Bladderwrack, Blue flag, Burdock, Cleavers, Comfrey, Dandelion, Devil's claw, Echinacea, Elderflower, Eyebright, Garlic, Golden seal, Brahmi, Holy thistle, Liquorice, Marshmallow, Nettle, Oregon grape root, Poke root, Red clover, St John's wort, Sarsaparilla

Analgesic/Anodyne
California poppy, Chamomile, Hops, Passion flower, Skullcap, St John's wort, Valerian, Wild lettuce

Anthelmintic
Aloe vera, Garlic, Senna, Thyme, Walnut , Wormwood

Antibilious
Barberry, Dandelion, Golden seal, Vervain, Wild yam, Wormwood

Anticatarrhal
Bearberry, Boneset, Cayenne pepper, Coltsfoot, Elder, Elecampane, Eyebright, Garlic, Goldenrod, Golden seal, Hyssop, Marshmallow, Mullein, Sage, Thyme, Yarrow

Antiemetic
Cayenne pepper, Dill, Fennel, Lavender, Lemon balm, Meadowsweet

Anti-inflammatory
Chamomile, Devil's claw, Frankincense, Ginger, Liquorice, Marigold, St John's wort, Turmeric, Witch hazel

Antilithic
Bearberry, Corn silk, Couch grass, Gravel root

Antimicrobial
Bearberry, Cayenne, Clove, Coriander, Echinacea, Elecampane, Garlic, Liquorice, Marigold, Myrrh, Peppermint, Rosemary, Sage, St John's wort, Thyme, Wormwood

Antispasmodic
Black cohosh, Black haw, Chamomile, Cramp bark, Lime flower, Mistletoe, Motherwort, Pasque flower, Skullcap, Thyme, Valerian, Vervain

Aromatic
Cardamom, Chamomile, Chinese angelica, Cinnamon, Coriander, Dill, Fennel, Forskohlii, Ginger, Hyssop, Meadowsweet, Peppermint, Rosemary, Valerian, Wild celery, Wood betony

Astringent
Agrimony, Bayberry, Bearberry, Beth root, Cramp bark, Elecampane, Eyebright, Goldenrod, Ground ivy, Meadowsweet, Mullein, Myrrh, Raspberry, Rosemary, Sage, Vervain, Witch hazel leaf

Bitter
Barberry, Dandelion root, Devil's claw, Globe artichoke, Golden seal, Hops, Ho shou wu, Sweet Annie, White horehound, Wood betony, Wormwood, Yarrow

Cardiotonic
Astragalus, Forskohlii, Hawthorn, Motherwort

Carminative
Angelica root, Cayenne pepper, Chamomile, Cinnamon, Dill, Fennel, Ginger, Hyssop, Lavender, Lemon balm, Peppermint, Rosemary

Cholagogue
Barberry, Blue flag, Gentian, Globe artichoke, Peppermint, Yellow dock

Demulcent
Chickweed, Comfrey, Fenugreek, Liquorice, Marshmallow, Mullein, Plantain, Slippery elm

Diaphoretic
Angelica root, Bayberry, Boneset, Cayenne, Chamomile, Elderflower, Elecampane, Ginger, Goldenrod, Hyssop, Lemon balm, Lime flower, Peppermint, Pleurisy root, Prickly ash, Vervain, Yarrow

Diuretic
Astragalus, Buchu, Corn silk, Couch grass, Dandelion leaf and root, Globe artichoke, Goldenrod, Gravel root, Horsetail, Shatavari, Wild celery seed

Emetic
Boneset, Elderflower, Lemon balm

Emmenagogue
Beth root, Black cohosh, Black haw, Chamomile, Chaste tree, Cramp bark, Fenugreek, Gentian, Ginger, Golden seal, Holy thistle, Marigold, Motherwort, Pasque flower, Peppermint, Raspberry, Rosemary, St John's wort, Thyme, Valerian, Vervain, Wormwood, Yarrow

Emollient
Borage, Chickweed, Coltsfoot, Comfrey, Elecampane, Fenugreek, Liquorice, Marshmallow, Mullein, Plantain, Rose petals, Slippery elm

Expectorant
Angelica root, Elecampane, Fennel, Ground ivy, Hyssop, Liquorice, Marshmallow, Mullein, Pleurisy root, Thyme, Vervain, White horehound

Febrifuge
Boneset, Borage, Cayenne pepper, Elderflower, Holy thistle, Hyssop, Lemon balm, Marigold, Peppermint, Plantain, Pleurisy root, Prickly ash, Raspberry, Thyme, Vervain

Galactogogue
Chaste tree, Fennel, Fenugreek, Goat's rue, Vervain, Shatavari

Hepatic
Agrimony, Aloe vera, Barberry, Blue flag, Cleavers, Dandelion, Elecampane, Fennel, Gentian, Globe artichoke, Golden seal, Hyssop, Kalamegha, Lemon balm, Motherwort, Prickly ash, Rosemary, Schisandra, Wild celery, Wild yam, Wormwood, Yarrow, Yellow dock

Hypnotic
California poppy, Hops, Mistletoe, Passion flower, Skullcap, Valerian

Laxative
Aloe vera resin, Barberry, Blue flag, Burdock, Chinese angelica, Cleavers, Dandelion leaf and root, Liquorice, Senna, Slippery elm, Yellow dock

Mucilage
Comfrey, Fenugreek, Marshmallow, Slippery elm

Nervine
Black cohosh, Bacopa, Brahmi, Chamomile, Cramp bark, Ginseng, Hops, Ho shou wu, Lavender, Lemon balm, Mistletoe, Motherwort, Pasque flower, Passion flower, Peppermint, Red clover, Rosemary, Skullcap, St John's wort, Schisandra, Thyme, Valerian, Vervain, Wild oats, Wormwood

Oxytocic
Beth root, Golden seal, Schisandra

Pectoral
Chinese angelica, Coltsfoot, Comfrey, Elder, Elecampane, Garlic, Golden seal, Hyssop, Liquorice, Marshmallow, Mullein, Pleurisy root, Vervain, White horehound

Rubefacient
Cayenne pepper, Garlic, Ginger, Nettle, Peppermint, Rosemary,

Sedative
Black cohosh, Black haw, Bladderwrack, Chamomile, Cramp bark, Hops, Motherwort, Pasque flower, Passion flower, Red clover, Skullcap, St John's wort, Saw palmetto, Valerian, Wild yam

Sialogogue
Blue flag, Cayenne pepper, Gentian, Ginger, Prickly ash

Stimulant
Bayberry, Bladderwrack, Cardamom, Cayenne pepper, Chinese angelica, Cinnamon, Dandelion, Garlic, Gentian, Ginseng, Gravel root, Ground ivy, Marigold, Peppermint, Prickly ash, Rosemary, White horehound, Wild yam, Wormwood, Yarrow

Styptic
Horsetail, Marigold, Nettle, Witch hazel leaf, Yarrow

Tonic
Agrimony, Bayberry, Bearberry, Beth root, Boneset, Buchu, Burdock, Chamomile, Cayenne pepper, Chinese angelica, Cleavers, Coltsfoot, Comfrey, Couch grass, Dandelion, Echinacea, Elecampane, Eyebright, Garlic, Gentian, Ginseng, Golden seal, Gravel root, Ground ivy, Hawthorn, Horse chestnut, Hyssop, Lemon balm, Liquorice, Marigold, Mistletoe, Motherwort, Myrrh, Nettle, Poke root, Raspberry, Red clover, Sarsaparilla, Skullcap, Thyme, Vervain, Wild oats, Wild yam, Wood betony, Yarrow

Vulnerary
Aloe vera, Burdock, Cleavers, Comfrey, Elder, Elecampane, Fenugreek, Garlic, Golden seal, Horsetail, Hyssop, Marigold, Marshmallow, Mullein, Myrrh, Plantain, Poke root, St John's wort, Slippery elm, Thyme, Witch hazel, Wood betony, Yarrow

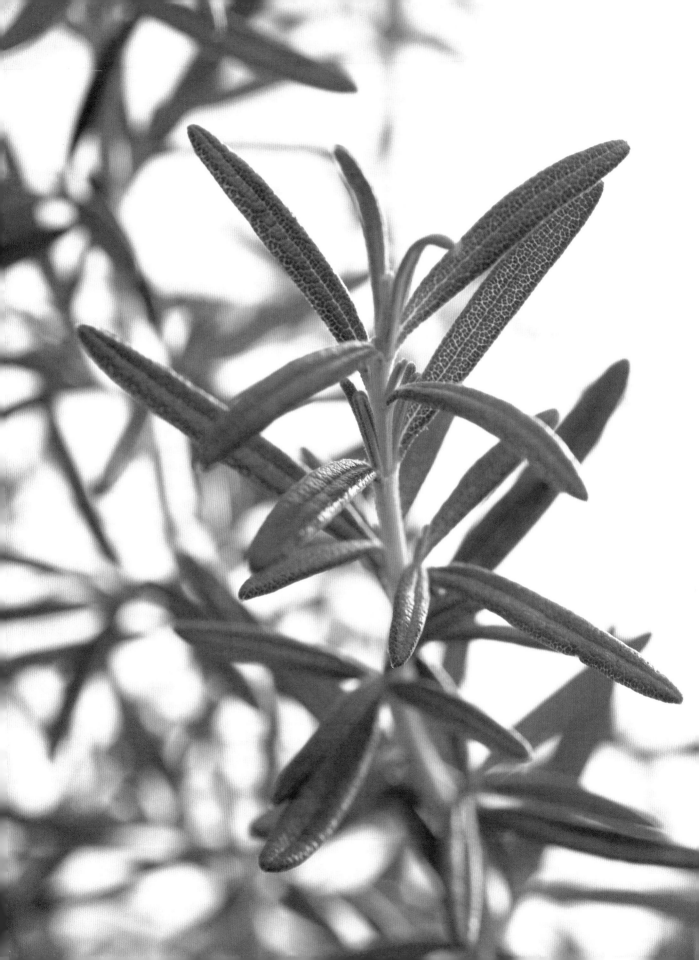

The herbal consultation

Before you make a diagnosis, prescribe remedies and prepare herbal medicines, it is essential to understand the concepts of holism and homeostasis, and how plants can enhance the body's innate healing processes. Treating underlying causes and not simply addressing symptoms forms the basis of a herbalist's practice, and every consultation, treatment plan and herbal prescription is tailored to individual patients with the aim of bringing positive and lasting results.

Healing the whole person

Modern medical herbalism is a synthesis of ancient and modern theories and practices, and its underlying philosophy is that health is intimately connected to the harmony of body, mind and spirit, which enables a balance of natural forces in the body. In a clinical context, the herbalist will interpret symptoms of ill health as a disturbance of this balance and consider them in the context of the patient as a whole and their lives, both inner and outer.

As Dr Edward Bach, famed for his flower remedies, said: '...disease of the body itself is nothing but the result of the disharmony between the soul and mind' and '...health is therefore the true realization of what we are; we are perfect; we are children of God.'

The now-familiar World Health Organization's definition of health as: 'The condition of perfect bodily, spiritual and social wellbeing, and not solely the absence of disease and injury' is a lofty aim, but certainly one that the herbal practitioner aspires to. We are not here solely to relieve symptoms. Bearing this in mind, in addition to redressing specific imbalances, herbalists should ideally prescribe plant remedies in order to attend to the deeper causes of that imbalance, setting their treatments within a framework of life-affirming lifestyles and eating habits.

In his or her 'holistic' approach, the herbalist recognizes that our bodies are made up of a complex organization of tissues and cells that operate on a molecular level, and yet the human organism is so much more than this. Behind the physical manifestation that is the body is the existence of subtle energy, which is recognized by mythology and religion but largely denied by modern science. It is known throughout the world by different names: life force, vital force, 'qi' and 'prana'. We can neither see it nor define it, but it is there and we are animated by this living force on every level of existence – physical, emotional, mental and spiritual. Through this we have an inherent ability to regulate the functions of the body and to heal ourselves, which is known in the West as homeostasis. When this life force is disturbed on any level, the health of the whole person is affected and illness results. Body, emotion, mind and spirit form one interrelated system and an imbalance in one creates disharmony in another. Symptoms of ill health in the

Qi, or life force, flows along energy channels, or meridians. This manuscript depicts the Conception Vessel meridian.

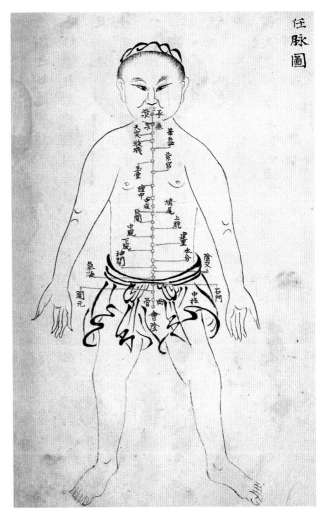

body represent the attempt by the organism to correct the imbalance and heal itself. If these symptoms are suppressed, as they are by modern drugs, the energy of the vital force is depleted, our healing ability dwindles and finally chronic illness results. The body needs to be permitted to express its symptoms as far as possible, and any treatment should be aimed at augmenting the efforts of the vital force, to enhance its healing energy and not work against it. The task of the herbalist is to analyse a patient's presenting symptoms in this respect and to support the body's homeostatic mechanisms through counselling, the use of herbs and foods and lifestyle guidance. A maxim of natural therapy is that medicine cannot change the workings of the body; it can only help them. One of the oldest medical teachings is '*Medicus curat, natura sanat*' – 'The doctor treats, but nature heals'.

Using herbs as medicines

Herbalists use the leaves, flowers, bark, berries, roots or seeds of medicinal plants as their therapeutic tools. By definition, a herb is any plant that has a medicinal action in the body, and this includes most fruits and vegetables. In fact, herbs act very much like foods, and many common foods are used for their medicinal actions:

carrots are good for skin and urinary problems; oats are a great tonic for the nervous system; garlic fights infection, regulates blood pressure and cholesterol; and Blueberries/Bilberries combat free radicals, strengthen blood vessels and help prevent urinary tract infections.

Plants absorb vital nutrients from the soil and then process and store them, providing raw materials – close in chemical composition to those that make up the human body, for growth and repair of bodily tissues – that are easily digested and assimilated. Their vitamins, minerals and trace elements are vital for health and recovery, while other medicinal substances they contain, such as tannins, volatile oils, phenols and saponins have affinities with particular tissues and systems, and act more specifically to promote homeostasis and healing. Clearly then, herbs operate at the level of biochemical reactions in the body, but they are capable of much more. They certainly provide us with a wealth of wonderful chemicals, but their healing power goes far beyond the physical to the realms of the vital force. When herbs work in the body, they enhance the healing action of the vital force, and as they do this, they may also heal our hearts and minds, for they help to restore harmony to an integrated whole.

A Chinese pharmacist explains how a patient should use the herbs she is prescribed.

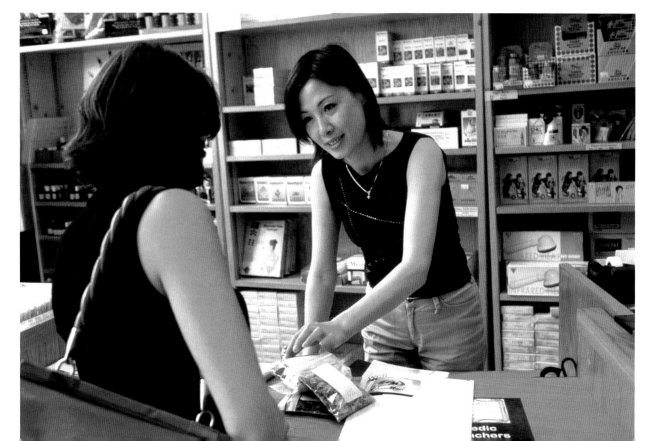

The first visit

It is worth recommending to patients that they prepare for a first visit by compiling lists of present symptoms, past medical and drug history, illnesses and operations as far back as infancy. Their immediate family may provide extra information that has been forgotten, for example breast-feeding and illness in early childhood.

Medical reports from other health consultants, as well as blood profiles, urine analyses, allergy tests and X-ray or scan reports, can provide important information. A diary of food eaten over the previous weeks will also be helpful to the practitioner when analysing the diet. A herbalist will always enquire into mento-emotional realms and some people may find it helpful to prepare for this, since it may be challenging for them to talk about painful experiences or they may not be accustomed to talking about themselves.

Individual evaluation

The consultation begins the minute patient meets practitioner. Consciously or unconsciously, the practitioner will be assessing the patient. The hue and tone of the skin, the brightness of the eyes and hair, the colour of the lips, the expression on the face, the tone of voice, general appearance and dress sense all begin to tell the story. Then there is body language: the expression in the face, the level of tension in the muscles, gait and posture all convey important messages. During the consultation the patient is given time and opportunity to describe his or her concerns in detail. Each person is evaluated as an individual by the herbalist, who records and analyses current presenting symptoms in relation to the person's complete medical history in order to understand the underlying causes and contributing factors that have made the patient seek help.

A case history includes:
- main presenting symptoms
- other symptoms that occur from time to time
- detailed past medical history
- lifestyle, including daily diet, sleep, exercise and relaxation
- temperament, stress levels and mento-emotional concerns

- bodily systems review
- appetite, digestion and elimination
- thirst and sweat
- body temperature; intolerance of heat or cold
- sleep
- energy
- other medicines being taken
- cautions, such as pregnancy or lactation

Through questioning, the practitioner will systematically go through the bodily systems, and the status of his or her functions will all contribute to the analysis of the total health picture of the patient. This will be followed by necessary and relevant physical examinations, which may include tongue, urine and pulse diagnoses, blood pressure, listening to the heart or chest, palpating the abdomen, examining the nails, eyes and skin.

CASE HISTORY

'I consulted a herbalist who combined Western herbal medicine with Ayurvedic techniques. She took a detailed record of my diet and daily routines, and within minutes I began to understand why I was lacking in energy, felt tearful and sensitive and why my digestion needed attention. Then the herbalist took notes on the condition of my skin, hair, eyes and nails. I was already feeling better before I had even been prescribed any herbs. I felt that the hour's consultation was relaxed, yet I had gained a deep and comprehensive understanding of myself as an individual.'

Name	Date of birth
	Occupation
Address	
Telephone E-mail	Date

| Main presenting symptoms | Other symptoms |

Past medical history	Orthodox medication
	Supplements

Family history

Bowel movements/ Appetite/thirst	Sweat Respiratory
Digestion	
	Sleep Hot/cold
Menstruation	Energy level
Genito urinary	
Circulation	

Temperament	Prakruti
	Vikruti
	Pulse
	Tongue

Diet and lifestyle

Aim of treatment

Treatment

The treatment of most ailments begins at home. Many people are almost unwittingly using herbal medicine in common household remedies like salt gargles for sore throats, hot lemon and honey drinks for colds and catarrh, Chamomile tea for sleep, Peppermint to settle the stomach, vinegar for wasp stings and Dock leaves for nettle stings.

The more you can learn about simple remedies that could be sitting in your larder or growing in your garden or wild in the hedgerows, the more opportunity you will have to treat the first signs of acute infections and minor ailments avoiding the necessity for drugs like antibiotics, and thereby help to prevent the development of more serious disorders. Herbs used in this way make excellent preventive medicines and can enhance general wellbeing when taken in conjunction with a healthy diet and lifestyle. For more chronic or serious disorders, it is advisable to consult a professional herbalist who uses herbs in the context of a holistic approach to healing, where physical symptoms are viewed in relation to other factors, including temperament, stress, social, domestic and working environment, relationships, diet, relaxation and exercise. All play a part in the emergence of an individual pattern of symptoms.

Types of patient

Most people consult a herbalist with chronic disorders because either they have been treated unsuccessfully elsewhere or they are seeking a more natural alternative or complement to allopathic drugs from their doctor. Frequently, it is those whose symptoms do not fit into a classic 'disease' picture or who have symptoms for which there is little in the way of allopathy to remedy their situation. Allergies such as eczema, urticaria and conjunctivitis, and hormonal, nervous and immune problems, are good examples of these. Often people come after years of coping with health problems, in which case it may take some time to return them to health. Herbal treatment can be taken alongside allopathic drugs in many instances, and a herbalist will check for any possible herb–drug interactions before prescribing.

For those battling with long-term problems such as heart disease and autoimmune disease, working with a herbalist will help improve general health, energy and

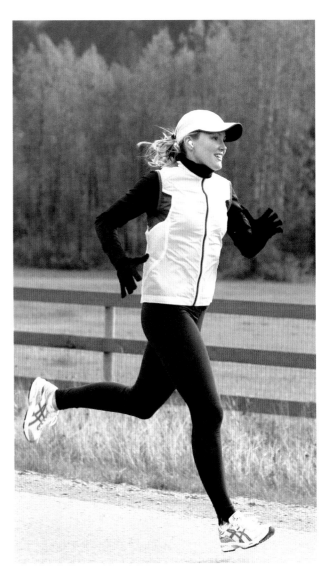

Plenty of exercise, rest and good food enhances wellbeing and makes preventive herbal remedies more effective.

joie de vivre so that the patient is better able to cope with their problems.

As people are becoming more health aware in the holistic sense, they are looking to alternative or complementary health models as a first line of treatment. They may simply feel under the weather, tired or run-down with vague symptoms that they would like to understand and resolve before they progress further. In many cases they may just need to have time to talk, to be heard and understood, and to activate their own self-healing mechanisms with the support of a herbal practitioner. The role of the herbalist is often that of counsellor.

Scheduling visits and fees

Generally, medical herbalists do not hold open surgery, as appointments tend to be lengthy and so need to be booked in advance. First appointments are likely to last about an hour and follow-up visits 30–45 minutes. Many herbalists operate a sliding scale of charges for the consultation and the herbal medicines prescribed, and for students, pensioners, the unemployed or those experiencing hard financial times, fees may be reduced.

Example patient

To illustrate, a patient who presents with chronic ear infections may not require antibiotics to provide an effective and lasting cure. Examination of past medical history may show that there is a history of digestive problems, eczema, asthma or hay fever, and several courses of antibiotics may have been prescribed. Questioning about a patient's diet may reveal chronically sluggish bowels, a tendency to bloating and abdominal discomfort, a high intake of milk products, white bread and sugary foods and drinks, and not enough fruit and vegetables. It is likely that the underlying problem here lies in the gut. Poor digestion and elimination suggested by the sluggish bowels and wind indicate that food is not being digested adequately, resulting in poor absorption, a low nutritional profile and some degree of dysbiosis, leading to food intolerance and toxicity. Food intolerances, most likely to wheat or gluten and dairy produce, as well as high refined carbohydrate and sugar intake, tend to lower immunity and cause accumulation of mucus and chronic congestion in the Eustachian tube that leads from the throat to the ear, predisposing to ear infections. Courses of antibiotics further aggravate the dysbiosis and lower immunity, and the cycle continues.

Diet and lifestyle advice

The herbalist will take time to make detailed dietary changes, recommending that the patient avoids dairy products and wheat or gluten, refined sugar and carbohydrates, and eats more fresh fruit and vegetables (organic wherever possible) combined with culinary herbs and spices that help combat intestinal dysbiosis, such as Oregano, Thyme, Rosemary, Garlic, Ginger, Turmeric and Long pepper. The importance of regular aerobic exercise and the right balance of activity and rest would be discussed. Mental pressures and emotional difficulties would also be gently brought out into the open, as these play a significant role in the digestive system and immunity. Then the herbal prescription would be made. This could consist of herbs in the form of tinctures, teas, tablets or capsules, or powders for internal use or creams, lotions or oils for external application. A follow-up appointment would be made to review progress and the treatment may then be modified if necessary. It is always preferable if a patient continues treatment until he or she feels better or the herbalist has taught the patient how to continue with his or her care at home. The role of the herbalist is definitely one of educator.

Herbal teas may be prescribed as part of dietary changes, replacing caffeinated drinks that may aggravate health problems.

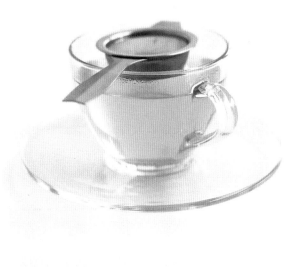

Formulating a herbal prescription

Herbal prescriptions are generally tailor-made for each individual depending on their specific needs. They need to address a variety of different issues. Digestion and elimination are absolutely central to good health, and poor digestion, dysbiosis and toxicity are underlying factors in a whole range of different illnesses, including gut problems, lowered immunity, allergies, autoimmune disease, obesity and cancer.

Herbs that improve digestion and clear toxicity from the bowel are, therefore, the first considerations. Then there are herbs that need to be added for the constitutional imbalance of the system of the body affected, whether it is the nervous system in the case of anxiety and insomnia or the respiratory system in the case of bronchitis. Finally, herbs need to be included that are specific to the actual symptoms or disease, such as Frankincense for arthritis and Bearberry for urinary tract infections.

In short, the following factors need to be addressed when formulating a prescription:
- digestion
- toxicity
- constitution
- system involved
- disease

Example prescription

In the example given on page 53 of chronic ear infection, a herbalist might prescribe antimicrobial herbs such as Garlic, Turmeric, Ginger, Golden seal, Neem and Cinnamon to combat infection and dysbiosis. The herbs chosen may be combined with immune-enhancing herbs such as Andrographis, Thyme, Echinacea and Pau d'arco. Decongestant herbs like Peppermint, Elderflower, Yarrow and Ginger can be given in teas (hot infusions work better than tinctures in this case) to clear excess mucus. Diluted essential oils of Lavender, Chamomile or Thyme can be used in ear drops or for massage around the ear and throat to relieve congestion in the Eustachian tube.

Many people ask how long it will take for them to recover, and of course this depends very much on the nature of their illness and how long the symptoms have been apparent, as well as on the age, constitution and strength of the patient. A person treated with herbs may not necessarily 'recover' as quickly as someone who has

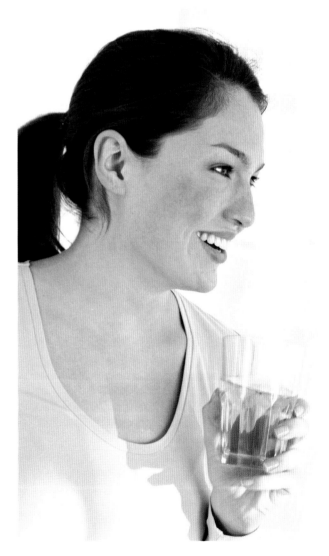

Hot infusions are more effective than tinctures for treating skin complaints, fevers, colds and catarrh.

been treated with conventional allopathic drugs, but once better, the patient will generally feel stronger than after taking a course of orthodox medicine. By increasing the patient's general health and the efficiency of weak organs or body systems, herbal medicine helps raise resistance to further illness and also helps to prevent chronic disease.

The method of administering herbs and the length of treatment needed by a patient will vary considerably according to the condition being treated, which herbs are used, the patient's age, build and constitution, and even the time of year. The dosage, the herbs chosen for the prescription and the timing of administration all need to be determined. A largely built person with big bones and muscles and a comparatively sluggish metabolism will generally require herbs to be given in larger doses and over a longer period of time than a small-framed, lightweight person with a more sensitive body and a faster metabolism.

Dosage for adult patients can also vary according to the practitioner and which kind of herbal medicine he or she practises. A standard dose of tincture can vary from a few drops to 5 ml (1 teaspoon). Teas are generally taken a cupful at a time, powders are taken in doses of ¼–1 teaspoon and syrups may require being taken a dessertspoonful or tablespoonful at a time. For dosage instructions for children, see the box below.

Chronic and acute conditions

When treating chronic conditions, generally mild herbal remedies are taken 3 times daily, over months at a time if necessary. It may be that the first prescription and dietary advice is intended to improve digestion and absorption, and to clear toxins from the system, which is necessary in so many cases. This will be followed up by more nourishing tonic medicines until the patient is better. Acute conditions may require stronger herbs given up to every 2 hours. For example, Ashwagandha is nourishing and strengthening and is taken 2–3 times a day over a few weeks or months to improve energy, vitality and immunity and enhance resilience to stress, while Echinacea and Wild indigo are taken every 2 hours to enhance immunity and combat acute infections.

Appropriate administration

Hot preparations are needed in fevers, colds, catarrh and problems associated with cold, such as poor circulation and menstrual cramps, while urinary problems and conditions associated with heat, such as hot flushes and acne, are better suited to cool preparations. Skin problems may improve more rapidly using herbal teas

as opposed to tinctures, but tinctures may be preferable when more concentrated medicines are needed, as when treating a virulent infection.

The herbs chosen may also indicate their best method of administration. When giving teas, the aerial parts of a plant are prepared as infusions, while roots, barks and seeds are better suited to decoctions. Nourishing tonics are best taken as powders stirred into warm milk or water, and warming spices to clear catarrhal congestion and coughs can be taken as powders mixed with honey and taken off a spoon.

Generally, herbs are taken either side of or during a meal. When using herbs to enhance appetite, digestion and absorption, they can be taken before a meal; for problems associated with heat, acidity and inflammation, they can be taken with a meal, otherwise they can be taken immediately after eating. Tinctures need to be diluted with water, otherwise they can taste unpleasant and irritate a delicate stomach.

CHILD'S DOSAGE GUIDELINES

When it comes to dosage for children, there are two rules that are employed by some practitioners:

Young's method: child's dosage = adult dose (generally 5 ml/1 teaspoon) x age divided by age +12

Cowling's method: child's dosage = adult dose x age divided by 24

Alternatively, dosage can be calculated according to weight: child's dosage = adult dose x child's weight divided by 68 kg (150 lb).

Safety issues

The question of possible side effects and toxicity has arisen more recently as herbs are increasingly under the scrutiny of the scientific eye. However, adverse reactions to herbal medicines seldom occur in practice, and those that do occur generally consist of mild rashes or bowel changes. A herbal practitioner would not normally expect 'healing crises', with an exacerbation of symptoms before they start to recede.

There are two main sources of information about the efficacy and safety of herbal medicines: ancient folklore and modern science. The empirical evidence gathered by herbalists over thousands of years, which is now being increasingly justified by scientific research, means that patients may be assured that their herbal prescriptions are based on reliable foundations. Many herbs form the basis of modern orthodox medicines and it may be surprising to learn that the pharmaceutical industry harvests huge plantations of herbs for use in the production of drugs each year. It also grows herbs for further research activities.

It is the herbalist's view that the use of whole-plant medicines as opposed to isolated active ingredients helps to prevent adverse side effects. The many types of substances in medicinal plants work synergistically together and probably all have important roles to play in the healing process. The primary healing agents are the active constituents that were isolated by the early chemists and developed into modern drugs, but the importance of the other, apparently secondary, constituents should not be ignored, as they are vital for determining the efficacy of the primary healing agents. Some secondary synergistic substances make the active constituents more easily assimilated and available in the body, while others will buffer the action of other potent plant chemicals, preventing possible side effects. It is largely the combination of both types of substance occurring in the whole plant that determines the potency and safety of herbal medicine.

Potential adverse reactions

Having said this, with the huge range of biochemical constituents that occur in herbs, it is possible that, though generally safe, some could potentially cause allergic reactions and idiosyncratic responses in the same way that foods do. Most of these can be avoided by herbalists who are generally familiar with the chemistry of herbs they are prescribing and prescribe herbs that are formulated to suit the specific needs of the patient in appropriate doses only after taking a detailed case history. Certain people are more likely to have hypersensitive reactions to herbs than others, particularly those who already have a history of food allergy or intolerance, or chemical sensitivity. This is more likely if they suffer from digestive problems, and specifically from imbalances in the intestinal flora, intestinal dysbiosis and leaky gut syndrome, which actually lend themselves very well to herbal treatment.

The risk of adulteration of herbs supplied to herbalists is one that is obviously a concern. Adverse effects have occurred on occasions due to adulteration with toxic herbs as well as bad labelling. When buying herbs it is vital that the sources of herbs are known to be reputable and preferably organic, as adverse reactions to pesticides and preservatives are hard to quantify and could be confused with reactions to a plant itself. Indian and Chinese herbs are considered more of a safety problem than European herbs, although the use of pesticides in Eastern Europe has also attracted negative attention.

Herb–drug interactions

This is a relatively new science, and very few herb–drug interactions have been recorded. Available information on the subject (much of which may be speculative rather than empirical) is growing all the time. Although herbs have been taken for thousands of years, they have been used in combination with nutritional supplements and allopathic drugs on a widespread basis for only approximately the last 30 years. The concern is not so much that the reaction between a herb and a drug is toxic, rather that it is possible that certain herbs can affect

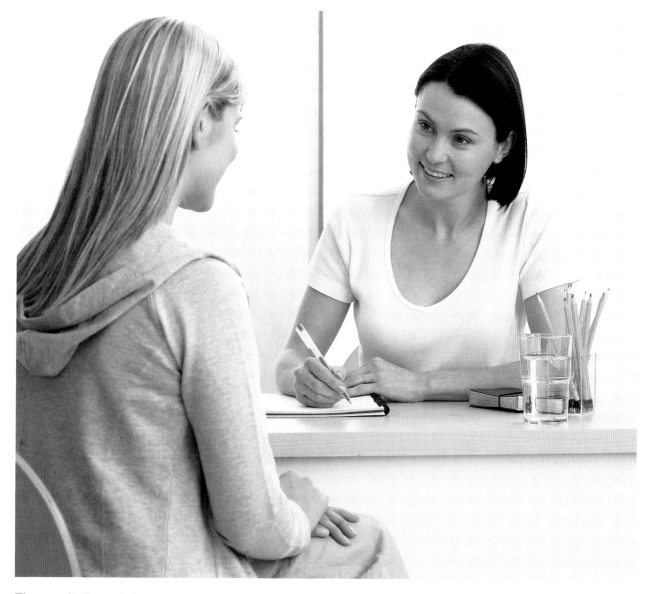

The consultation is the herbalist's tool for determining the right course of herbal treatment for the patient.

the bioavailability of drugs and nutrients, and cause an increase or decrease in levels of drugs in the blood. This is an especially important consideration for the herbal prescriber if patients are taking specific doses of powerful drugs, such as cardiac medication and anticlotting agents or drugs given prior to surgery.

Herbs high in mucilage or fibre, such as Slippery elm or Psyllium seeds, or herbs rich in tannins that could bind up drugs in the intestines, may inhibit absorption. Warming digestive herbs such as Cayenne pepper, Long pepper and Black pepper can increase the absorption of medicine, while herbs that act on liver enzyme systems may affect the breakdown of certain drugs and inhibit its elimination, effectively raising the drug dosage, which could cause side effects. Care needs to be taken with insulin-dependent diabetics, as certain herbs lower blood sugar. Interestingly, in China where the herbal tradition has remained unbroken and there is less suspicion about herbs than there is in the West, herbs are often combined with drugs for intentional effects, either to reduce side effects of drugs or to enhance their effects.

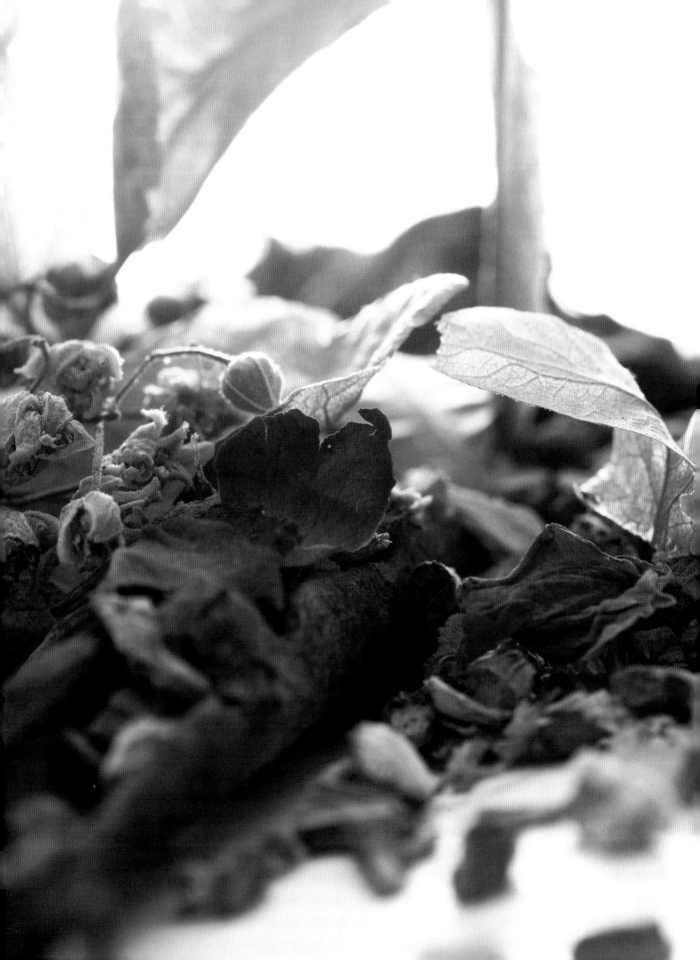

The herbal pharmacy

There are many ways to prepare beneficial herbal remedies so that they will be absorbed by the body and exert their effects. Depending on the condition being treated and the health or age of the patient, a herbalist might choose to prescribe a tea, a syrup, or an ointment to apply to the skin. Here are step-by-step instructions for preparing these remedies, as well as tinctures and decoctions, honeys, poultices and fragrant baths. Dosage instructions are included.

Preparing herbs

Collecting wild herbs or growing them in your garden and harvesting them for making medicines can be very rewarding and uplifting. For those who do not have access to fresh plants, dried herbs are available from many suppliers. Try to use organic herbs as pesticides may disrupt the therapeutic effect or cause adverse reactions.

Methods of preparation

Herbs can be prepared as medicines in a variety of ways. What is important is that they are absorbed into the body so that they can exert their maximum benefit. Internal preparations such as infusions, decoctions, tinctures, syrups, honeys and tablets and capsules are swallowed so that they pass through the digestive tract and into the bloodstream. Many people are unconsciously taking remedies in their food on a daily basis, for not only do all the culinary herbs and spices add flavour to our diet but at the same time they contain volatile oils, which have digestive and antimicrobial effects among many other benefits. As the foods are absorbed from the digestive tract, so the therapeutic constituents of the herbs enter the bloodstream and then circulate round the body.

When used externally, herbs can be applied to the skin, as in aromatherapy or rubbing a Dock leaf onto a nettle sting, or used in herbal baths, compresses and poultices. Once in contact with the skin they are absorbed into tiny capillaries under the surface and then circulated around the body. The conjunctiva of the eye also absorbs herbal preparations. A Chamomile eyebath or a Marigold compress will relieve sore and inflamed eyes. Inhalations are another very good therapeutic pathway and a main one that is utilized by aromatherapists. By inhalation into the nose, which is lined with nerve endings, the messages from the herbs are carried directly to the brain and to the lungs, where they are absorbed with oxygen into the bloodstream and circulated throughout the body.

Infusions

Herbal teas, often known as infusions, are simple water-based preparations that extract the medicinal properties of herbs, used either fresh or dried. They can be drunk as teas or used externally as skin washes, eyebaths, compresses and douches, or added to baths or sitz baths.

To make an infusion

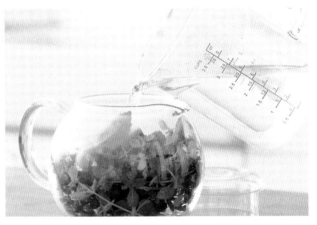

1 Take 50 g (2 oz) fresh herb per 600 ml (1 pint) water or 2 teaspoons of herb per cupful of water. Halve the amount of herbs if they are being used dried. Place the herbs in a warmed teapot and pour on boiling water.

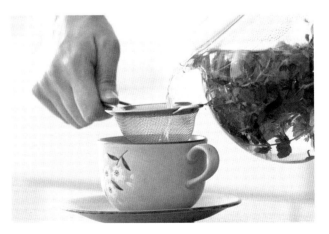

2 Cover to prevent oils escaping into the atmosphere. Leave to infuse for 10–15 minutes, strain and drink.

Infusions are prepared like a normal cup of tea using the soft parts of plants, leaves, stems and flowers. Generally, infusions are best drunk when still hot, especially when treating fevers, colds and catarrh, but need to be taken lukewarm to cool for problems of the urinary tract. If necessary, they can be covered and stored in the refrigerator for up to 2 days. Some herbs need to be prepared as cold infusions, as their therapeutic components are likely to be destroyed by high temperatures. These include herbs that have a high proportion of mucilage, such as Marshmallow and Comfrey leaf. They are prepared in the same way (as shown on page 60), but using cold water and left to infuse for 10–12 hours.

Dosage

Generally, infusions are taken by the cupful 3–6 times a day, depending on whether the ailment being treated is chronic or acute. It may come as a surprise to some who are used to the delightful taste of culinary herbs such as Basil and Rosemary that many herbs are found by our pampered palates to taste strange, often even unpleasant. Although the bitters in some herbs need to be tasted to be effective, the bitter taste is generally not something we relish. However, it is possible to combine several herbs together in an infusion so that aromatic, pleasant-tasting herbs such as Peppermint, Fennel, Lemon balm and Lavender can disguise less-palatable herbs while not reducing their effect. Liquorice and Aniseed also make excellent herbs for flavouring. Infusions can be sweetened with honey if necessary.

Herbal tea bags are sold in health-food stores and supermarkets (buy organic if you can) and normally comprise the more aromatic, pleasant-tasting herbs like Lime flower, Fennel and Peppermint.

Decoctions

The hard, woody parts of plants have tough cell walls that require greater heat to break them down before they will release their constituents into the water. Bark, seeds, roots, rhizomes and nuts all need to be prepared as decoctions.

Use the same proportion of herbs to water as you do when preparing an infusion (see page 60), but just add a little more water to make up for losses during boiling.

Dosage

As for infusions (see above).

To make a decoction

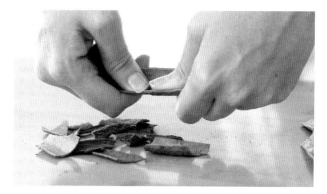

1 Break the herb up into small pieces, crush with a pestle and mortar or smash with a hammer if very hard.

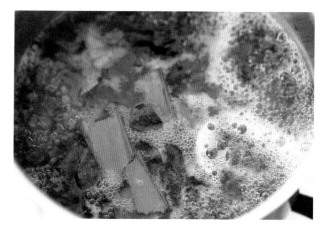

2 Place the herbs in a stainless steel or enamel saucepan and cover with cold water. Bring to the boil, then reduce the heat, cover and simmer for 10–15 minutes.

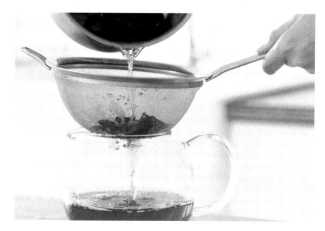

3 Strain and drink in the same way as an infusion (see page 60).

Tinctures

Tinctures are concentrated extracts of herbs made with a mixture of water and alcohol, which acts to extract the constituents of the plants and also as a preservative. According to herbal pharmacopoeias there is a correct ratio of water and alcohol to plant matter for each herb, depending on the constituents that need extracting. This can range from 25 per cent alcohol for simple glycosides and tannins to 90 per cent for resins and gums such as those in Marigold flowers. Herbs can be used in a ratio of 1 part fresh herbs to 2 parts liquid, or 1 part dried herbs to 5 parts liquid.

As an example, to make 1 litre (1¾ pints) Chamomile tincture, use 200 g (7 oz) dried flowers and 1 litre (1¾ pints) fluid. Chamomile requires a 45 per cent alcohol solution, so neat brandy or vodka would be perfectly adequate. If you have 100 per cent alcohol, use 450 ml (¾ pint) alcohol to 550 ml (18 fl oz) water.

Vinegar- and glycerol-based tinctures

Tinctures can also be prepared using neat cider vinegar, as the acetic acid acts as a solvent and preservative. Raspberry vinegar, for example, is a traditional remedy for coughs and sore throats. Glycerol-based tinctures have a sweet, syrup-like taste that makes them a good medium for children's medicines. Pour 80 per cent of glycerol and 20 per cent of water over the herbs in the same proportion of herb to liquid as for alcohol tinctures (see above). Peppermint, Lemon balm, Lavender, Rose, Holy basil, Elderflower and Mint are well suited to this method.

Dosage

Because they are concentrated, only small amounts of tincture need to be taken at regular intervals through the day. The dose will vary from 5–10 drops to 1 teaspoon, taken in a little warm water, fruit juice or herbal tea, 3–6 times daily, depending on whether the condition is chronic or acute. Tinctures can also be added to bath water, mixed with water for compresses, mouthwashes or gargles, or stirred into a base to make ointments or creams. Tinctures require more preparation time, but they have several advantages. They are easy to store, do not deteriorate in cold or damp conditions, take up relatively little storage space, are easy to carry around and keep almost indefinitely, although they are best taken within 2 years.

To make a tincture

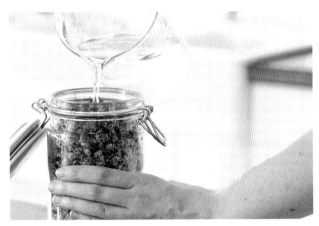

1 Place the chopped herb in a large, clean jar and pour the water and alcohol mixture over it so that the plant is immersed. Place an airtight lid on the jar and leave it to macerate away from direct sunlight for no less than 2 weeks, shaking the jar well about once a day.

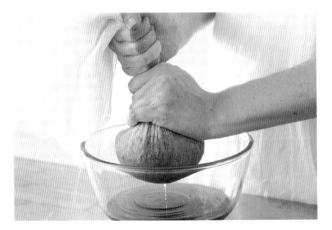

2 Once the tincture has macerated, use a press such as a wine press to extract as much of the fluid as possible. Alternatively, squeeze it through muslin, which is much harder work but possible. Discard the herbs, then transfer the tincture to a clean, dark, lidded bottle, label with the name of the herb and date and store in a cool, dark place.

Syrups

This type of herbal remedy is designed to make herbal preparations more palatable. Bitter herbs such as Dandelion, Burdock, Rosemary, White horehound, Yellow dock, Vervain and Motherwort are particularly suited to this method when these herbs are being prescribed for children.

Expectorant herbs for coughs, asthma and chest infections including Thyme, Hyssop, Elecampane, White horehound, Elderberry, Coltsfoot and Mullein are are often prepared as syrups, particularly when honey is included in the ingredients. Syrups can also be added to other herbal preparations to mask their more unpleasant tastes. These remedies will keep for up to 2 years.

Dosage

Generally, 1–2 dessertspoonfuls should be taken 3–4 times a day for chronic problems and every 2 hours in acute cases.

To make a syrup

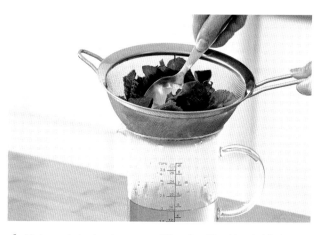

1 Make an infusion (see page 60) using 25 g (1 oz) dried herb to 600 ml (1 pint) boiling water. Double the amount of herbs if they are being used fresh. Leave to macerate in water for 6–8 hours. Strain the liquid, press as much residual water from the herb before discarding it and measure how much fluid is left.

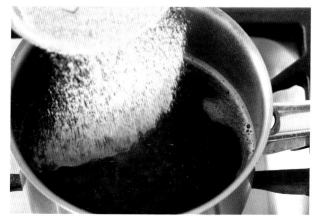

3 Add 400 g (13 oz) sugar or 350 ml (12 fl oz) honey (or other sweetener of your choice) and bring to the boil until the sugar has dissolved.

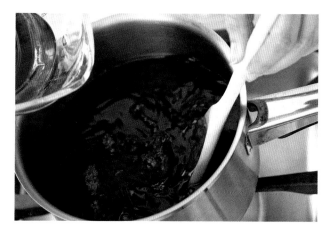

2 Pour the infusion into a saucepan and bring to the boil. Cover and simmer over a low heat until the liquid is reduced by half, which may take several hours.

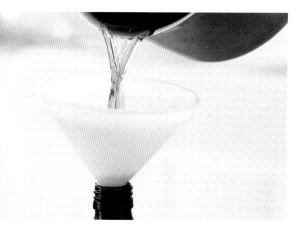

4 Pour into a sterilized bottle and leave to cool. If desired, add 5 per cent of the same tincture to preserve the syrup for longer. Label the bottle and store in a cool, dark place.

Honeys

Honey has been used for healing for thousands of years. It is hydroscopic, which means that it absorbs the water-soluble constituents and volatile oils of the plant. Honey has antibacterial, expectorant and healing properties, so herbal honeys can be used to treat sore throats, coughs, chest infections and asthma, and can also be used externally to heal or soothe skin problems such as cuts and grazes, burns and varicose ulcers. Honey makes an excellent medium for antimicrobial herbs such as Garlic, Onion, Thyme, Hyssop, Oregano and Rosemary.

Honey is also highly nutritive, rich in easily digestible sugars and energy giving, and it enhances the immune system. It contains pollen, which is rich in protein, vitamins, minerals and fatty acids and helpful in the treatment of allergies and asthma, and propolis, which is a powerful antimicrobial. Thyme honey from Greece is renowned for its health-giving properties, as is Manuka honey from New Zealand, which is often used as an antibacterial.

Dosage
Take 1 tablespoon of herbal honey in a little hot water or simply off the spoon. Do not give to children under the age of 1 due to the risk of botulinus.

Other uses for honey
You can also simply give freshly chopped herbs in a teaspoon of honey. Sweets and throat lozenges can be made by rolling powdered herbs in honey to make a paste that can be rolled into balls and then again in the powder to prevent stickiness for handling and storing. Store in a tightly fitting tin.

Tablets and capsules

Many herbs are available from herbal suppliers in tablet or capsule form and this is a convenient way to take herbs, but it bypasses the taste buds on the tongue, which may reduce the therapeutic effects in some cases. However, only standard preparations will be available as commercial pills, so should you require a specific combination of herbs they can be made up in gelatin capsules. Capsules can be filled with mixtures of the appropriate herbs using a capsule maker.

Dosage
Two main sizes of capsule are used by medical herbalists: size 0, which holds 0.35 gm powder, and size 00, which holds about 0.5 gm; 1–2 size 0 capsules can be taken once daily and 1 size 00 capsule 3 times daily.

To make a honey

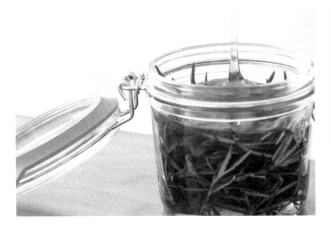

Place your chosen herbs, coarsely chopped or bruised, in a clean, sterilized jar, cover with honey and stir well. Seal with an airtight lid, label clearly and leave to macerate for at least 4 weeks but preferably several months. Store in a cool, dark place or in the refrigerator.

To make capsules

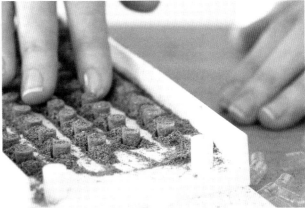

Fill a capsule maker with open capsules, cover them with your chosen combination of powdered herbs and make sure each capsule is packed tightly. Add the capsule lids and then remove the capsules from the maker. Place in a clearly labelled container with an airtight lid and store in a cool, dark place.

Ointments and creams

Ointments and creams can be applied to the skin not only for treatment of skin problems but also for the treatment of less superficial ailments, such as inflamed joints and headaches. Any fresh or dried herb can be made into an ointment using the recipe below.

Creams can be made easily by stirring tinctures, decoctions or a few drops of essential oil into a cream base such as aqueous cream. Many types of eczema can be effectively treated, for example, by mixing 2–3 drops of Chamomile oil (*Chamomilla Recutita*) into 50 g (2 oz) of base cream that can be purchased from most herbal suppliers.

Dosage

Apply ointments and creams to the affected areas 2–3 times daily in chronic conditions, or more frequently if necessary in acute problems.

To make an ointment

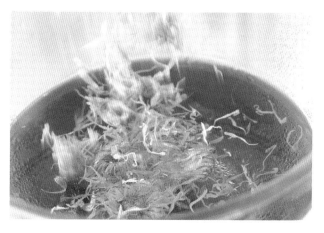

1 Melt 50 g (2 oz) beeswax with 450 ml (¾ pint) olive oil in a Pyrex bowl over a saucepan of boiling water, or a double boiler. Add as much herb as possible. Leave to macerate for a few hours over a low heat.

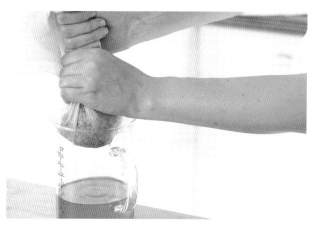

3 Squeeze the muslin to press out as much of the mixture as possible and discard the herb.

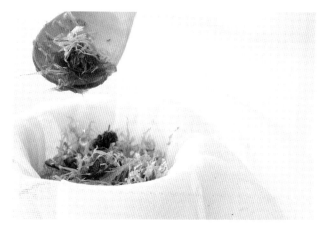

2 Spoon the macerated herbs into a piece of muslin placed over a jug. Allow the liquid to strain through the fabric.

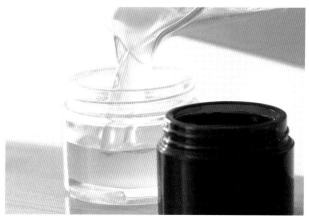

4 While warm, pour into clean ointment jars to solidify quickly. Seal with an airtight lid, label and store in a cool, dark place.

Compresses

A clean cloth or flannel can be soaked in either a hot or cold infusion (see page 60), a decoction (see page 61), a dilute tincture (see page 62), or water with a few drops of diluted essential oil (see below), then wrung out and applied to the affected part. This can help relieve symptoms such as headaches, abdominal colic, backache, boils and painful joints. The treatment needs to repeated several times for good effect.

Poultices

These are similar to compresses but involve using the herb itself rather than an extract of the herb. Some herbs can be applied directly to the skin, such as Comfrey. They need to be softened first by removing any hard stalks or ribs and immersing them briefly in hot water to prevent any discomfort to the skin. Once applied, they can be secured in place by a light bandage and left overnight.

Liniments

A rubbing oil or liniment consists of extracts of herbs in an oil or tincture, or a mixture of both. The oils can be infused oils or essential oils diluted in a base such as sesame oil (see below). They are used in massage to relax or stimulate muscles and ligaments or to soothe away pain from inflammation or injury. They are intended to be absorbed by the skin to reach the affected part and so they often contain a stimulating essential oil such as Ginger or Black pepper and are therefore not suitable for use on delicate baby skins.

Oils

Essential oils need to be used with care, especially with children and babies. They can be used diluted in a base oil such as sesame oil (1–2 drops of essential oil per 5 ml/1 teaspoon of base oil) for massage and use in the bath. They can also be used neat in burners to permeate the atmosphere or in inhalations for a variety of symptoms such as colds, catarrh, coughs, insomnia and anxiety.

While essential oils are extracted from aromatic plants professionally by steam distillation, infused oils can easily be prepared at home. Place finely chopped, preferably fresh herbs (make sure they are not wet) in a jar with a tight-fitting lid, cover them with an oil such as almond, coconut, olive or sesame, pouring it up to the top of the jar, and then stir well. Add the lid, label the jar with the name of the herb and the date, then place the jar on a sunny windowsill to macerate for approximately 4–8 weeks. Be aware that if there is any moisture on the plant or jar, or if it is left for longer than the specified time, the oil may go mouldy.

To make a poultice

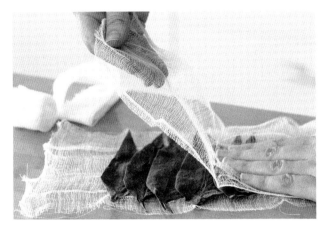

1 Place the fresh or dried herb between 2 pieces of gauze. If you use fresh leaves, stems or roots, they need to be bruised before being applied. If the herbs are dry, add a little hot water to powdered or finely chopped herbs to make a paste.

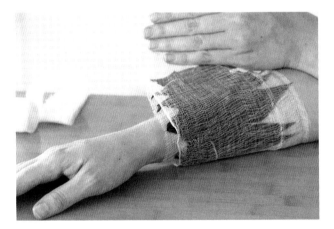

2 Use a light cotton bandage to bind the gauze poultice to the affected part and keep it warm with a hot water bottle. Replace after 4 hours and apply about 3 times daily.

The oil gradually takes up the plant constituents; you can see this in action if you macerate St John's wort in oil. In minutes the oil will turn deep red. This oil is a useful remedy for healing cuts and sores, and when massaged over the affected part can relieve painful nerve conditions such as trigeminal neuralgia and shingles. After 2 weeks, filter the oil through muslin, squeezing to extract all the oil. Store in a clean, dark, labelled bottle with an airtight lid in a cool, dark place.

Herbal baths

A fragrant hot bath makes a very pleasant and simple way to take herbs. There are various ways of adding herbs to bath water: you can dilute essential oils (1 drop of essential oil per 5 ml of base oil such as sesame oil) and add them into the bathwater; hang a muslin bag containing fresh or dried aromatic herbs under the hot tap as you draw the bath; or pour 600 ml (1 pint) of strong herbal infusion (double the standard dose given on page 60) into the water. Soak in the warm bath for 10–20 minutes.

When herbs are used in this way, the essential oils from the plants are taken in via the pores of the skin, which are opened up by the warmth of the water. The oils are also carried on the steam, which is simultaneously inhaled via nose and mouth into the lungs and from there into the bloodstream. From the nose, messages are carried from the oils via nerve pathways to the brain. Herbal medicines are assimilated quickly and directly in this way, bypassing the lengthy process of digestion necessary when herbs are taken by mouth. They are particularly useful for relaxing and soothing the nervous system and for easing mental and emotional strain.

Lavender, Lemon balm, Holy basil, Rose and Chamomile are not only wonderfully fragrant but also relaxing, calming tension and anxiety and helping to ensure restful sleep. Chamomile is excellent for fractious children, particularly when they are unwell, for not only does it possess antimicrobial properties but it also helps induce sleep – nature's best way to ward off infection and enable self-healing. Rosemary baths, while also relaxing, have a stimulating edge, as they enhance blood flow to the head and enable greater alertness and concentration.

Herbal sitz baths can be very useful for soothing the pain and irritation of cystitis, vaginal infections or haemorrhoids. Simply fill a large, shallow bowl with about 1 litre (1¾ pints) of strained, strong infusion, enough to reach the necessary areas, sit in it and relax for 10–15 minutes.

Hand and foot baths

Mustard foot baths were historically used for all afflictions of cold and damp climates, from colds and flu to poor circulation and arthritis. The ancient tradition of hand and foot baths was popularized by the famous French herbalist Maurice Mességué, who has written several books on herbal therapy based simply on this form of treatment. He recommends foot baths for 8 minutes in the evening and hand baths for 8 minutes in the morning. The hands and feet are, according to Mességué, highly sensitive areas of the skin, rich in nerve endings, and despite some thickening of the skin from use, the constituents pass easily from the skin into the body. To try this, add 1 tablespoon of mustard powder to a bowl of warm water and sit with your feet in it for 8–10 minutes.

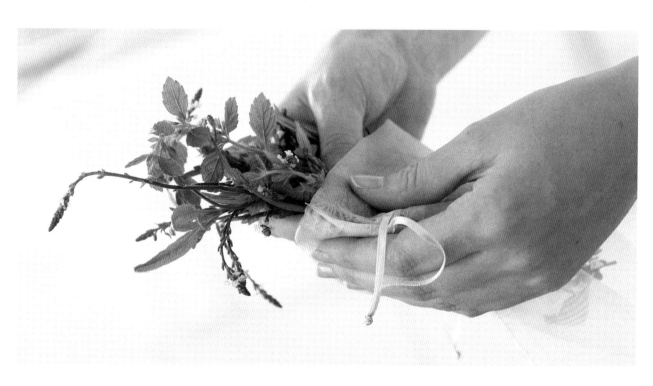

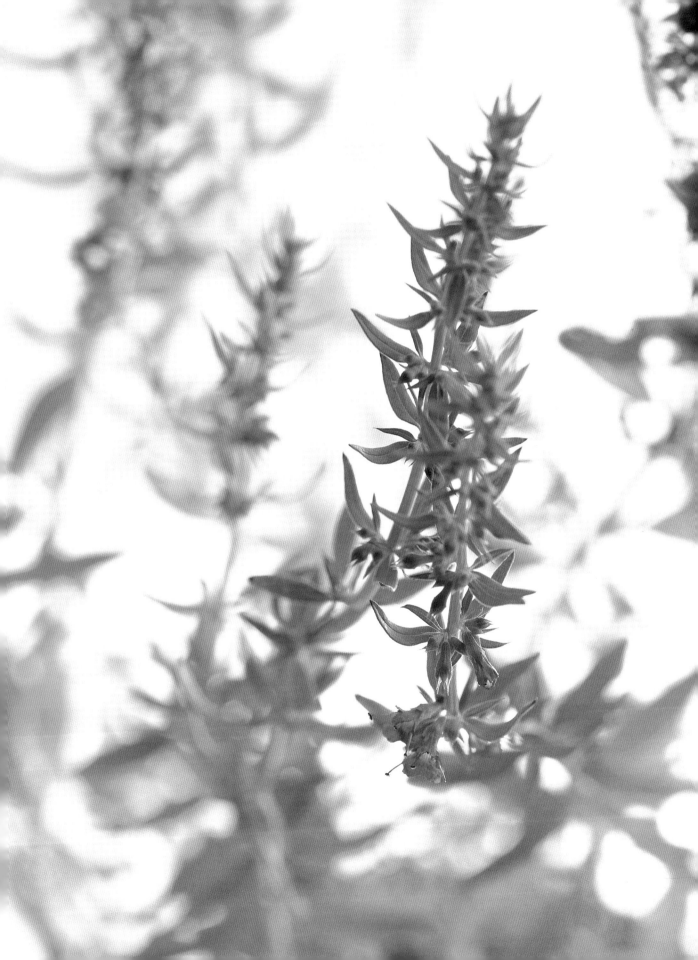

The materia medica

A materia medica is a compendium of medicinal herbs used for their therapeutic effects, and traditionally describes each herb's pharmacological properties and medicinal actions. The first such collection of knowledge on healing plants appeared in India around 700 BCE, compiled by the scholar Charaka, and a similar manual was assembled in China around 1000 CE. The term *materia medica* is Latin and has been used since Roman times when Dioscorides wrote a five-volume book in Greek *'De Materia Medica'* that was subsequently translated into Latin around 60 CE. Dioscorides' book was a commentary on around 500 medicinal plants.

How to use the materia medica

The materia medica is the heart of this book. It is a comprehensive directory of the 150 herbs most commonly used by modern Western herbalists. They are all easily available from most herbal suppliers, and because this book is intended for use by lay people as well as students and practitioners of herbal medicine, none of them is a 'Schedule 3' herb, that is herbs whose dosage is restricted by law due to the presence of powerful constituents, often alkaloids, that require caution in their use.

The materia medica is divided into two parts. The first part is a photographic identification guide. The herbs are grouped in botanical families, which can be a helpful way of classifying them, not only because of their botanical resemblances but also because there are often similarities in the actions of herbs in the same family. Take the rose family, for example, which includes Rose, Agrimony, Lady's Mantle, Meadowsweet and Hawthorn. All of these herbs contain tannins that have an astringent effect in the body, drying excess secretions and protecting mucous membranes from infection and inflammation. Many of the mint family (Lamiaceae) are rich in essential oils and are important as culinary herbs, while a number of herbs in the daisy family (Asteraceae) are good for healing wounds and stopping bleeding.

If you intend to use this part of the materia medica to identify fresh herbs you have gathered from the wild, it is very important that you make doubly sure you are picking the correct herb before using it by verifying it with someone familiar with the plant.

The second part of the materia medica is a detailed herbal directory, organized alphabetically by Latin name. Each entry includes the common name, family, parts used, major constituents and the actions of the plant. It then lists the herb's indications for use in treatment according to the systems of the body, including recent scientific research information. This makes for easy cross-reference to the 'Treating common ailments' chapter (see pages 176–231) so that you can be informed about the herbs that you choose.

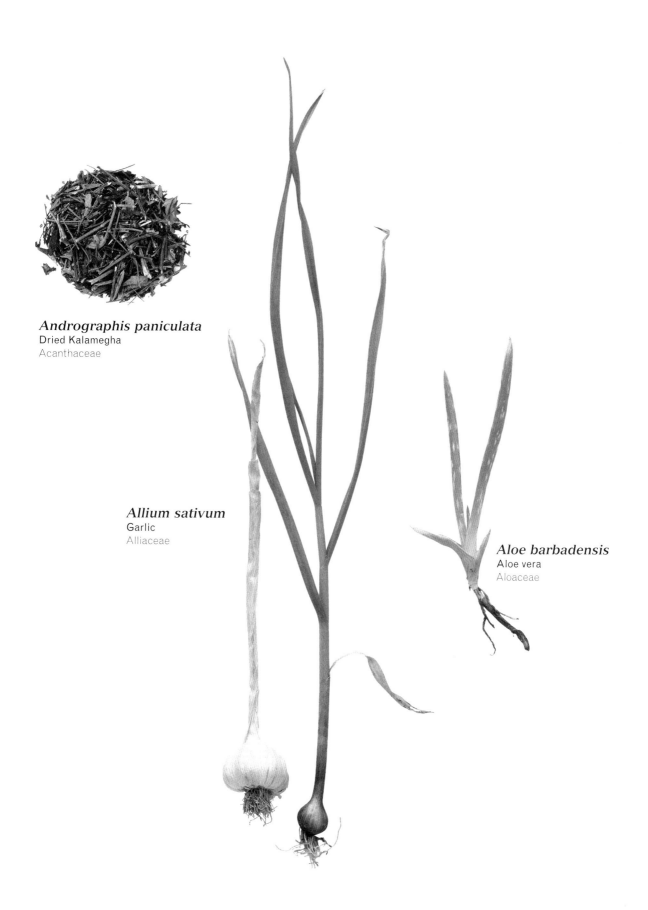

Andrographis paniculata
Dried Kalamegha
Acanthaceae

Allium sativum
Garlic
Alliaceae

Aloe barbadensis
Aloe vera
Aloaceae

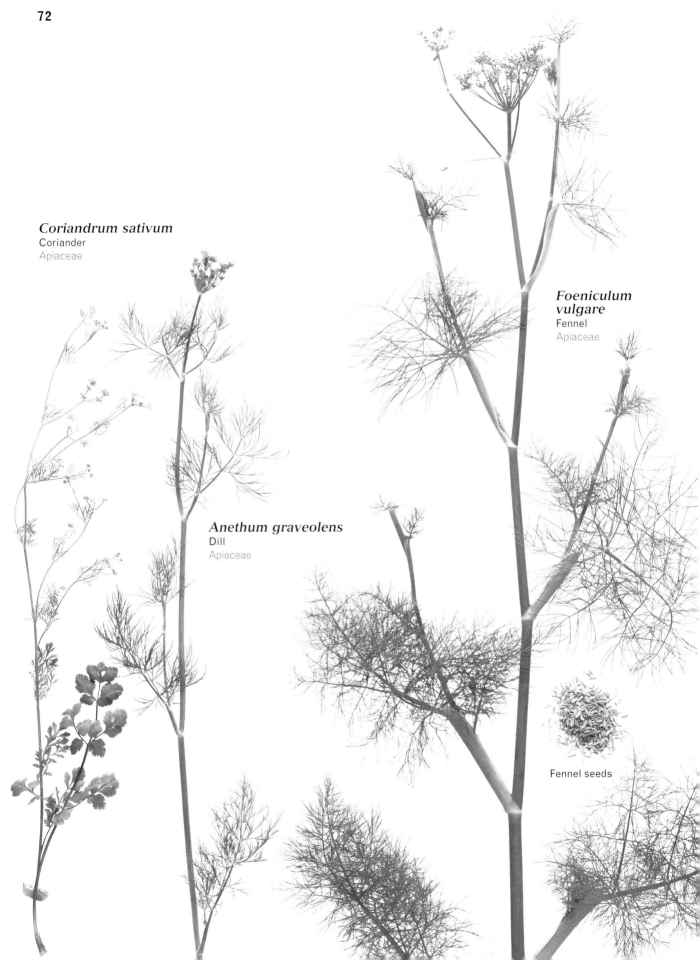

Coriandrum sativum
Coriander
Apiaceae

Foeniculum vulgare
Fennel
Apiaceae

Anethum graveolens
Dill
Apiaceae

Fennel seeds

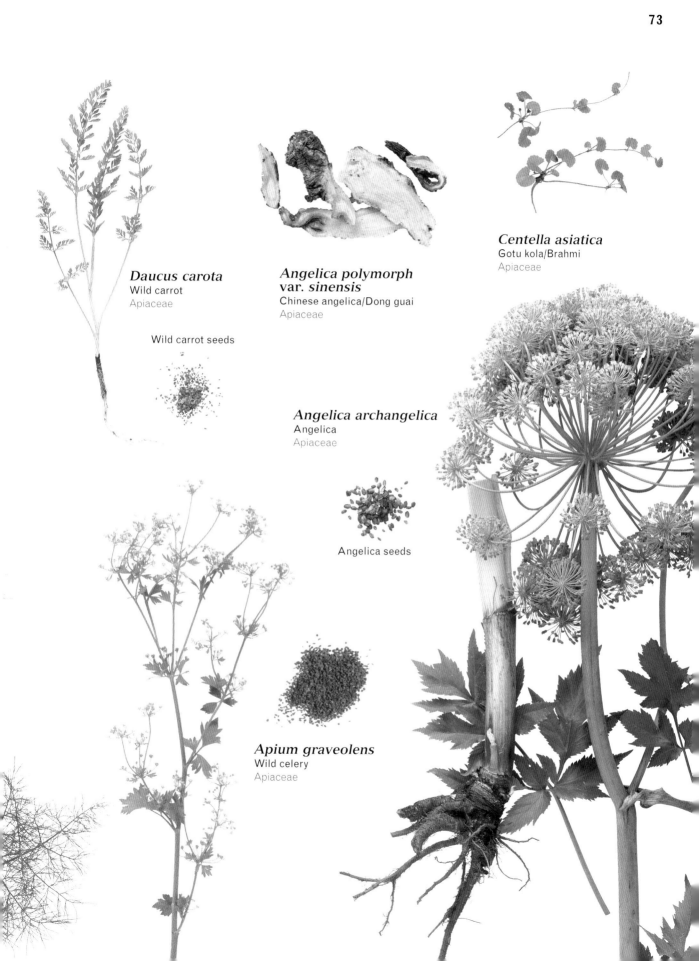

Daucus carota
Wild carrot
Apiaceae

Wild carrot seeds

Angelica polymorph
var. sinensis
Chinese angelica/Dong guai
Apiaceae

Centella asiatica
Gotu kola/Brahmi
Apiaceae

Angelica archangelica
Angelica
Apiaceae

Angelica seeds

Apium graveolens
Wild celery
Apiaceae

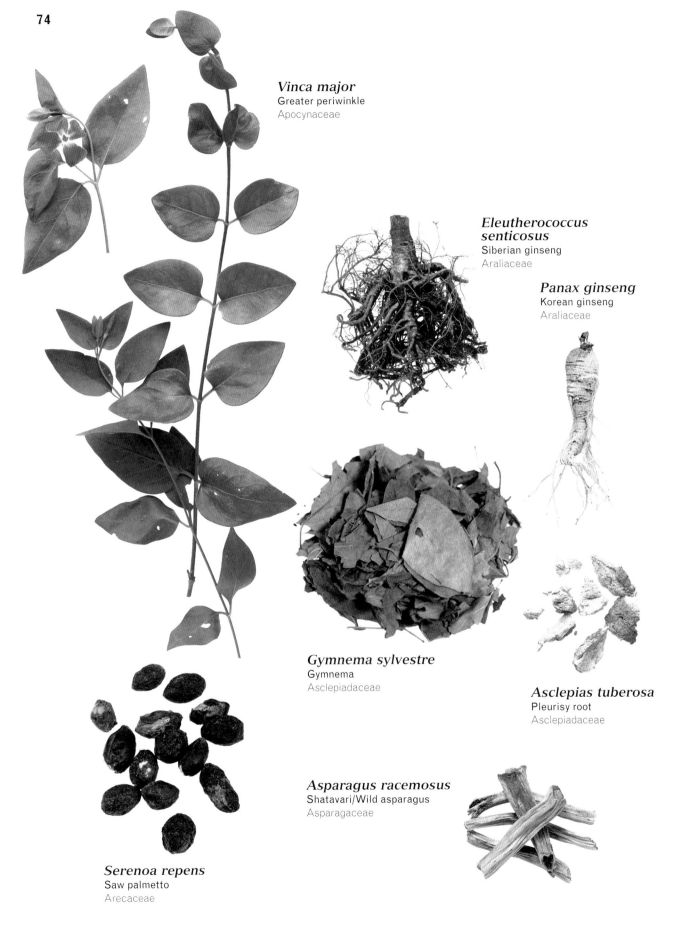

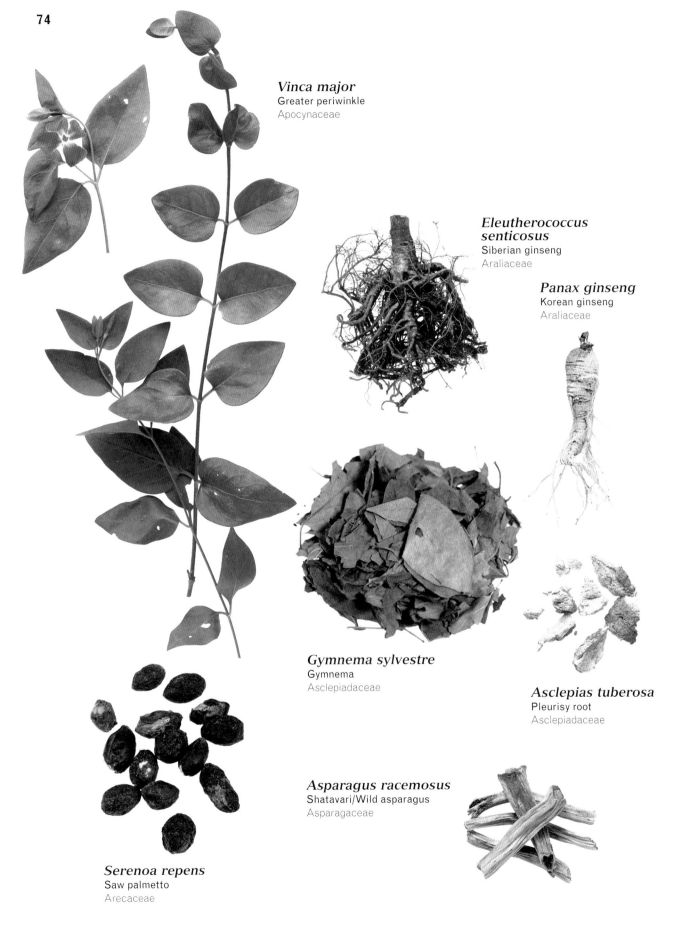

74

Vinca major
Greater periwinkle
Apocynaceae

Eleutherococcus senticosus
Siberian ginseng
Araliaceae

Panax ginseng
Korean ginseng
Araliaceae

Gymnema sylvestre
Gymnema
Asclepiadaceae

Asclepias tuberosa
Pleurisy root
Asclepiadaceae

Asparagus racemosus
Shatavari/Wild asparagus
Asparagaceae

Serenoa repens
Saw palmetto
Arecaceae

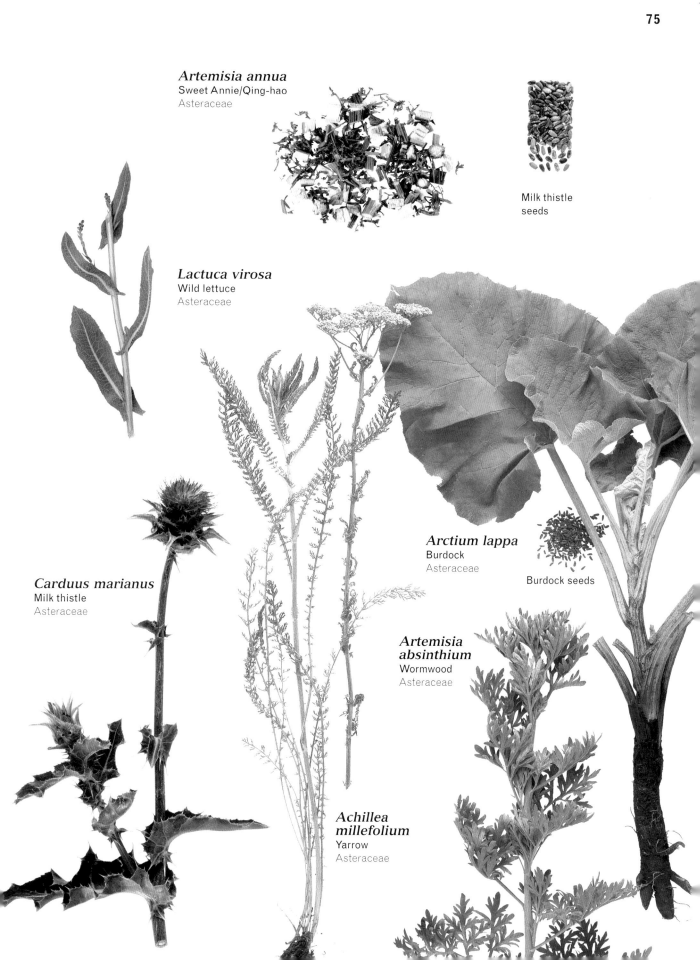

Artemisia annua
Sweet Annie/Qing-hao
Asteraceae

Milk thistle
seeds

Lactuca virosa
Wild lettuce
Asteraceae

Arctium lappa
Burdock
Asteraceae

Burdock seeds

Carduus marianus
Milk thistle
Asteraceae

**Artemisia
absinthium**
Wormwood
Asteraceae

**Achillea
millefolium**
Yarrow
Asteraceae

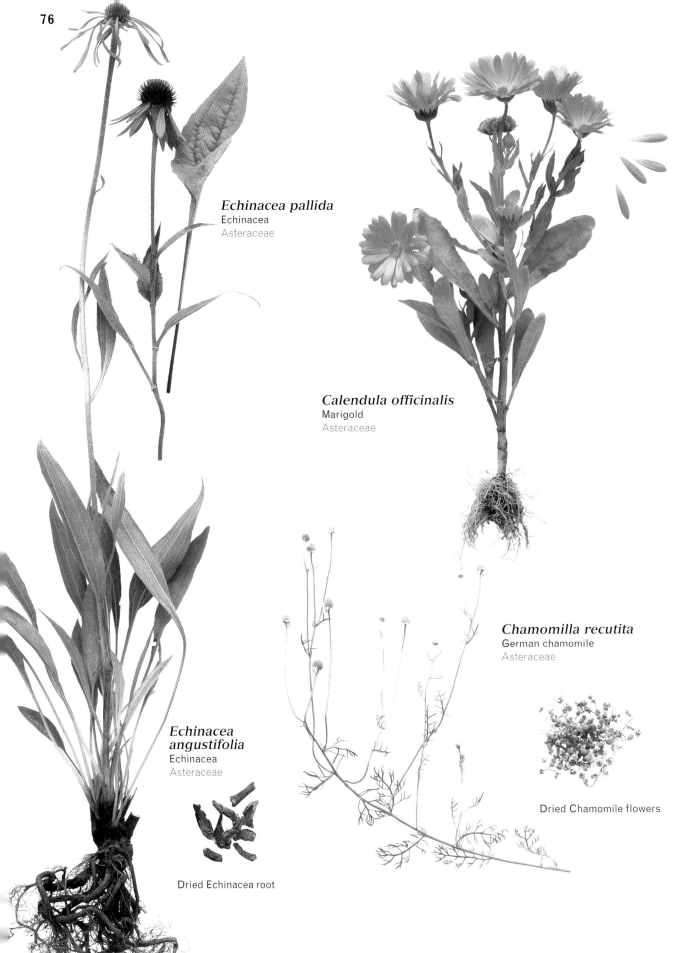

76

Echinacea pallida
Echinacea
Asteraceae

Calendula officinalis
Marigold
Asteraceae

Chamomilla recutita
German chamomile
Asteraceae

Echinacea angustifolia
Echinacea
Asteraceae

Dried Chamomile flowers

Dried Echinacea root

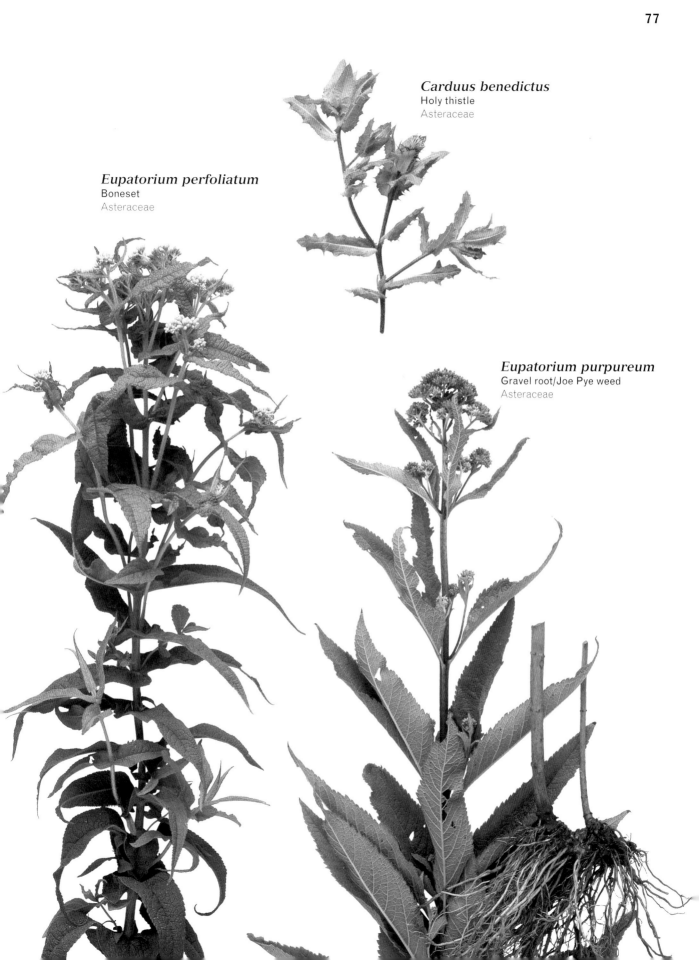

Carduus benedictus
Holy thistle
Asteraceae

Eupatorium perfoliatum
Boneset
Asteraceae

Eupatorium purpureum
Gravel root/Joe Pye weed
Asteraceae

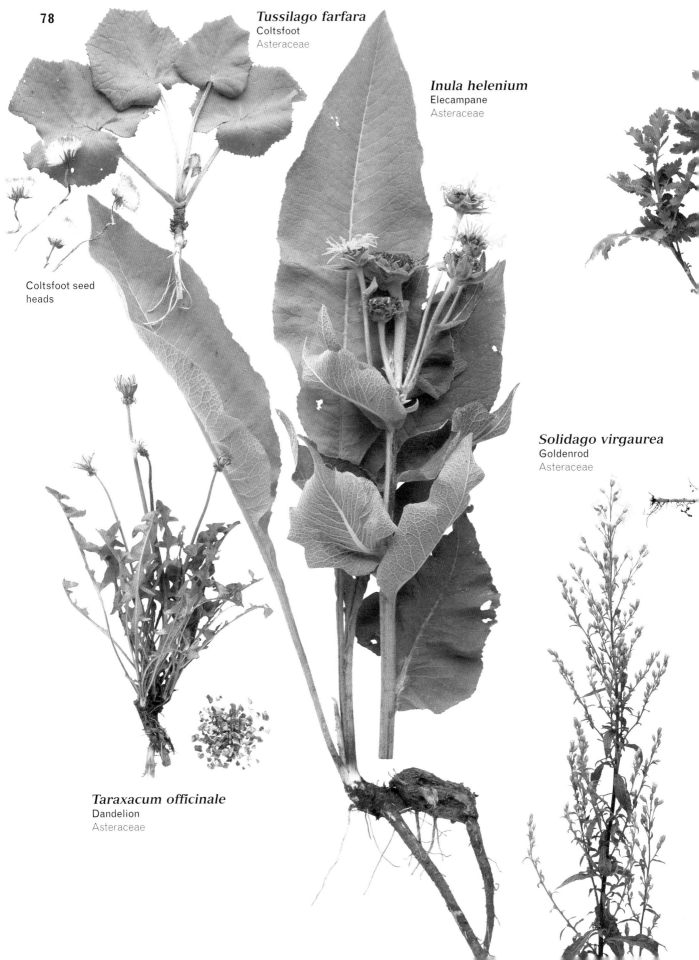

78

Tussilago farfara
Coltsfoot
Asteraceae

Inula helenium
Elecampane
Asteraceae

Coltsfoot seed
heads

Solidago virgaurea
Goldenrod
Asteraceae

Taraxacum officinale
Dandelion
Asteraceae

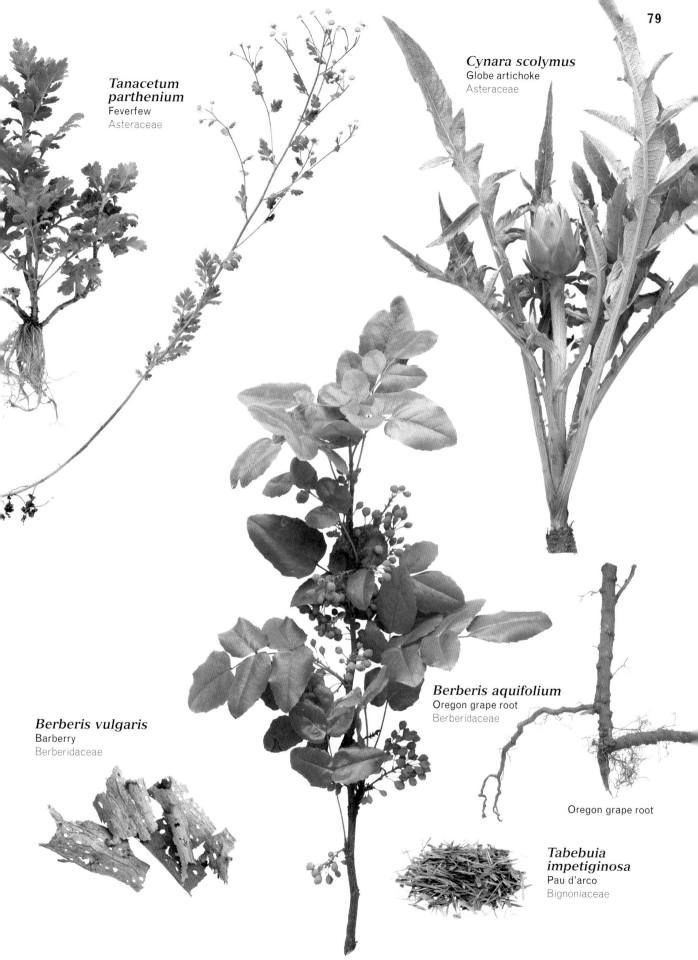

Tanacetum
parthenium
Feverfew
Asteraceae

Cynara scolymus
Globe artichoke
Asteraceae

Berberis aquifolium
Oregon grape root
Berberidaceae

Oregon grape root

Berberis vulgaris
Barberry
Berberidaceae

Tabebuia
impetiginosa
Pau d'arco
Bignoniaceae

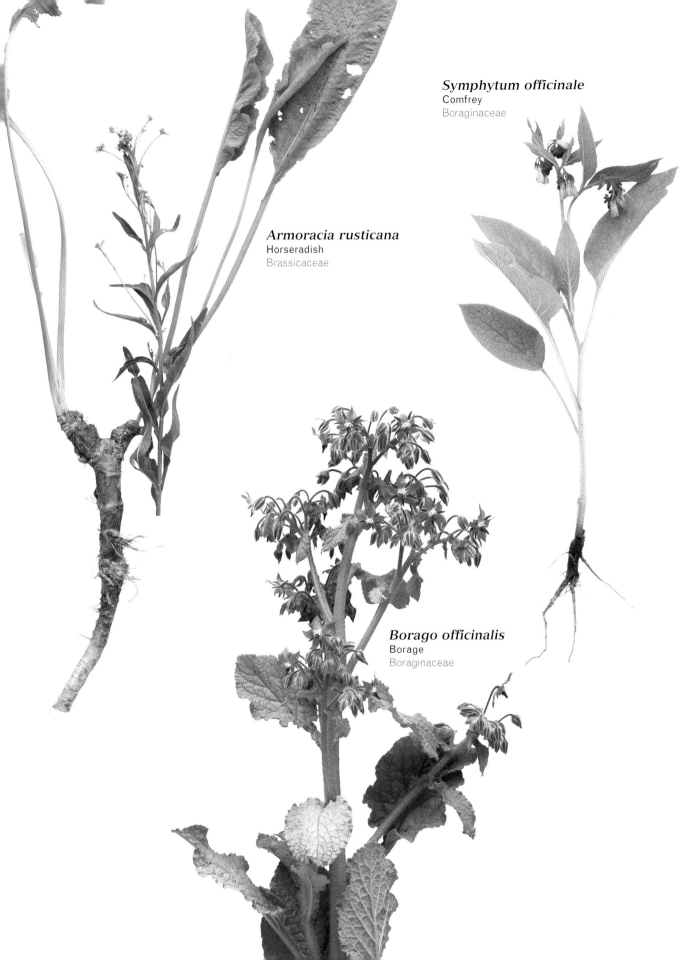

Symphytum officinale
Comfrey
Boraginaceae

Armoracia rusticana
Horseradish
Brassicaceae

Borago officinalis
Borage
Boraginaceae

Boswellia serrata
Frankincense
Burseraceae

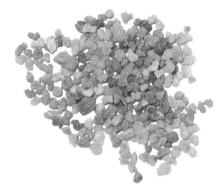

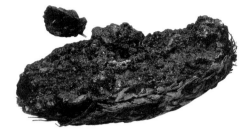

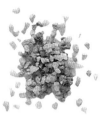

Commiphora mukul
Guggulu
Burseraceae

Commiphora molmol
Myrrh
Burseraceae

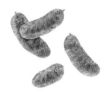

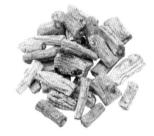

Cassia senna
Senna
Caesalpiniaceae

Codonopsis pilosula
Codonopsis
Campanulaceae

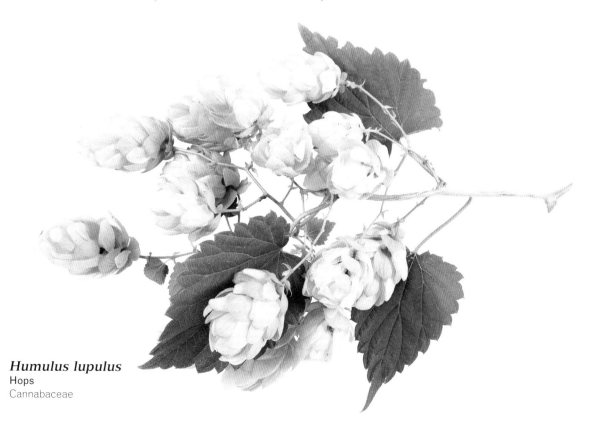

Humulus lupulus
Hops
Cannabaceae

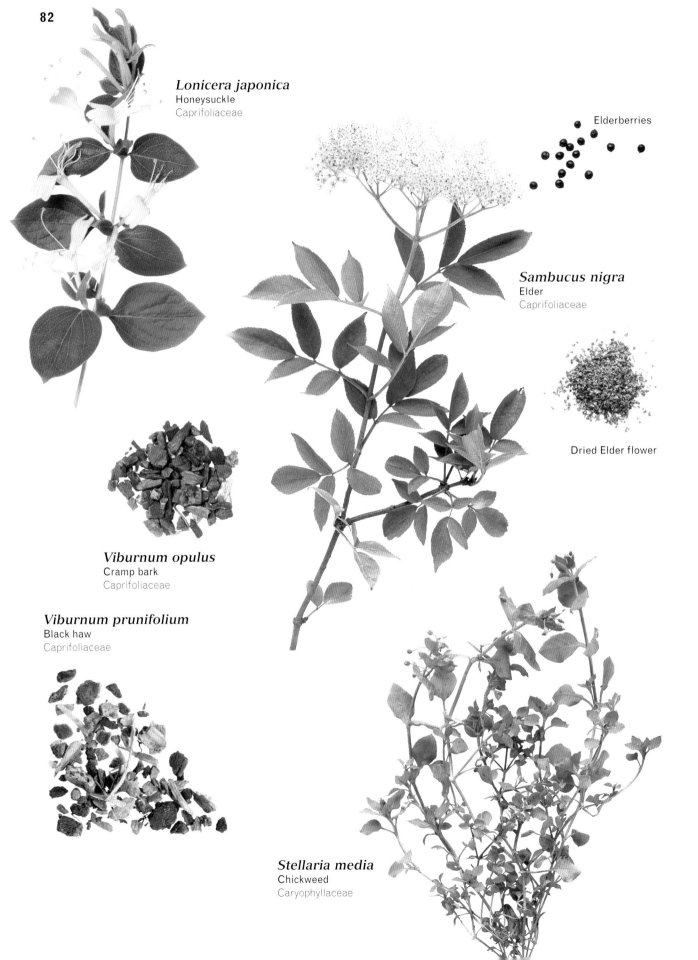

Lonicera japonica
Honeysuckle
Caprifoliaceae

Elderberries

Sambucus nigra
Elder
Caprifoliaceae

Dried Elder flower

Viburnum opulus
Cramp bark
Caprifoliaceae

Viburnum prunifolium
Black haw
Caprifoliaceae

Stellaria media
Chickweed
Caryophyllaceae

Hypericum perforatum
St John's wort
Clusiaceae

Rhodiola rosea
Rhodiola
Crassulaceae

Dioscorea villosa
Wild yam
Dioscoreaceae

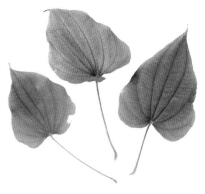

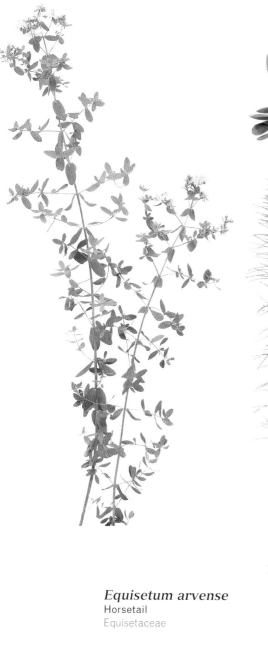

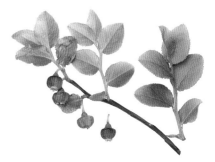

Vaccinium myrtillus
Blueberry/Bilberry
Ericaceae

Equisetum arvense
Horsetail
Equisetaceae

Arctostaphylos uva ursi
Bearberry
Ericaceae

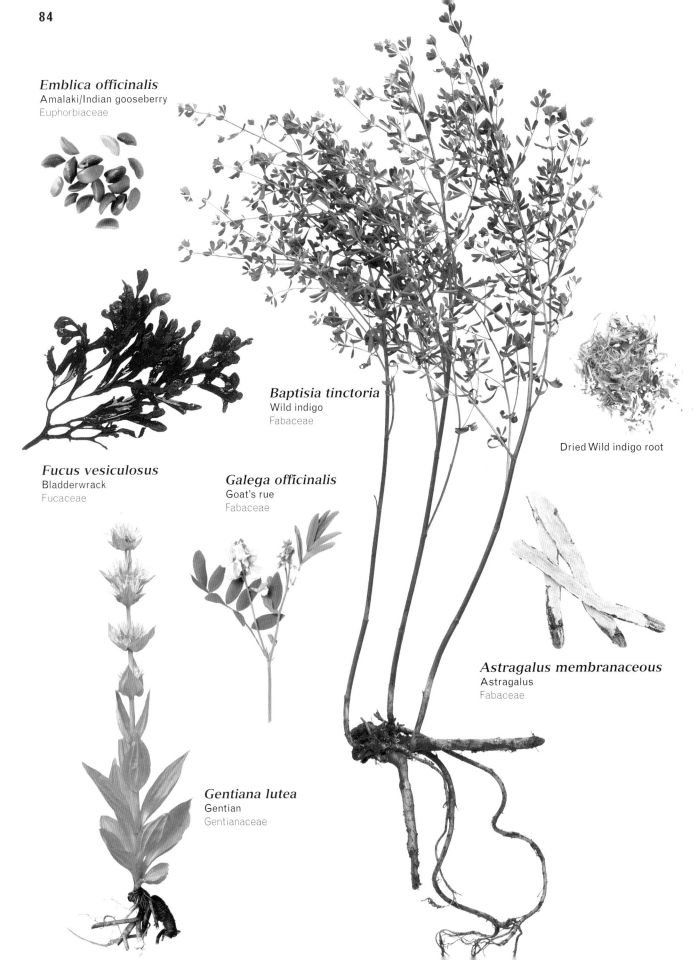

Emblica officinalis
Amalaki/Indian gooseberry
Euphorbiaceae

Fucus vesiculosus
Bladderwrack
Fucaceae

Baptisia tinctoria
Wild indigo
Fabaceae

Dried Wild indigo root

Galega officinalis
Goat's rue
Fabaceae

Astragalus membranaceous
Astragalus
Fabaceae

Gentiana lutea
Gentian
Gentianaceae

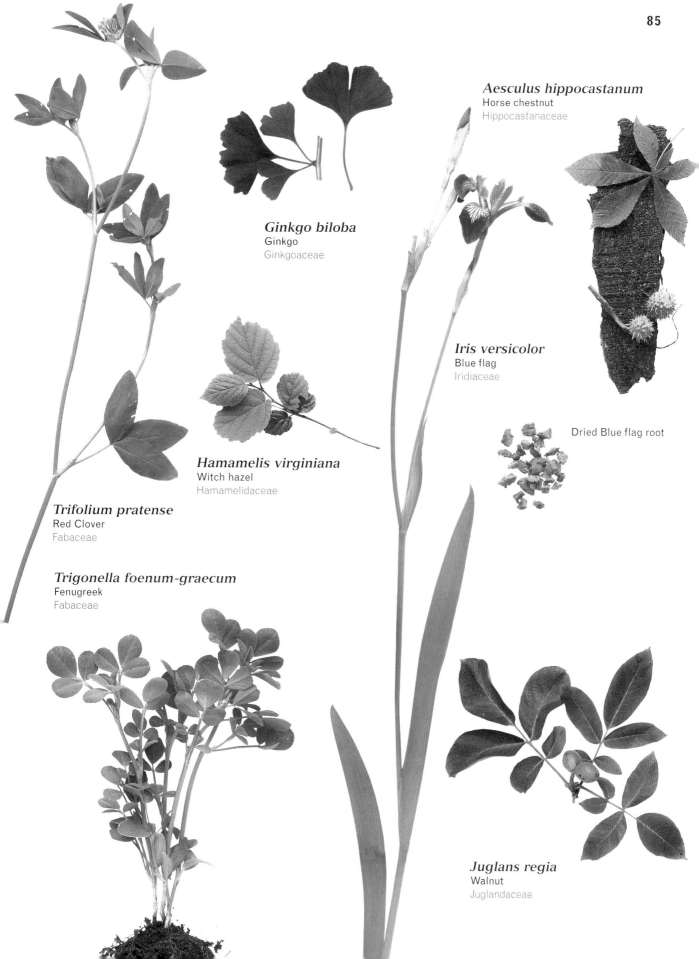

Ginkgo biloba
Ginkgo
Ginkgoaceae

Aesculus hippocastanum
Horse chestnut
Hippocastanaceae

Iris versicolor
Blue flag
Iridiaceae

Dried Blue flag root

Hamamelis virginiana
Witch hazel
Hamamelidaceae

Trifolium pratense
Red Clover
Fabaceae

Trigonella foenum-graecum
Fenugreek
Fabaceae

Juglans regia
Walnut
Juglandaceae

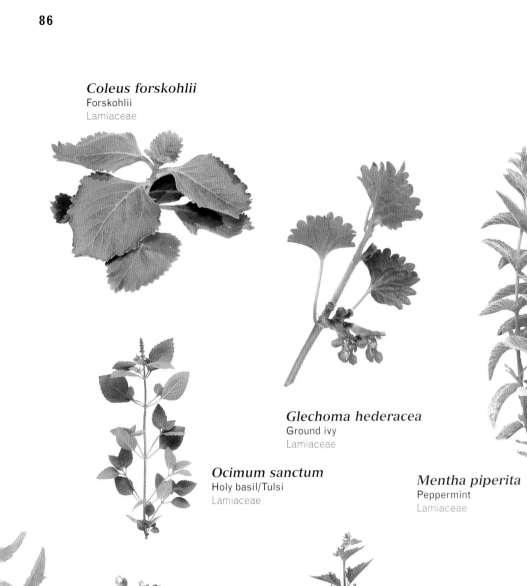

Coleus forskohlii
Forskohlii
Lamiaceae

Glechoma hederacea
Ground ivy
Lamiaceae

Ocimum sanctum
Holy basil/Tulsi
Lamiaceae

Mentha piperita
Peppermint
Lamiaceae

Origanum majorana
Sweet marjoram
Lamiaceae

Scutellaria baicalensis
Baikal skullcap/Huang qin
Lamiaceae

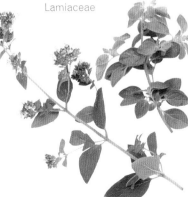

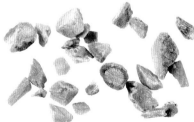

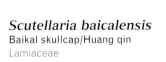

Baikal scullcap root

Scutellaria laterifolia
Skullcap
Lamiaceae

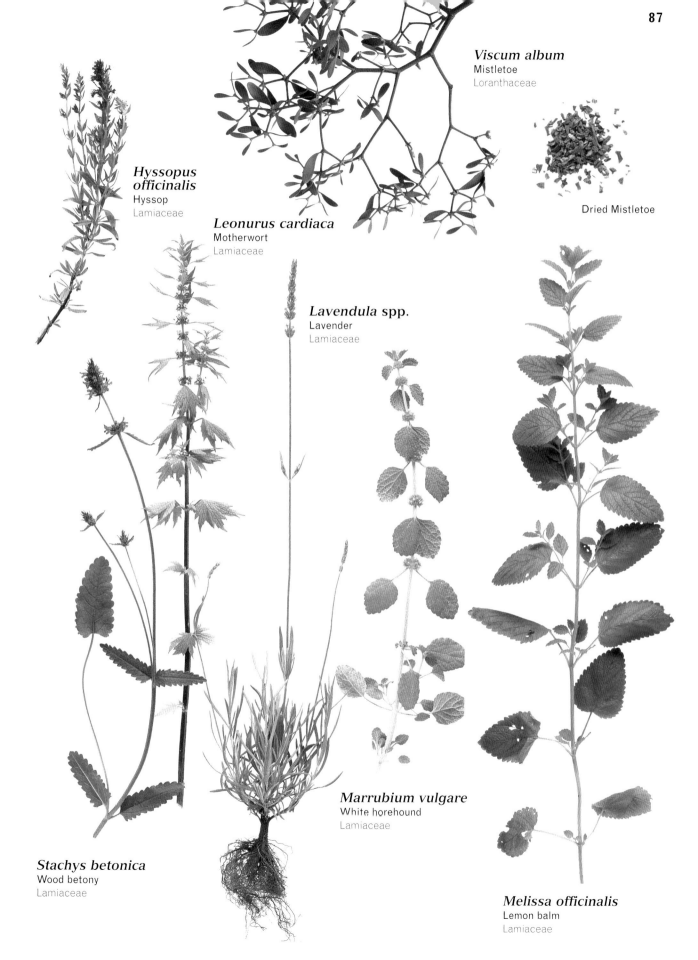

Hyssopus officinalis
Hyssop
Lamiaceae

Viscum album
Mistletoe
Loranthaceae

Dried Mistletoe

Leonurus cardiaca
Motherwort
Lamiaceae

Lavendula spp.
Lavender
Lamiaceae

Marrubium vulgare
White horehound
Lamiaceae

Stachys betonica
Wood betony
Lamiaceae

Melissa officinalis
Lemon balm
Lamiaceae

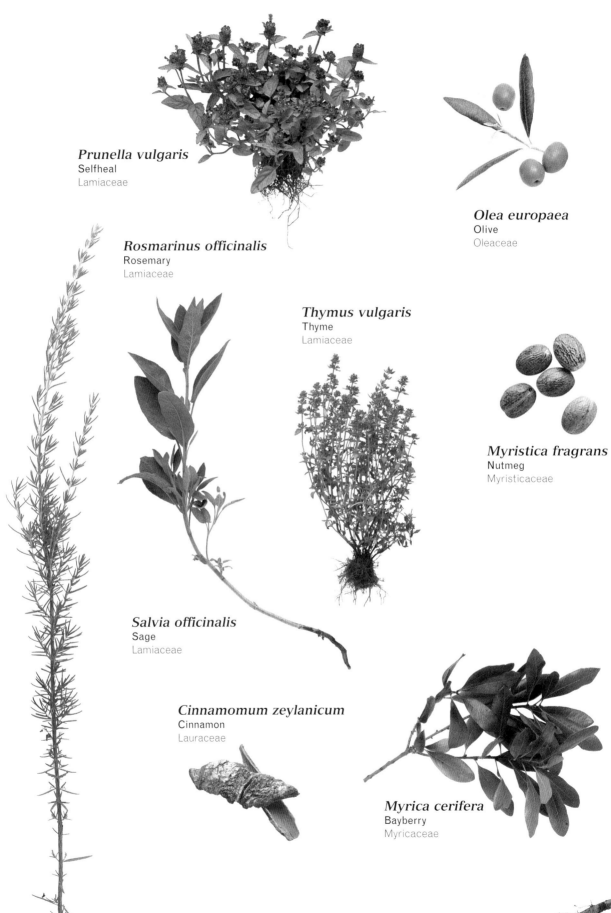

Prunella vulgaris
Selfheal
Lamiaceae

Olea europaea
Olive
Oleaceae

Rosmarinus officinalis
Rosemary
Lamiaceae

Thymus vulgaris
Thyme
Lamiaceae

Myristica fragrans
Nutmeg
Myristicaceae

Salvia officinalis
Sage
Lamiaceae

Cinnamomum zeylanicum
Cinnamon
Lauraceae

Myrica cerifera
Bayberry
Myricaceae

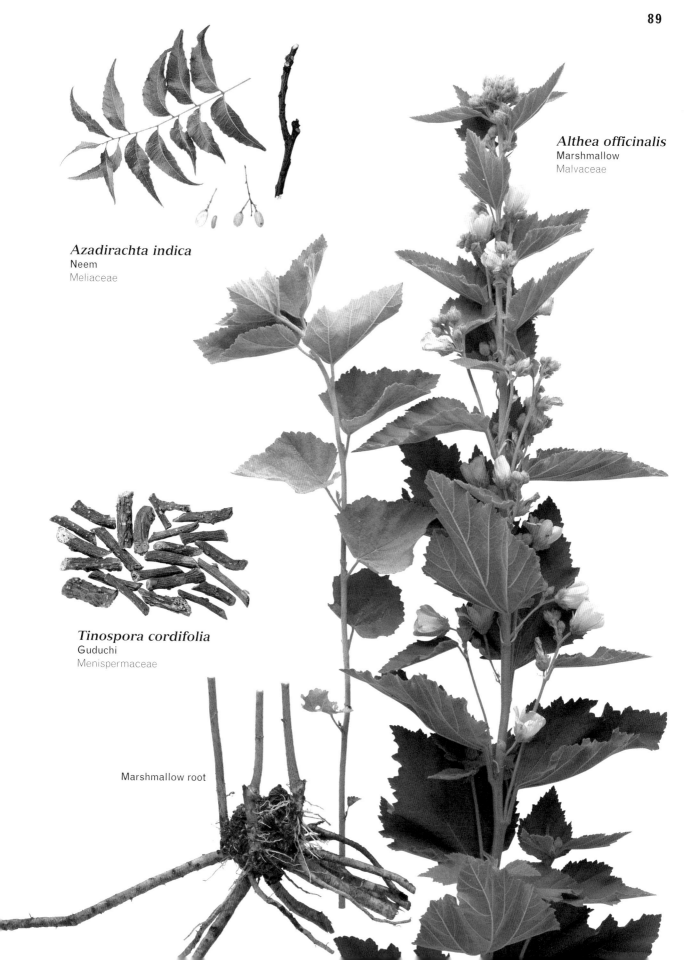

Azadirachta indica
Neem
Meliaceae

Tinospora cordifolia
Guduchi
Menispermaceae

Althea officinalis
Marshmallow
Malvaceae

Marshmallow root

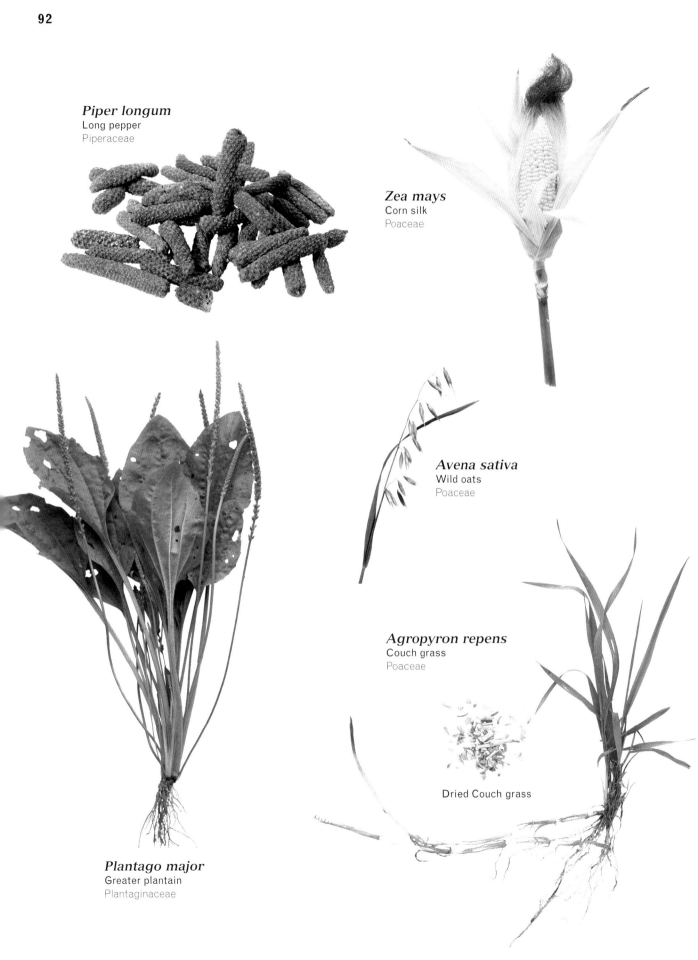

Piper longum
Long pepper
Piperaceae

Zea mays
Corn silk
Poaceae

Avena sativa
Wild oats
Poaceae

Agropyron repens
Couch grass
Poaceae

Dried Couch grass

Plantago major
Greater plantain
Plantaginaceae

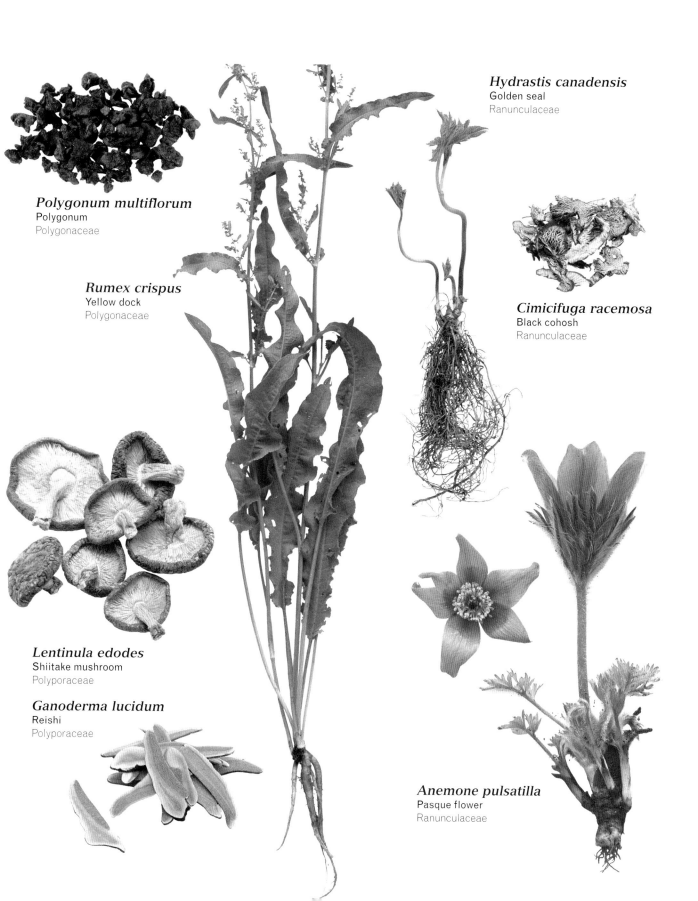

Polygonum multiflorum
Polygonum
Polygonaceae

Rumex crispus
Yellow dock
Polygonaceae

Lentinula edodes
Shiitake mushroom
Polyporaceae

Ganoderma lucidum
Reishi
Polyporaceae

Hydrastis canadensis
Golden seal
Ranunculaceae

Cimicifuga racemosa
Black cohosh
Ranunculaceae

Anemone pulsatilla
Pasque flower
Ranunculaceae

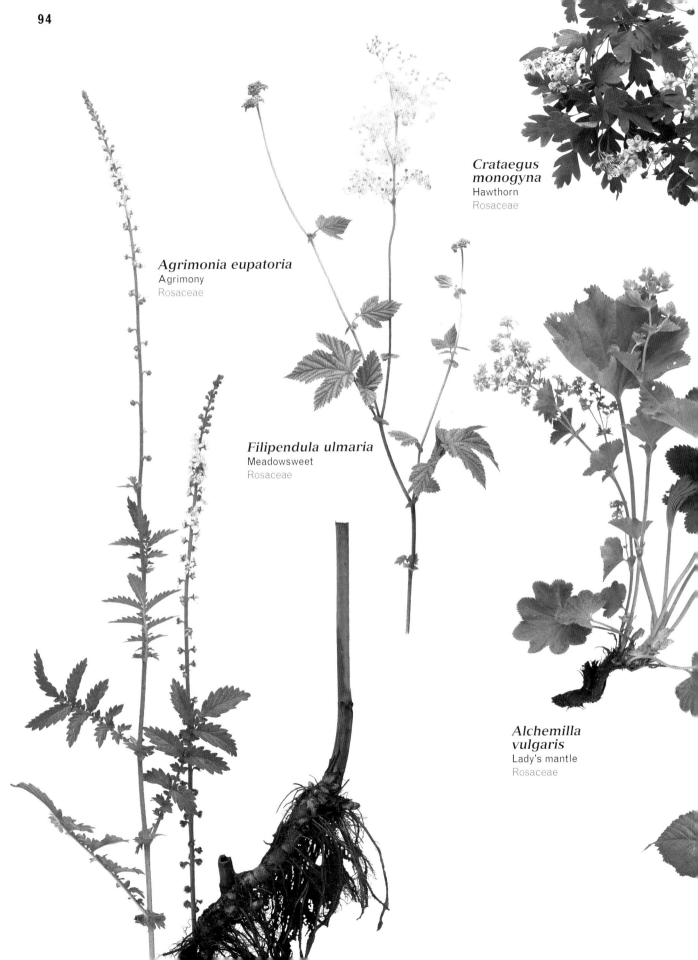

94

Crataegus monogyna
Hawthorn
Rosaceae

Agrimonia eupatoria
Agrimony
Rosaceae

Filipendula ulmaria
Meadowsweet
Rosaceae

Alchemilla vulgaris
Lady's mantle
Rosaceae

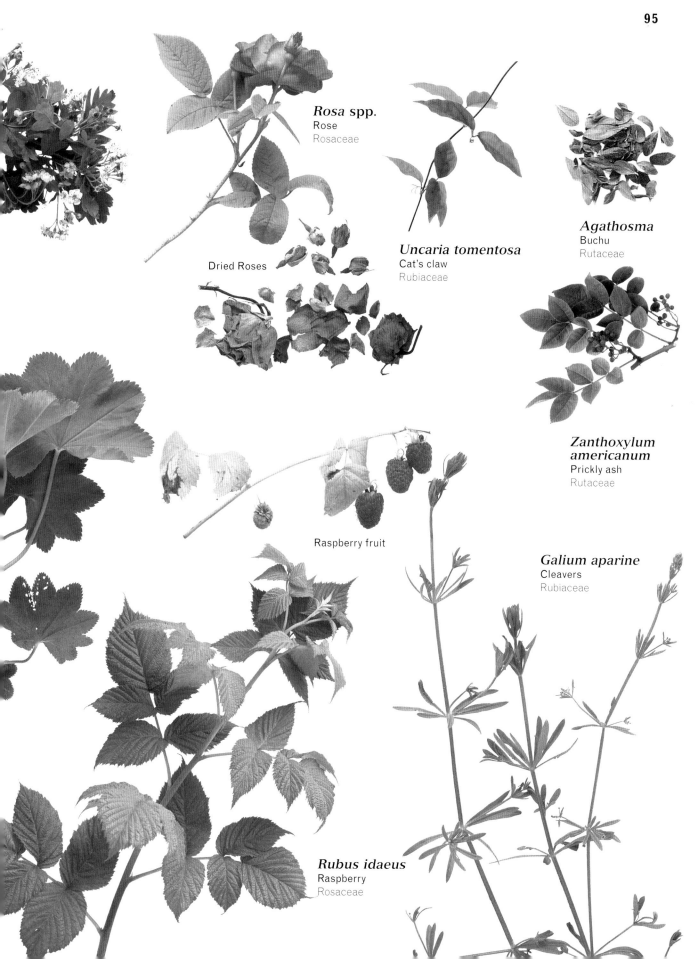

Rosa spp.
Rose
Rosaceae

Dried Roses

Uncaria tomentosa
Cat's claw
Rubiaceae

Agathosma
Buchu
Rutaceae

*Zanthoxylum
americanum*
Prickly ash
Rutaceae

Raspberry fruit

Galium aparine
Cleavers
Rubiaceae

Rubus idaeus
Raspberry
Rosaceae

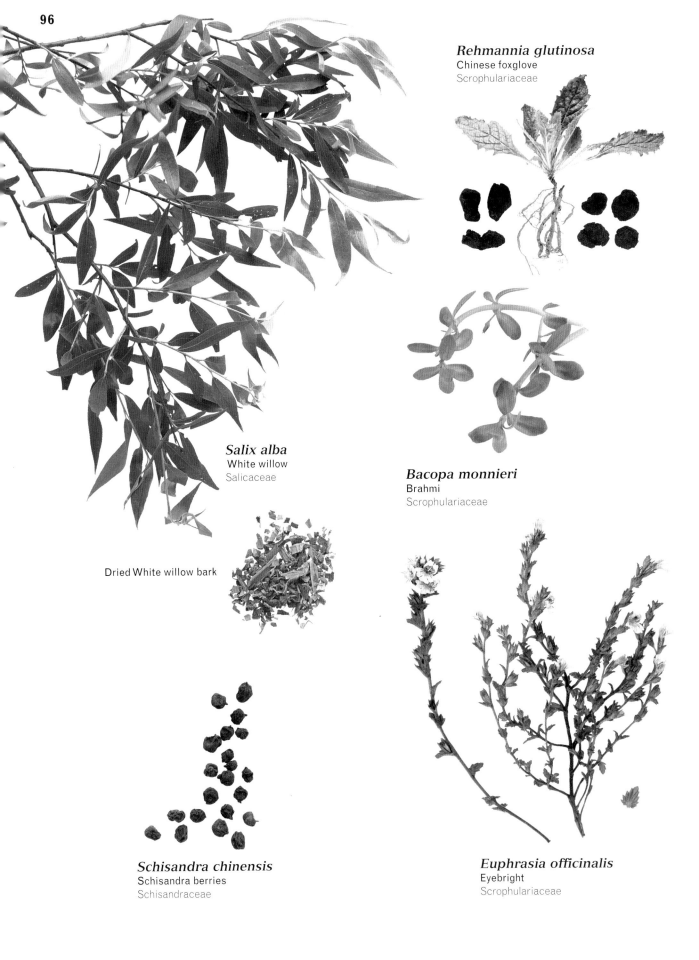

Rehmannia glutinosa
Chinese foxglove
Scrophulariaceae

Salix alba
White willow
Salicaceae

Dried White willow bark

Bacopa monnieri
Brahmi
Scrophulariaceae

Schisandra chinensis
Schisandra berries
Schisandraceae

Euphrasia officinalis
Eyebright
Scrophulariaceae

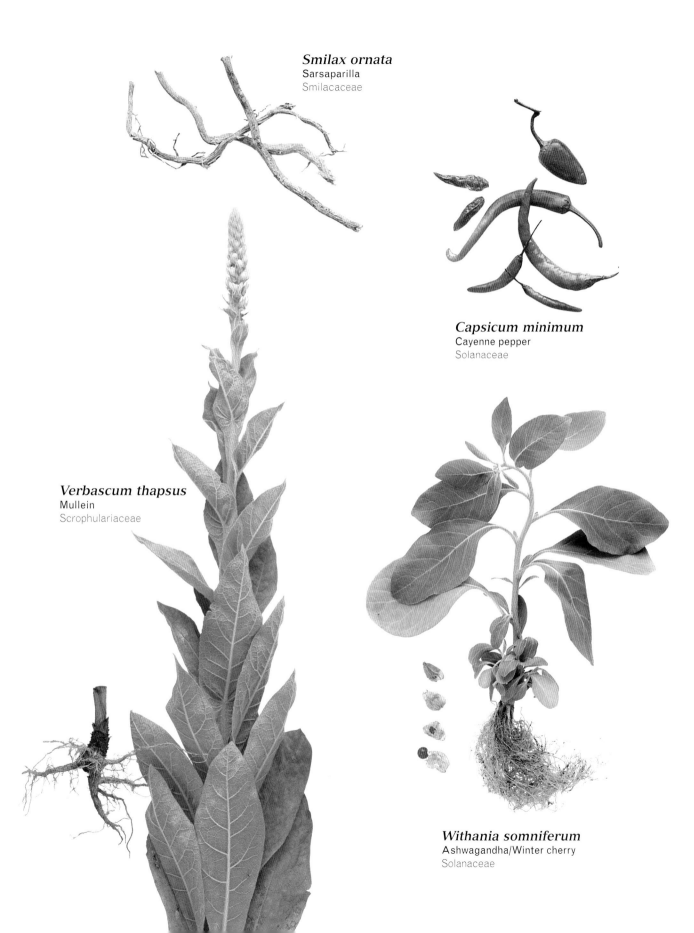

Smilax ornata
Sarsaparilla
Smilacaceae

Capsicum minimum
Cayenne pepper
Solanaceae

Verbascum thapsus
Mullein
Scrophulariaceae

Withania somniferum
Ashwagandha/Winter cherry
Solanaceae

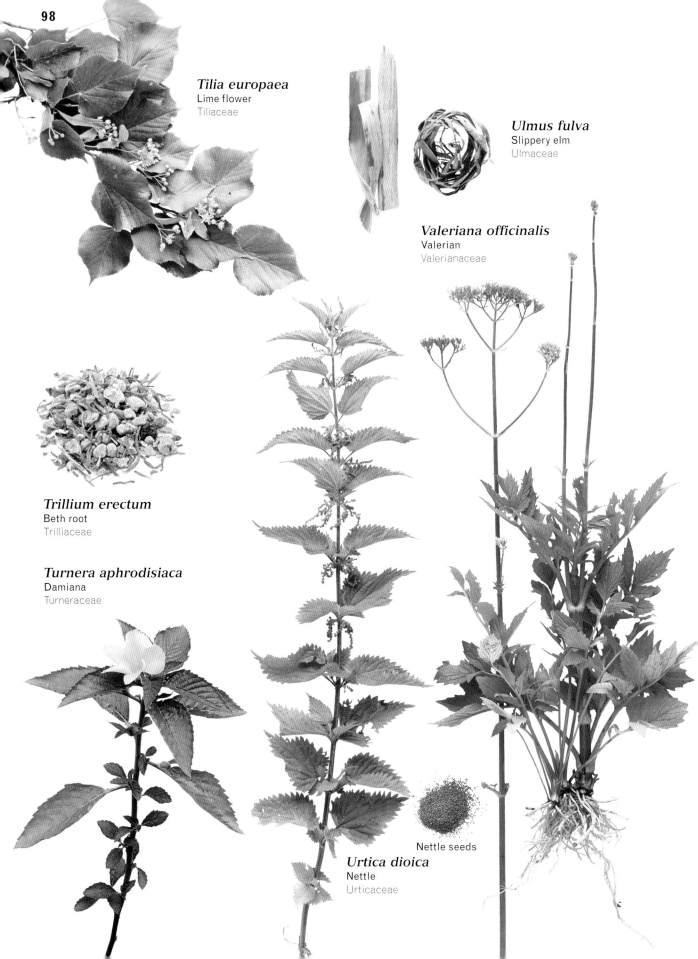

98

Tilia europaea
Lime flower
Tiliaceae

Ulmus fulva
Slippery elm
Ulmaceae

Valeriana officinalis
Valerian
Valerianaceae

Trillium erectum
Beth root
Trilliaceae

Turnera aphrodisiaca
Damiana
Turneraceae

Nettle seeds

Urtica dioica
Nettle
Urticaceae

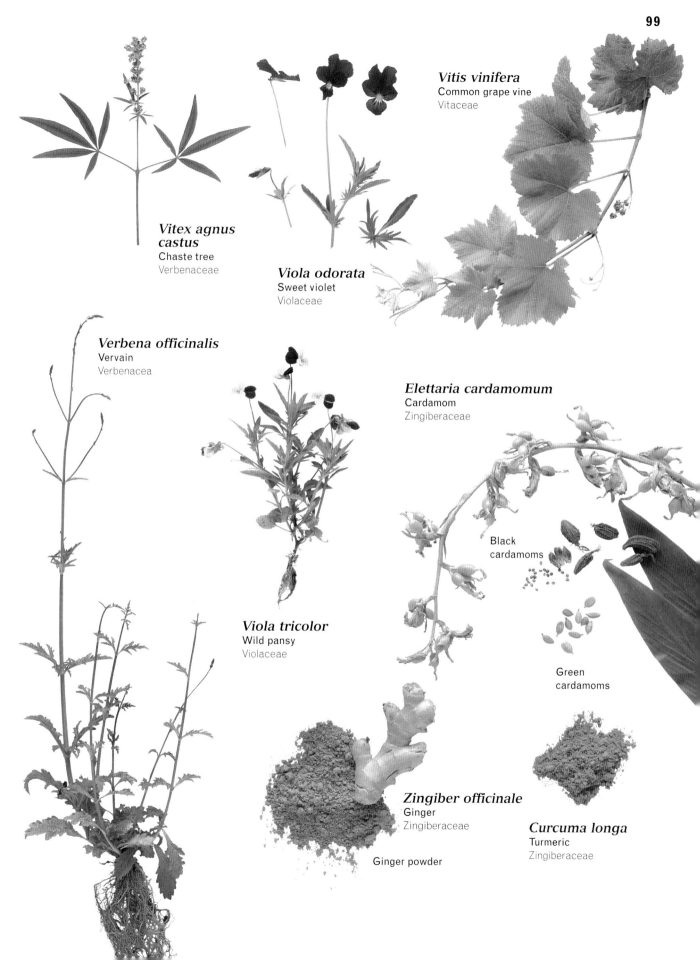

Vitex agnus castus
Chaste tree
Verbenaceae

Viola odorata
Sweet violet
Violaceae

Vitis vinifera
Common grape vine
Vitaceae

Verbena officinalis
Vervain
Verbenacea

Viola tricolor
Wild pansy
Violaceae

Elettaria cardamomum
Cardamom
Zingiberaceae

Black cardamoms

Green cardamoms

Zingiber officinale
Ginger
Zingiberaceae

Ginger powder

Curcuma longa
Turmeric
Zingiberaceae

Herb directory

The entries in this directory of commonly used herbs
are arranged alphabetically by their botanical name, followed
by their common name. A brief introduction to the native
region and key therapeutic effect of each plant is followed
by details of its chemical constituents and their actions. To
find out more about each one, turn to the explanation of
constituents on pages 40–43. Further information on the
efficacy of each herb for common ailments is broken down
by body system. For a brief overview of the workings of
each system, turn to pages 178–231. For full instructions on
preparing herbal medicines, see pages 60–67.

Achillea millefolium
Yarrow

Yarrow is a perennial herb native to Europe and Asia. It has been valued for stopping bleeding since the time of the ancient Greeks.

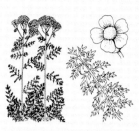

FAMILY   Asteraceae
PARTS USED   Aerial parts
CONSTITUENTS   Volatile oil, flavonoids, sesquiterpenes, silica, sterols, bitters, tannins, salicylic acid, amino acids (including lysine), coumarins, fatty acids (including linoleic, palmitic and oleic).
ACTIONS   Diaphoretic, diuretic, astringent, digestive, bitter tonic, antimicrobial, decongestant, anti-inflammatory, antispasmodic, analgesic, antihistamine, emmenagogue, expectorant, haemostatic, alterative.

Digestion • Stimulates appetite, aids digestion and absorption. • Relieves wind, spasm, IBS and indigestion. • Astringent tannins protect the gut from irritation and infection; helpful in diarrhoea and inflammatory problems.
Circulation • Taken in hot tea it promotes sweating and reduces fevers. • Lowers blood pressure, improves circulation and relieves leg cramps and varicose veins.
Respiratory system • Taken in hot tea with mint and elderflower it relieves colds and congestion. • Antihistamine effect is useful in treating allergies.
Immune system • Volatile oils and luteolin have anti-inflammatory and antioxidant effects[1]; relieve arthritis, allergies and autoimmune problems. • Stimulates blood flow to the skin and brings out the rash in eruptive infections such as measles and chickenpox. • Clears toxins by aiding elimination via the skin and kidneys.
Urinary system • Diuretic, relieves irritable bladder. Tightens muscles, helping incontinence.
Reproductive system • Regulates menstrual cycle, relieves PMS and heavy bleeding.
Externally • Tannins and silica speed healing of cuts, wounds, ulcers, burns, varicose veins, haemorrhoids and skin conditions. • Infusion used as a vaginal douche, skin lotion and mouthwash for gingivitis.

CAUTION   Avoid in pregnancy and if allergic to Asteraceae. Can cause contact dermatitis and photosensitivity.
Drug interactions   Avoid with anticoagulants.

Aesculus hippocastanum
Horse chestnut

This magnificent tree is native to western Asia and was brought to Europe in the mid-17th century. It is also found in North America. The extract of the seeds has long been valued in the treatment of vascular problems.

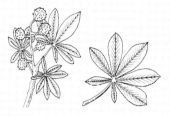

FAMILY   Hippocastanaceae
PARTS USED   Seeds, bark
CONSTITUENTS   Sterols, triterpene saponin glycosides (including aescin), fatty acids, flavonoids, coumarins, allantoin, tannins.
ACTIONS   Astringent, anti-inflammatory, febrifuge, anticoagulant, expectorant.

Digestion • Bark is rich in astringent tannins, useful for treating diarrhoea.
Circulation • Aescin strengthens blood vessel walls and enhances their elasticity, improving blood flow and venous return, and preventing pooling of blood causing piles and varicose veins. • Reduces oedema, cramps and pain and tension in the legs. • Reduces inflammation in blood vessels. • Relieves pressure on the heart and high blood pressure. • Anticoagulant properties reduce blood clotting.
Immune system • Saponin aescin has anti-inflammatory effects, helpful in easing joint pain. • Hot decoction reduces fevers; a traditional substitute for Peruvian Bark (*Cinchona*) for treating malaria and intermittent fevers.
Externally • Contracts blood vessels and reduces fluid and swelling around areas of trauma, useful after surgery. • Creams or gels are excellent for treating varicose veins and ulcers, phlebitis and haemorrhoids, as well as cellulite. Can relieve the pain and swelling of arthritis, neuralgia, sunburn, bruises, sprains and other sports injuries.

CAUTION   Avoid in pregnancy, lactation and children. All parts are toxic when raw; use pre-treated preparations and avoid large doses.
Drug interactions   Avoid with anticoagulants and salicylates.

Agathosma betulina (also known as *Barosma betulina*)
Buchu

This woody evergreen shrub native to South Africa has highly aromatic leaves. It was used by the indigenous people to ward off insects and as an antiseptic for urinary tract infections, digestive problems, arthritis and gout.

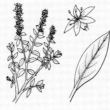

FAMILY Rutaceae
PARTS USED Leaves
CONSTITUENTS Volatile oils (including diosphenol, d-pulegone, iso-menthone and menthone), flavonoids (diosmin, hesperidin, quercitrin and rutin), coumarins, mucilage, vitamin C, betacarotene, calcium, chromium, magnesium, zinc.
ACTIONS Antimicrobial, urinary antiseptic, diuretic, stimulating tonic, digestive, antilithic, anti-inflammatory, depurative, astringent, carminative, diaphoretic, uterine stimulant, vulnerary.

Digestion • Antimicrobial for treating infections such as gastroenteritis, diarrhoea and dysentery. • Relieves bloating, flatulence, stomach cramps and colic[2]. • Helps regulate blood sugar.
Circulation • May reduce blood pressure.
Immune system • Anti-inflammatory and cleansing; helps the elimination of uric acid. Used in treating arthritis, gout, rheumatism and muscle aches. • Aids resistance to colds and flu; taken at onset of acute infections, chills and fevers.
Urinary system • Effective diuretic, often included in formulae for PMS to relieve fluid retention. • Improves circulation to the urinary system. • Antibacterial and anti-inflammatory, used for treating urinary tract infections, cystitis, irritable bladder, stones, dysuria and haematuria. • Reduces acute and chronic inflammation and infection of the prostate.
Externally • Infusion mixed with vinegar traditionally used as a lotion for bruises and sprains[3]. • The oil is used as an insect repellent. • Used as a vaginal douche it allays yeast infections and leucorrhoea.

CAUTION Avoid in cases of acute inflammation of the liver and kidneys, and during pregnancy.
Drug interactions Avoid with warfarin and other anticoagulants.

Agrimonia eupatoria
Agrimony

This perennial plant native to Europe and northern Asia has spikes of yellow flowers and is named after the ancient Greek king Mithridates VI Eupator, who used it for treating liver problems and poisoning. It was valued on medieval battlefields for stopping bleeding.

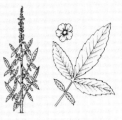

FAMILY Rosaceae
PARTS USED Aerial parts
CONSTITUENTS Tannins, agrimonim, flavonoids, furanocoumarins, polysaccharides, bitters, volatile oil, vitamins B1, K and C, silica.
ACTIONS Astringent, analgesic, anti-inflammatory, antispasmodic, antilithic, antibacterial, digestive tonic, vulnerary, cholagogue, diuretic, emmenagogue, febrifuge, haemostatic.

Digestion • Protects the gut lining from irritation and inflammation and counteracts infection. Used for peptic ulcers, gastritis, colitis and diarrhoea. • Bitters stimulate digestive juices and bile from the liver and gall bladder, enhancing digestion and absorption, improving bowel function. Used for gallstones and cirrhosis of the liver. • Lowers blood sugar.
Mental and emotional • Flower remedy for those who hide pain and anguish behind a brave face and try to keep others happy.
Respiratory system • Antispamodic for asthma and coughs. • Antibacterial for infections and bronchitis.
Immune system • Combats bacterial and viral infections. • Helps inhibit growth of tumours.
Urinary system • Astringent diuretic for bed-wetting and incontinence, bladder irritation, cystitis and kidney stones. • Aids elimination of uric acid, helpful for gout and arthritis.
Reproductive system • Astringent for heavy periods.
Externally • Gargle/mouthwash for sore throats, laryngitis and inflamed gums; eyebath for inflammatory eye problems; douche for vaginal infections such as trichomonas. • Stems bleeding, speeds healing of cuts and wounds, bruises, sprains and varicose veins, and relieves aching muscles and skin problems.

Drug interactions Avoid with blood thinners such as warfarin; monitor with diabetic drugs and antihypertensives.

Agropyron repens (also known as *Triticum repens* and *Elymus repens*)
Couch grass

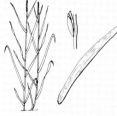

This perennial grass is native to Europe and North America. The rhizomes are a valuable remedy for urinary problems and can be ground into flour and roasted to make coffee.

FAMILY Poaceae
PARTS USED Rhizomes
CONSTITUENTS Polysaccharides (triticin), mannitol, inositol, mucilage, saponins, essential oil, vanillin, silicic acid, vitamins A and B complex, iron, potassium, zinc.
ACTIONS Demulcent, emollient, diuretic, antilithic, anti-inflammatory, antimicrobial, antifungal.

Digestion • Soothes mucous membranes throughout the gut. • Clears heat and inflammation in the stomach, intestines, liver and gall bladder.
Circulation • Reduces harmful cholesterol.
Respiratory system • Soothing, antimicrobial and anti-inflammatory for irritating coughs, bronchitis and laryngitis. • Clears catarrhal congestion through its soothing effect on mucosa in the nose, throat and bronchi. • Silica has a healing effect on the lungs.
Musculoskeletal system • Diuretic actions clear toxins, wastes and uric acid and helps relieve arthritis and gout. • Anti-inflammatory action is helpful in treating joint disease.
Immune system • A traditional spring tonic, eliminates accumulated wastes via the kidneys. • Clears heat and reduces fevers.
Urinary system • Abundant mucilage soothes the urinary tract. • Mannitol acts as an osmotic diuretic, saponins and vanillin are also diuretic, aiding the excretion of wastes including excess sodium and uric acid. • Used for treating infections and inflammatory conditions such as cystitis, irritable bladder, dysuria, haematuria, urethritis, prostatitis (acute and chronic) and benign enlargement of prostate. • Prevents and remedies stones and gravel. • Silicic acid is healing and strengthening to the urinary tract and sphincters, used for bed-wetting and urinary incontinence.
Externally • Gargle used for sore throats, laryngitis, tonsillitis; soothing wash for inflammation, eczema, cuts and grazes. • Silica speeds the healing of wounds.

Alchemilla vulgaris
Lady's mantle

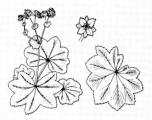

Lady's mantle is a distinctive perennial native to Europe and northern Asia. It was traditionally dedicated to the Virgin Mary, as the leaves are thought to resemble her cloak, and was a favourite of medieval alchemists for the dew drops that exude from the leaves, which they believed were invaluable in their search for the 'philospher's stone' or enlightenment.

FAMILY Rosaceae
PARTS USED Root, leaves, flowers
CONSTITUENTS Salicylic acid, ellagitannins (pedunculagin, agrimoniin and alchemillin), bitters, flavonoids (quercitrin), saponins, volatile oils, phytosterols.
ACTIONS Astringent, haemostatic, anti-inflammatory, diuretic, emmenagogue, nervine, vulnerary, febrifuge.

Digestion • Astringent for diarrhoea and inflammatory problems such as gastritis, colitis and gastroenteritis.
Urinary system • Cools heat and inflammation and relieves cystitis.
Reproductive system • Astringent and anti-inflammatory for heavy, painful and irregular periods, prolonged bleeding due to fibroids or during menopause. • Used to promote fertility. • Toning for weak pelvic floor muscles, helps prevent miscarriage and good for treating prolapse. • Used to aid contractions during childbirth, speed recovery and regulate hormones and strengthen muscles after miscarriage and childbirth. Taken a few days prior to birth helps prevent post-partum bleeding. • Cooling and balancing remedy during menopause. • For fibroids, genito-urinary infections, endometriosis and pelvic inflammatory disease.
Externally • Astringent fresh root/leaves stop bleeding and promote healing. • Gargle/mouthwash used for mouth ulcers and sores, sore throats and laryngitis. • Lotion used for skin problems such as inflamed cuts and abrasions, pimples or rashes; eyewash for conjunctivitis. • Douche used for vaginal irritation and infections such as candida and after-antibiotic treatment for infection such as trichomonas, when the vaginal flora has been disturbed.

CAUTION Avoid during pregnancy, except in the last few weeks.

Allium sativum
Garlic

This excellent antimicrobial herb has been prescribed since the 1st century CE by Ayurvedic doctors for infections. Its antibiotic activity was noted by Louis Pasteur and employed by Albert Schweitzer in Africa for amoebic dysentery.

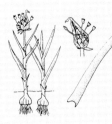

FAMILY Alliaceae
PARTS USED Bulb
CONSTITUENTS Sulphur-containing compounds (including alliin), lipids, quercetin, kaempferol, glycosides, scordinins, tellurium compounds, amino acids, volatile oil, mucilage, germanium, glucokinins.
ACTIONS Carminative, expectorant, alterative, immunostimulant, antimicrobial, anthelmintic, hypocholesterolaemic, hypotensive, antitumour, rejuvenative, circulatory stimulant, digestive.

Digestion • Stimulates digestion and absorption.
• Antimicrobial; restores gut flora after infection/antibiotics via probiotic effects of fructo-oligosaccharides[4]. • May benefit type 2 diabetes.
Circulation • Increases circulation and reduces blood pressure. Used for cramps and disorders such as Raynaud's disease. • Lowers harmful cholesterol and triglyceride levels. • Reduces tendency to clotting and reduces the risk of heart attacks and strokes.
Respiratory system • Antimicrobial for chest infections, colds and flu. • Expectorant and decongestant; clears catarrh, sinusitis, coughs, asthma, hay fever and rhinitis.
Immune system • Antibacterial, antifungal, antiviral and antiparasitic[5], particularly for the respiratory, digestive and urinary systems. Active against viruses, including influenza B and herpes simplex type 1 and 2. • Powerful antioxidant[6]; slows ageing process. • Sulphur compounds have antitumour activities[7] and protect against pollution and nicotine.
Externally • Oil/ointment used for cuts, wounds, arthritis, sprains, unbroken chilblains, athlete's foot, stings and warts. • Eardrops used for middle ear infection.

CAUTION Avoid large doses during pregnancy. May cause gastrointestinal upset. Applied to skin can cause dermatitis.
Drug interactions Avoid large doses with warfarin and antihypertensives.

Aloe barbadensis
Aloe vera

Indigenous to East and South Africa, this perennial succulent grows happily in most tropical places. Aloe juice is made by mixing the clear mucilaginous gel inside the leaves with water, which is used for problems associated with excess heat and inflammation.

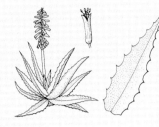

FAMILY Aloaceae
PARTS USED Gel of inner leaves
CONSTITUENTS Polysaccharides (acemannan and glucomannans), enzymes, vitamins A, B, C and E, amino acids, minerals, saponins, sterols, salicylic acid.
ACTIONS Demulcent, immunostimulant, anti-inflammatory, alterative, analgesic, antihistamine, antibacterial, antiviral, antiseptic, anthelmintic, digestive, rejuvenative, antioxidant, hypoglycaemic, diuretic.

Digestion • Mild laxative; clears toxins and heat from the bowel. • Combats pathogenic micro-organisms.
• Enhances the secretion of digestive enzymes and balances stomach acid. • Regulates sugar and fat metabolism. • Soothes and protects the gut lining; used for colitis, peptic ulcers, IBS and inflammatory bowel disease.
Musculoskeletal system • Anti-inflammatory and detoxifying for arthritis.
Immune system • Acemannan enhances immunity, is antiviral and stimulates activity of B- and T-lymphocytes, helping to destroy malignant cells. • Sterols have an anti-inflammatory action. • Antiviral for herpes simplex and zoster (shingles). • Used as a probiotic to treat candida.
Reproductive system • Increases blood to the uterus.
• Reduces hot flushes during menopause. • Used to treat PMS.
Externally • Soothes and heals burns, sunburn, wounds, haemorrhoids and skin conditions such as acne, eczema and psoriasis. • Antibacterial, antifungal and antiviral.
• Rejuvenates skin and reduces wrinkles. • Excellent for sensitive and allergic skin conditions.

CAUTION **Drug interactions** Possible interaction with cardiac glycosides and steroids.

Althea officinalis
Marshmallow

This stately perennial grows in marshes by the sea in Europe and western Asia. An abundance of mucilage makes Marshmallow the most soothing of medicines, cooling irritation and inflammation – ideal for treating sore or inflamed mucous membranes.

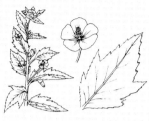

FAMILY Malvaceae
PARTS USED Root, leaf, flower
CONSTITUENTS Mucilage (glucans, arabans and galacturonic rhamnans), tannins, pectin, sterols, coumarins, phenolic acidasparagin, flavonoids (quercitrin, kaempferol and scopoletin), sugars.
ACTIONS Emollient, demulcent, vulnerary, anti-inflammatory, analgesic, antiseptic, antitussive, expectorant, diuretic, antilithic, immune enhancer, galactogogue.

Digestion • Anti-inflammatory for ulcerative colitis, gastritis and peptic ulcers. • Mucilage soothes heartburn, IBS and constipation from dryness. • Reduces peristalsis and relieves diarrhoea; larger doses have a mild laxative effect.
Respiratory system • Mild expectorant and immune enhancer. Soothes harsh, dry coughs, sore throats, laryngitis, bronchitis and croup; clears catarrh and alleviates inflammation.
Immune system • Antimicrobial against *Proteus vulgaris*, *Pseudomonas aeruginosa* and *Staphylococcus aureus*[8]. • Stimulates production of white blood cells.
Urinary system • Soothing diuretic, relieving cystitis, urethritis and irritable bladder. Eases passing of gravel and stones.
Reproductive system • Traditionally added to prescriptions to ease childbirth. • Stimulates flow of breast milk.
Externally • Leaves are applied to irritation and inflammation from insect bites and wasp and bee stings. • Used with lavender and flax oil for treating scalds and burns and sunburn. • Soothes and heals inflamed skin in sore nipples, acne and eczema. • Warm poultice used to draw out splinters and for mastitis, boils and abscesses. • Mouthwash/gargle used to treat sore throats and inflamed gums.

Andrographis paniculata
Andrographis

Native to India and cultivated in China, this annual has a very bitter taste and is highly valued in Ayurvedic medicine for enhancing immunity and combating acute infection.

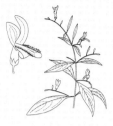

FAMILY Acanthaceae
PARTS USED Aerial parts
CONSTITUENTS Diterpenoid lactones (andrographolides), flavones (oroxylin and wogonin).
ACTIONS Immunostimulant, antimicrobial, choleretic, hepatoprotective, febrifuge, anodyne, antiparasitic, anthelmintic.

Digestion • Antiviral, antiprotazoal, antifungal, antiparasitic and anthelmintic. Helps re-establish normal gut flora and combat acute infections, bacillary dysentery, enteritis, worms, parasites and candida. • Antibacterial against *Staphylococcus aureus*, *Pseudomonas aeruginosa*, *Proteus vulgaris*, *Shigella dysenteriae* and *E. coli*[9]. • Bitter and cooling, it enhances digestion, stimulates bile flow from the liver and protects the liver from damage by toxins, alcohol and infections such as hepatitis[10]. • Anti-inflammatory for indigestion, heartburn, acidity, flatulence, gastritis, colitis and peptic ulcers.
Respiratory system • For throat and ear infections, coughs, colds, flu, acute bronchitis and chest infections with fever[11]. • Reduces phlegm; helpful in asthma[12]. • Used in Ayurvedic medicine for pneumonia[13].
Immune system • Immune enhancing; excellent for the prevention and treatment of infections such as colds, flu, coughs, sinusitis, mouth ulcers, shingles, otitis media, sore throats, laryngitis, tonsilitis and septic conditions of the blood[14]. • Useful for leptospirosis[15], high fevers and malaria. • Protects the liver and inhibits platelet aggregation[16].
Urinary system • For heat and infection of the urinary tract from dysuria, haematuria and proteinuria[17].
Externally • Used as a wash/cream for inflamed and infected skin problems such as acne, eczema, spots and boils.

Anemone pulsatilla
Pasque flower

The Pasque flower, with its silky purple flowers and silvery hairs, followed by feathery seed heads, is one of the most beautiful wild flowers of Europe. Despite its delicate appearance it is remarkably resilient, flowering in early spring but often in very wintery weather.

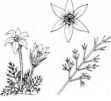

FAMILY Ranunculaceae
PARTS USED Dried aerial parts
CONSTITUENTS Glycoside (ranunculin in the fresh plant, which is poisonous, producing anemonin on drying), tannins, saponins, resin, volatile oil, chelidonic acid, flavonoids.
ACTIONS Analgesic, sedative, antispasmodic, decongestant, febrifuge.

Circulation • Improves venous circulation; for varicose veins and nosebleeds.
Mental and emotional • Excellent relaxant and nerve tonic. Promotes relaxation and sleep and facilitates recovery when run-down by conserving energy. • Used for nervous exhaustion, depression, insomnia, nightmares, irritability, weepiness, clinginess and fear of being alone. • Used for PMS, overexcitement, weepiness, depression after childbirth and during menopause.
Respiratory system • Astringent and antibacterial; used for colds, acute and chronic catarrh and coughs.
Musculoskeletal system • Relieves spasm and excellent for reducing pain; used for colic, period pain, headaches, asthma and neuralgia.
Immune system • In hot infusion relieves fevers, brings out rash in eruptive infections such as measles and speeds recovery.
Reproductive system • Specific for pain and inflammation in men and women • Good analgesic for childbirth. • Used for afterpains and post-natal depression. • Tonic and relaxant properties help regulate contractions. • Used for PMS and menopausal depression.
Eyes and ears • Used for painful inflammatory eye conditions including scleritis, iritis, glaucoma and cataracts. • Used for otitis media and earache.

CAUTION Avoid during pregnancy.

Anethum graveolens
Dill

This highly aromatic annual is originally from the Mediterranean. Its name is said to come from the Saxon word *dilla*, meaning 'to lull', due to its ability to relax babies and children into a restful sleep.

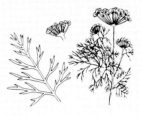

FAMILY Apiaceae
PARTS USED Leaf, seed
CONSTITUENTS Volatile oil (including limonene and carvone), flavonoids (including quercitrin, kaempferol and vincenin), coumarins, triterpenes, magnesium, iron, calcium, potassium, vitamin C.
ACTIONS Carminative, alterative, expectorant, diuretic, antispasmodic, galactogogue, vermifuge, analgesic, relaxant, digestive, sedative, anti-inflammatory, antioxidant, antimicrobial.

Digestion • Stimulates appetite and digestion. • Releases tension and spasm; used for colic, wind, indigestion, nausea, constipation and diarrhoea. • Important ingredient in gripe water for babies' colic. • Used as a vermifuge in India.
Mental and emotional • Helps alleviate tiredness from disturbed nights and enhances concentration and memory. • Relaxant for insomnia and stress-related digestive disorders such as wind, colic and constipation.
Respiratory system • Antispasmodic and expectorant for harsh, dry coughs and asthma.
Musculoskeletal system • Volatile oil in the leaves and seeds relaxes smooth muscle. Good for relieving tension and pain.
Immune system • Research has confirmed its antibacterial[18] and anticandida properties[19]. • May inhibit cancer formation.
Urinary system • It has diuretic effects.
Reproductive system • Used for painful periods. • Emmenagogic properties regulate menstruation. • In the East it is given to women prior to childbirth to ease childbirth. • Increases milk in breast-feeding women.
Externally • Analgesic and anti-inflammatory properties relieve pain and swelling. • Essential oil in massage oils and liniments used to treat abdominal pain, colic, arthritis and earache.

Angelica archangelica
Angelica

This statuesque biennial, native to parts of Europe, was historically valued for its protection against poisoning, contagion and witches. Its healing properties were reputedly revealed to a monk during a plague epidemic by the Archangel Michael or Gabriel – hence its Latin name.

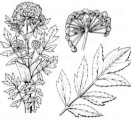

FAMILY Apiaceae
PARTS USED Dried root, leaf, stem, seed
CONSTITUENTS Essential oil, coumarins, resins, sugars, starch.
ACTIONS Antibacterial, antifungal, alterative, anti-inflammatory, carminative, diaphoretic, digestive, diuretic, nervine, tonic, circulatory stimulant, antispasmodic, expectorant, emmenagogue.

Digestion • Stimulates digestion; used for weak digestion, hypochlorhydria, nausea, indigestion, wind and colic. • Inhaling the crushed leaves relieves travel sickness. • Improves appetite, metabolism and absorption. • Taken regularly it is traditionally thought to reduce the desire for alcohol; excellent for alcoholics.
Circulation • Warming circulatory tonic; stimulates blood flow to the periphery; excellent for problems with poor circulation such as Raynaud's disease and Buerger's disease. • Calcium-channel blocker in the heart; useful for high blood pressure, angina and heart arrhythmias[20]. • Used to treat anaemia.
Mental and emotional • Strengthening nerve tonic; aids inspiration. • Mood elevating in depression. • Enhances mental clarity.
Respiratory system • Warming expectorant and decongestant for coughs, acute bronchitis, asthma, sore throats, colds and catarrh. • Hot tea helps to relieve fevers.
Immune system • Antimicrobial and cleansing; aids detoxification and enhances immunity. • Anti-inflammatory for arthritis and gout.
Reproductive system • Regulates menstrual cycle and relieves period pain and PMS.
Externally • Used in massage oils or baths to relieve muscle tension and joint stiffness and pain.

CAUTION Avoid fresh root during pregnancy. May cause photosensitivity.

Angelica polymorph var. *sinensis*
Chinese angelica/Dong guai

This perennial herb is found in the mountain forests of China, Japan and Korea. It is an important blood and liver tonic in Traditional Chinese Medicine, used to treat anaemia and vitiligo.

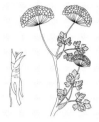

FAMILY Apiaceae
PARTS USED Root
CONSTITUENTS Volatile oils, vitamin B12, coumarins, sterols, ferulic acid, polysaccharides.
ACTIONS Emmenagogue, antiviral, antibacterial, antifungal, antispasmodic, circulatory stimulant, digestive, hypotensive, alterative, analgesic, anti-inflammatory, decongestant, diuretic, immunostimulant, post-partum tonic, uterine tonic, rejuvenative.

Digestion • Warming digestive stimulant; increases appetite and digestion. Used for constipation.
Circulation • Decreases blood pressure, regulates the heart, inhibits platelet aggregation, reduces atherosclerosis, enhances circulation and dilates coronary arteries. • Used for angina, arrhythmias, palpitations, atrial fibrillation, Buerger's disease, Raynaud's syndrome and cramps.
Mental and emotional • Mild analgesic for headaches, neuralgia and shingles pain. • Strengthening tonic for exhaustion. • Relaxant for insomnia.
Respiratory system • Clears catarrh and asthma.
Immune system • Stimulates formation of white blood cells, lymphocytes and phagocytes. • For herpes infections and malaria. • May have an anticancer effect by increasing tumour necrosis. • Protects the liver. • Inhibits immunoglobulin E antibodies in allergies.
Urinary system • Diuretic; relieves fluid retention. Useful for dispelling premenstrual fluid accumulation.
Reproductive system • Balances hormones. • Renowned women's tonic for menstrual irregularities, dysmenorrhoea, PMS and heavy periods. • Enhances fertility. • Aids contractions during childbirth. • Used for menopausal symptoms such as night sweats, hot flushes, depression and mood swings.
Eyes • May decrease intraocular pressure.

CAUTION Avoid during pregnancy.
Drug interactions Avoid with anticoagulants.

Apium graveolens
Wild celery

This aromatic biennial, native to the Mediterranean, is believed to be the original celery. It has been popular since Roman times for relieving aches and pains, as a digestive and for overweight and fluid retention.

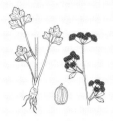

FAMILY Apiaceae
PARTS USED Seeds
CONSTITUENTS Volatile oils, apiol, sulphur, alkaloids, furanocoumarin, flavonic glycoside (apigenin), alpha lipoic acid, flavonoids, phenols, resin, fatty acids, calcium.
ACTIONS Diuretic, urinary antiseptic, antioxidant, hypotensive, depurative, antibacterial, antifungal, sedative, antispasmodic, uterotonic, antineoplastic, anti-inflammatory, immunostimulant, galactogogue, analgesic.

Digestion • Antispasmodic and digestive; enhances appetite, digestion and absorption and relieves spasm, colic, wind, halitosis, indigestion, hiccups, heartburn and nausea. • May help to regulate metabolism and blood sugar levels.
Circulation • Reduces circulating dopamine, norepinephrine and epinephrine, helping to reduce blood pressure[21]. • Antiplatelet effects; reduces the formation of clots and helps prevent heart attacks and strokes.
Mental and emotional • Calming and uplifting; used for stress-related headaches, mental and physical tiredness, insomnia, depression, agitation and panic. • Releases muscle tension and spasm.
Musculoskeletal system • Excellent anti-inflammatory for arthritis, rheumatism and gout. • A diuretic that dissolves and excretes uric acid. • Relieves muscle pain, tension and spasm. • Reduces neuralgia and sciatica.
Immune system • Enhances immunity; antimicrobial effects help ward off colds, flu, asthma and bronchitis. • May have antitumour properties.
Urinary system • Apiol is a urinary antiseptic. • Relieves fluid retention and cystitis; helps to eliminate toxins. • Prevents the formation of stones and gravel.
Reproductive system • Enhances milk supply in lactating mothers. • Uterine stimulant; brings on periods and stimulates contractions in childbirth.

CAUTION Avoid in pregnancy and with kidney inflammation.

Arctium lappa
Burdock

A biennial native to temperate Europe and northern Asia, respected for its detoxifying and antiseptic properties. The root is generally favoured in Western medicine, while the seeds are also used in Asian medicine.

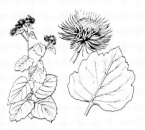

FAMILY Asteraceae
PARTS USED Root, seed, leaf
CONSTITUENTS Root: inulin, mucilage, pectin, polyacetylenes, volatile acids, sterols, tannins, bitters, aldehydes, flavonoid glycosides (quercetin and kaempferol), asparagin, polyphenolic acid; seed: fixed oils, bitter glycoside (arctiin), flavonoids, chlorogemc acid; leaves: terpenoids, sterols, triterpenols, arctiol, fulcinone, taraxasterol, mucilage, essential oil, tannin, inulin.
ACTIONS Alterative, diaphoretic, demulcent, diuretic, astringent, bitter tonic, digestive, mild laxative, antimicrobial, hypoglycaemic, antitumour, probiotic.

Digestion • Enhances digestion and liver function, mild laxative and depurative. Relieves wind, distension and indigestion. • Hypoglycaemic action; helpful for diabetes[22]. • Mucilaginous fibres absorb toxins from the gut and enhance their elimination from the bowel. • Used for bacterial and fungal infections; fructooligosaccharides in the root have a probiotic effect[23].
Respiratory system • Enhances immunity to infections. • Used for sore throats, swollen glands and tonsils.
Immune system • Antibacterial, antifungal and antitumour. • In hot decoction it reduces fevers, clears toxins via the skin, brings out eruptions and speeds recovery from measles and chickenpox. • Cleansing for chronic inflammatory conditions such as gout, arthritis and rheumatism and skin problems.
Urinary system • Aids elimination of toxins via urine. • Used for cystitis, water retention, stones and gravel.
Reproductive system • Root stimulates the uterus, aids liver function and the breakdown of hormones and helps regulate periods. • Traditionally used for prolapse. • Imparts strength before and after childbirth.
Skin • Used for chronic skin disease such as acne; improves action of the sebaceous glands.

CAUTION Avoid in pregnancy.
Drug interactions Avoid with antidiabetic drugs as it may have hypoglycaemic effects.

Arctostaphylos uva ursi
Bearberry

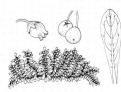

This trailing evergreen shrub is native to Europe, Asia and North America. Popular since the Middle Ages, Bearberry became an official medicine in England in 1788, listed in the *London Pharmacopoeia* as an effective medicine for kidney-related problems, including nephritis and gout.

FAMILY Ericaceae
PARTS USED Leaf
CONSTITUENTS Hydroquinones (arbutin and methylarbutin), flavonoids (quercetin and myricitrin), tannins, triterpenes, allantoin, phenolic acids, volatile oil, resin.
ACTIONS Urinary antiseptic, diuretic, antimicrobial, anti-inflammatory, astringent, antihaemorrhagic, oxytocic, antifungal, astringent, antilithic, parturient.

Immune system • Effective against *E. coli, Streptococcus faecalis, Proteus vulgaris, Staphylococcus aureus, Salmonella typhi, Candida albicans*[24], *Mycoplasma hominis* and *Shigella sonnei.* • Quercetin and phenolic acids are anti-inflammatory.
Urinary system • Specific for chronic irritation/infection in the genitourinary tract; antibacterial properties (probably due to arbutin) reach maximum activity within 3–4 hours after taking it. Used for cystitis, urethritis, pyelonephritis, prostatitis and stones and gravel[25]. • Relieves fluid retention and aids the elimination of toxins and uric acid. • Its astringent properties and allantoin tone and heal inflamed and irritated urinary passages. • Used for bed-wetting and incontinence.
Reproductive system • Uterine tonic, reduces heavy periods, tones muscles in bladder, reduces uterine prolapse and vaginal laxity[26], and stimulates contractions in childbirth. • For gynaecological infection and inflammation such as endometritis and vaginal infections.
Externally • Applied via tampon, pessary or douche for cervical erosion and vaginal discharge/thrush. • Lotion used for haemorrhoids.

CAUTION Drug interactions May increase the effects of non-steroidal anti-inflammatory drugs.

Armoraca rusticana (also known as *Cochlearia armoracia*)
Horseradish

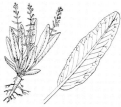

Native to south-eastern Europe and western Asia, this perennial herb has a white tapered root that when cut or grated releases its strong aroma and powerfully acrid properties. It needs to be preserved in vinegar or cream, otherwise it quickly loses its potency.

FAMILY Brassicaceae
PARTS USED Fresh root
CONSTITUENTS Sinigrin (a glucosinolate that is broken down by enzymes, released when cut or grated, to produce allyl isothiocyanate – mustard oil), vitamin C, resin, flavonoids (quercitrin and kaempferol), coumarins (aesculetin, caffeic acid and scopoletin), asparagin.
ACTIONS Circulatory stimulant, decongestant, digestive, antimicrobial, expectorant, alterative, anthelmintic, diuretic, anti-inflammatory.

Digestion • Enhances appetite, digestion and absorption. • Traditionally used as horseradish sauce to accompany roast beef because it stimulates the flow of gastric juices that break down heavy, indigestible foods and prevents indigestion.
Circulation • Horseradish is a powerful stimulant, improving circulation and useful in disorders such as Raynaud's disease and Buerger's disease.
Respiratory system • Stimulates mucous membranes; acts as a decongestant and expectorant, clearing catarrh and blocked sinuses. • Antimicrobial properties help combat infection. • Relieves coughs, colds, fevers, flu, sinusitis and hay fever.
Musculoskeletal system • Hastens the elimination of toxins; recommended for gout and arthritis.
Immune system • Antibiotic properties; excellent for respiratory and urinary infections.
Urinary system • Asparagin is diuretic; relieves fliud retention and clears toxins via the kidneys.
Other • Stimulating, heating energy tonic, excellent in winter for warding off the cold.

CAUTION May irritate the eyes and skin when grating/cutting the fresh root. Avoid in pregnancy and with thyroid problems and symptoms characterized by heat such as gastritis and peptic ulcers.

Artemisia absinthium
Wormwood

This aromatic perennial is native to Europe, western Asia and North Africa. Intensely bitter and aromatic, it is strengthening and reviving, stimulating the stomach, gall bladder and liver. It is a key ingredient in bitter aperitifs and wines such as vermouth.

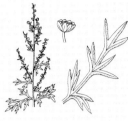

FAMILY Asteraceae
PARTS USED Aerial parts
CONSTITUENTS Flavonoids, phenolic acid, lignans, volatile oils (alpha and beta thujone, alpha pinene and linalool), bitter glycoside absinthe, sesquiterpene lactones, tannins, carotene, vitamin C.
ACTIONS Bitter tonic, digestive, anthelmintic, alterative, antiseptic, anti-inflammatory, anodyne, immunostimulant, nervine, antifungal, cholagogue, antiemetic, diuretic, antilithic, emmenagogue, insecticide.

Digestion • Stimulates the flow of hydrochloric acid and enhances appetite, digestion, absorption and liver function. • Used for heartburn, acidity, liver problems, halitosis, gastritis, indigestion, anorexia, flatulence, nausea, vomiting, diarrhoea and gastroenteritis.
• Taken on an empty stomach for treating pin worms.
• Antimicrobial for food poisoning.
Mental and emotional • Stimulates the brain.
• Traditionally used for neuralgia, depression and nervous exhaustion.
Musculoskeletal system • Anti-inflammatory for gout and arthritis.
Immune system • Volatile oils are strongly antibacterial. • Enhances immunity and clears toxins; good when run-down or recovering from illness. • Taken hot for fevers, colds and flu and to clear catarrh.
Reproductive system • Stimulates uterine muscles, brings on periods and aids contractions during childbirth. • Regulates the menstrual cycle, relieves painful periods and promotes fertility.
Externally • A wash used for fleas and lice[27]; lotion for skin problems such as nappy rash, athlete's foot, scabies and boils, and hair loss, bruises, sprains and arthritic pain.

CAUTION Avoid during pregnancy and breastfeeding. Low doses are recommended; for example, 0.25–1 ml of tincture 3 x daily or 1–2 g dried herb 3 x daily.

Artemisia annua
Sweet Annie

Native to Asia and eastern Europe, this annual feathery herb is found throughout temperate and subtropical areas. Artemisinin, a key active component, was first isolated by researchers in China in 1972 and has since become hugely popular as an effective remedy for malaria.

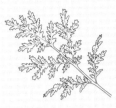

FAMILY Asteraceae
PARTS USED Leaf
CONSTITUENTS Essential oil, flavanoids, artemisinin (containing a peroxide), qinghaoic acid.
ACTIONS Bitter, carminative, digestive, antiparasitic, febrifuge, antimalarial, antiseptic, antibacterial, anti-inflammatory, digestive.

Digestion • Enhances appetite and digestion; relieves wind and indigestion. • Recommended for infections including salmonella, dysentery and diarrhoea.
Respiratory system • Infusion of the leaves is used to treat fevers, chills, colds and other infections.
Immune system • Clears heat; reduces fevers from infections and sunstroke. • Antimicrobial for TB and other infections. • Enhances immunity, reduces inflammation and may be helpful in autoimmune disease. Studies using 50 g herb or 0.3 g artemisinin daily have shown it to improve symptoms in systemic lupus erythematosus[28]. • Qinghaoic acid is antibacterial against, for example, *Staphylococcus aureus*, *E. coli* and *Salmonella typhosa*[29]. • Artemisinin releases free radicals once inside red blood cells that kill malaria parasites[30].
• Artemisinin is effective against drug-resistant *Plasmodium* spp. Research has shown its efficacy in treating malaria, but other constituents may contribute.
• May have anticancer properties, particularly in relation to breast and prostate cancer and leukaemia.
Externally • Poultice of the leaves is applied to nosebleeds, abscesses and boils. • In China the leaves are burned as a fumigant insecticide to kill mosquitoes.

CAUTION Avoid in pregnancy. May cause contact dermatitis.

Asclepias tuberosa
Pleurisy root

Native to North America, Pleurisy root was used by Native American tribes as a remedy for chest infections and externally to treat wounds. It became an official medicine in the *United States Pharmacopoeia* from 1820 to 1905 for fevers, respiratory infections and pleurisy.

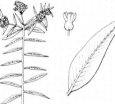

FAMILY Asclepiadaceae
PARTS USED Root
CONSTITUENTS Glycoside (asclepiadin, found mostly in the fresh herb), volatile oils, resins, mucilage, starch, tannin, mineral salts, flavonoids (kaempferol and quercetin), rutin, cardiac glycosides (cardenolides), amino acids, sterols.
ACTIONS Diaphoretic, vasorelaxant, febrifuge, antispasmodic, amphoteric, expectorant, nervine, anti-inflammatory, antiviral, antimicrobial, expectorant, carminative, cathartic, diuretic, emetic (large doses).

Digestion • Antispasmodic and soothing; relieves flatulence, colic and irritation of the gut lining that causes indigestion and diarrhoea.
Circulation • Traditionally used for pericarditis and to slow down a rapid pulse[31]. • Relaxes arteries, brings blood to the periphery and promotes sweating; relieves pressure in the heart and arteries.
Mental and emotional • Calms the nerves and relaxes tense muscles.
Respiratory system • Promotes sweating in fevers and flu. • Expectorant for coughs; helps clear catarrh. • Its antispasmodic properties are helpful in asthma and emphysema. • Relieves pain, infection and inflammation in bronchitis, laryngitis, croup, pneumonia, hoarsness[32] and chest infections including pneumonia. • Reabsorbs pleural effusion from the pleura; specific for pleurisy, pleuritic pain and dry, painful coughs.
Skin • Brings out rash in eruptive diseases including measles and chickenpox.

CAUTION Large doses may cause diarrhoea and vomiting. Avoid in pregnancy and breastfeeding.

Asparagus racemosus
Shatavari/Wild asparagus

This perennial is similar in appearance to cultivated asparagus, with thick, tuberous roots. Shatavari translates as 'she who possesses a hundred husbands' and is the most important rejuvenative tonic for women in Ayurvedic medicine.

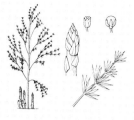

FAMILY Asparagaceae
PARTS USED Leaf, root
CONSTITUENTS Saponins, steroidal glycosides and aglycones, flavonoids (including quercetin, rutin and hyperoside), alkaloids, mucilage.
ACTIONS Female tonic, rejuvenative, galactogogue, adaptogen, antispasmodic, nervine, anti-inflammatory, demulcent, refrigerant, diuretic, aphrodisiac, tonic, expectorant, antibacterial, alterative, antitumour, antacid.

Digestion • Cooling and demulcent for dry, inflamed mucous membranes, dyspepsia, gastritis, peptic ulcers and inflammatory bowel problems such as Crohn's disease and IBS. • Relieves hyperacidity, diarrhoea and dysentery.
Mental and emotional • Valued in India for promoting memory and mental clarity. • For ADHD in children combined with brain tonics such as *Centella asiatica* (Gotu kola). • Reduces anxiety and stress. • Increases energy and strength.
Respiratory system • Soothes sore throats, dry coughs and irritated conditions.
Immune system • Adaptogen. • Enhances immunity, growth and development in babies and children. • Enhances the ability to fight infections and the production of immune-regulating messenger molecules • Protects blood-producing cells in the bone marrow, aiding recoverery after exposure to toxic chemicals[33]. • Antibacterial activity including *E. Coli*, *Shigella* spp., *Salmonella* spp. and *Pseudomonas*[34]; antiviral against herpes. • Anti-inflammatory for gout and arthritis.
Urinary system • Soothing and cooling for cystitis. • Dissolves stones and gravel. • Reduces fluid retention.
Reproductive system • Enhances fertility; used for low libido and sperm count. • Regulates hormonal imbalances; useful during menopause. • Increases milk production.
Externally • Used for swollen joints and muscle tension; ingredient of mahanarayan oil for joint and muscle pain.

Astragalus membranaceous
Astragalus

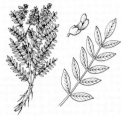

Native to Mongolia and China, Astragalus is a popular Chinese tonic herb used to increase vitality and strengthen immunity, excellent for enhancing endurance, promoting weight gain when weak and underweight and relieving debility, fatigue and chronic fatigue syndrome.

FAMILY Fabaceae
PARTS USED Rhizome (underground stem)
CONSTITUENTS Triterpenoid saponins (astragalosides), flavonoids, polysaccharides, asparagin, linoleic acid, linolenic acid.
ACTIONS Immune enhancing, tonic, adaptogen, adrenal tonic, digestive, vasodilator, cardiotonic, hypotensive, diuretic, antiviral, antibacterial.

Digestion • Improves digestion and absorption, nourishing and strengthening. • Used for stomach ulcers, lingering diarrhoea and rectal prolapse. • Helps regulate blood sugar.
Circulation • Antioxidant and diuretic. • Lowers blood pressure. • Improves heart function; beneficial in ischemic heart disease and heart conditions such as angina[36]. • Vasodilator; promotes blood flow, allowing blood through partially clogged arteries[37].
Immune system • Enhances immunity, antiviral and antibacterial. • Increases the production of antibodies and interferon, increasing white blood cell formation and the production of natural killer cells; useful in the treatment of cancer, chronic hepatitis, HIV and autoimmune disease. • Prophylactic against colds and upper respiratory infections[38]. • May speed recovery and enhance outcome of cancer patients undergoing chemotherapy and radiation therapy[39]. • Shown to increase survival rates in acute *coxsackie B3* viral myocarditis infections[40]. • Protects the liver against damage from drugs, chemicals and alcohol.
Urinary system • Traditionally used to strengthen kidney energy and to treat chronic kidney problems and night sweats. • Diuretic; reduces fluid retention.

CAUTION Avoid in acute infections.
Drug interactions Use cautiously with immunosuppressive drugs.

Avena sativa
Wild oats

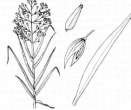

An annual grass native to Europe, Asia and North Africa, oats are highly nutritious, full of protein, calcium, magnesium, silica, iron and vitamins, which are strengthening to bones and teeth and vital to a healthy nervous system. They are an excellent energy-giving food and body builder.

FAMILY Poaceae
PARTS USED Whole plant, seed
CONSTITUENTS Saponins, polyphenols, sterol, monosaccharides, oligosaccharides, alkaloids, flavonoids, gluten, protein, fats, minerals, vitamin B.
ACTIONS Sedative, nervine, antidepressant, diuretic, antispasmodic, demulcent, laxative, nutritive, rejuvenative, antilipidemic, hypocholesterolaemic, antidiabetic.

Digestion • For constipation; help prevent bowel cancer by removing toxins from the bowel. • Since they lower blood sugar, they are useful for diabetics.
Circulation • Lower blood cholesterol and help combat cardiovascular problems; oat bran fibre binds to cholesterol and bile components to be excreted via the bowels.
Mental and emotional • Good tonic for the nervous system, supporting the body during times of stress, relieving depression, anxiety, tension and nervous exhaustion. • Worth taking when withdrawing from tranquillizers and antidepressants. Oat green tea is used for drug, alcohol and nicotine addiction. • May decrease the hypertensive effects of nicotine[41].
Reproductive system • Regulate hormones in the body, notably oestrogen.
Externally • Oatmeal makes a good facial scrub and soothing remedy for irritated and inflamed skin conditions.

Drug interactions May decrease the effects of morphine.

Azadirachta indica
Neem

This evergreen tree native to
South East Asia provides one
of the best-known antiseptic
and detoxifying herbs in
Ayurvedic medicine. It is
primarily used for combating
infections and inflammation.

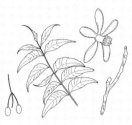

FAMILY Meliaceae
PARTS USED Flower, seed, leaf, bark
CONSTITUENTS Leaves: flavonoids, meliacins,
triterpenoids, phytosterols (campesterol, stigmasterol
and beta-sitosterol), omega-3, 6 and 9 fatty acids,
nimbidin tannins; bark: arginine, glutamic acid,
methionine, tryptophan, nimbinin, gallic acid,
epicatechin, polysaccharides.
ACTIONS Febrifuge, antiseptic, vulnerary, anthelmintic,
insecticidal, alterative, anti-inflammatory, expectorant,
hepatoprotective, hypoglycaemic, antimicrobial,
antimalarial, antifertility, alterative, antibacterial,
antifungal, antiviral, astringent, bitter, emmenagogue.

Digestion • Stimulates appetite, digestion and enhances
liver function. • Hepatoprotective activity protects the
liver from injury from toxins, drugs, chemotherapy
and viruses. • Regulates blood sugar in diabetes[42].
• Recommended for acidity, heartburn, gastritis, peptic
ulcers, nausea, vomiting and worms.
Circulation • Reduces serum cholesterol levels and
blood pressure and regulates the heart.
Mental and emotional • Reduces anxiety, stress, anger,
irritability, intolerance and depression. • Relieves pain.
Respiratory system • Decongestant, expectorant and
antimicrobial; clears infection and phlegm.
Immune system • Leaves and bark are antibacterial,
antifungal and antiparasitic[43]. • Used in the prevention and
treatment of malaria[44]. • Used for inflammatory arthritis.
Reproductive system • Stimulates uterine muscle; used
for delayed and painful childbirth and as a tonic after birth.
Skin • For skin disorders, eczema, acne, boils, psoriasis,
abscesses and haemorrhoids.
Externally • For infections such as chickenpox, head lice
and athlete's foot. Widely used in non-toxic insecticides.
• In liniments for joint pain and muscle aches.

CAUTION Avoid in pregnancy and lactation. May reduce
fertility and cause hypersensitivity reactions[45].
Drug interactions Use with care in patients on insulin.

Bacopa monnieri (also known as *Herpestis monniera*)
Brahmi

Native to India and other
tropical regions, Brahmi
derives its name from
Brahman, meaning 'pure
consciousness', because of
its ability to calm mental
turbulence and aid
meditation. It is often confused with Gotu kola (*Centella
asiatica*), which is also called Brahmi in northern India.

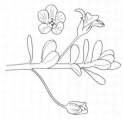

FAMILY Scrophulariaceae
PARTS USED Dried whole plant, mainly leaf and stalk
CONSTITUENTS Steroidal saponins, alkaloids brahmine
and herpestine, flavonoids, amino acids, d-mannitol,
beta-sitosterone.
ACTIONS Adaptogen, antidepressant, anxiolytic,
nervine tonic, diuretic, sedative, cardiotonic, rejuvenative,
antispasmodic, carminative, bronchial dilator,
anticonvulsant, immunostimulant, anti-inflammatory,
antiseptic, antifungal, antioxidant, antirheumatic, diuretic.

Digestion • Suppresses appetite; best combined with
warming digestive herbs such as Ginger and Cardamom.
• Astringent for stress-related diarrhoea and IBS.
Mental and emotional • Used in India and China to
enhance brain function and learning ability, improve
memory and concentration and calm anxiety and mental
turbulence. • Enhances neurotransmitter/synapse
function and increases serotonin production and brain
cell activity[46]. Helpful for ADD, ADHD, learning and
behavioural problems, hyperactivity, Alzheimer's disease,
epilepsy, mental illness, restlessness, insomnia and
anxiety. • Increases resilience to stress, combats nervous
exhaustion and relieves depression. • Hersaponin, one of
four saponins, has sedative and cardiotonic properties.
Respiratory system • For coughs and colds, bronchitis,
asthma and hoarseness. • Poultice of the boiled plant can
be applied to the chest for bronchitis and chronic cough.
Urinary system • Cooling diuretic; used for cystitis and
irritable bladder. • Nourishing kidney tonic.
Other • Relieves joint pain. • Helps chelate heavy metals
from the body.
Externally • Oil/fresh leaf juice is used for joint pain.
• Applied to the head to clear the mind and relieve
headaches.

Baptisia tinctoria
Wild indigo

This North American perennial plant has bright yellow flowers. It was popular among American physicians in the early 1900s as an 'epidemic remedy' to combat infections.

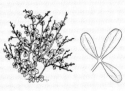

FAMILY Fabaceae
PARTS USED Root, leaf
CONSTITUENTS Coumarins, flavonoids, glycoproteins, polysaccharides, isoflavones, alkaloids (baptitoxin and cytosine), glycosides (bapin), oleoresin, coumarins.
ACTIONS Lymphatic, antipyretic, immune enhancing, alterative, antibiotic, anti-inflammatory, antiseptic, antiviral, astringent, emmenagogue, laxative, stimulant.

Digestion • Laxative; clears toxins and infection from the bowel. • Used for acute infections, gastroenteritis and bacterial dysentery. • Traditionally used for typhoid.
Respiratory system • Antibacterial and antiviral; helps ward off and treat infections of the ear, nose, throat and chest. • Useful for treating chronic bronchitis.
Immune system • Potent antimicrobial for acute and chronic infections. Polysaccharides stimulate phagocytosis, enhancing immunity. • Used at the onset of colds, flu, fevers, infections of the respiratory and digestive system, herpes, glandular fever, tonsillitis and laryngitis. • Good remedy for chronic fatigue syndrome. • Indicated in immunization reactions[47]. • May have antimalarial and anticancer activity.
Urinary system • Antimicrobial for chronic cystitis[48].
Skin • Cleansing and antimicrobial for infected skin problems including boils, abscesses, *Staphylococcus aureus* infections, warts and impetigo.
Externally • Poultice used for spots, boils, acne, eczema, *Staphylococcus aureus* infections, warts, cuts and wounds. • Mouthwash/gargle used for inflammation or infection of gums, mouth ulcers and sore throat. • Used as a douche for cervicitis, vaginal discharge, candida and vaginitis[49].

Berberis aquifolium (also known as *Mahonia aquifolium*)
Oregon grape root

Native to western North America, this evergreen shrub is popular among gardeners, with its yellow flowers and purple berries. The root was traditionally used by Native American tribes as a detoxifying herb for infections and skin problems.

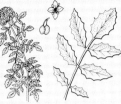

FAMILY Berberidaceae
PARTS USED Dried root, rhizome
CONSTITUENTS Alkaloids (berberine, berbamine, oxyacanthine and herbamine), tannin, resin, fats.
ACTIONS Alterative, bitter tonic, cholagogue, digestive, laxative, astringent, antiseptic, antitumour, diuretic, thyroid stimulant, antioxidant, antiproliferative, antipyretic.

Digestion • Excellent for the liver and gall bladder; used for treating hepatitis and gallstones. • Bitters stimulate the flow of saliva, digestive enzymes and bile. • Enhances appetite, digestion and absorption. • Clears toxins and relieves constipation. • Clears infections, diarrhoea, dysentery, *Shigella* spp., *Staphylococcus aureus*, *Salmomella* spp. and dysbiosis. • Used for headaches and malaise associated with toxicity. • Increases stamina.
Circulation • Reduces venous congestion; improves varicose veins and haemorrhoids. • Dilates blood vessels and reduces blood pressure. • For anaemia; releases stored iron from the liver.
Mental and emotional • Cooling remedy for fiery people who are critical, self-critical and dissatisfied.
Musculoskeletal system • Anti-inflammatory and depurative for gout, rheumatism and arthritis.
Immune system • Berberine enhances immunity against a wide range of microbes and inhibits tumour development.
Urinary system • Diuretic; aids cleansing by enhancing the elimination of toxins.
Reproductive system • Reduces uterine blood congestion that causes heavy periods and menstrual pain.
Skin • Clears toxins, heat and inflammation, acne, boils, herpes, eczema and psoriasis.
Externally • Compress or poultice used for boils and irritation of the skin. • Gargle used for sore throats.

CAUTION Avoid in hyperthyroidism and during pregnancy. Fresh roots/rhizomes are purgative. May cause flatulence.

Berberis vulgaris
Barberry

Native to temperate climates, this shrub is found growing wild in Europe and North America. One of the best cleansing herbs, the root was traditionally used by Native Americans and in European folk medicine for infections, liver and stomach ailments and as a general tonic during convalescence.

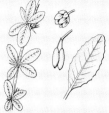

FAMILY Berberidaceae
PARTS USED Root, stem/bark
CONSTITUENTS Isoquinoline alkaloids (berberine, palmatine, oxyacanthine, magnoflorine, jatrorrhizine and columbamine), tannins, resin.
ACTIONS Antimicrobial, cholagogue, choleretic, antiemetic, bitter tonic, antiparasitic, probiotic.

Digestion • Maintains normal gut flora and combats infection in the gut including *E. coli* and amoebic dysentery, *Giardia*, *Blastocystis hominis* and *Dientamoeba fragilis*[50]. Inhibits endotoxins. • Bitters stimulate bile flow from the liver and help detoxify the body. • Indicated for viral liver infections and gall bladder problems.
Circulation • Regulates the heart and decreases ventricular arrhythmias and palpitations. • Increases platelets in thrombocytopenia[51].
Musculoskeletal system • Anti-inflammatory and detoxyifing remedy for arthritis, rheumatism and gout.
Immune system • Antioxidant; reduces oxygen free radicals[52] and helps protect against cancer. • Potent antimicrobial active against bacteria, fungi, viruses, worms and chlamydia. • Berberine is active against *Staphylococcus epidermidis*, *E. coli* and *Neisseria meningitides*[53]. • Indicated in acute bowel infection, diarrhoea, dysentery and cholera. • Decreases inflammation and has an antihistamine action, useful in infected skin conditions such as boils and abscesses and allergies, including hay fever, atopic eczema and asthma, and migraine.
Externally • Cream used for psoriasis[54]. • Used in a saline solution as eye drops[55].

Borago officinalis
Borage

Native to Europe, Asia and North Africa, borage is a perennial with bright blue flowers and leaves that smell like cucumber. The plant is good for cooling inflammation and clearing toxins, while the oil is rich in gamma-linoleic acid (GLA).

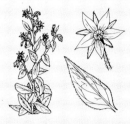

FAMILY Boraginaceae
PARTS USED Leaf, flower, seed oil
CONSTITUENTS Leaf and flower: mucilage, tannin, saponins, essential oil, pyrrolizidine alkaloids, potassium, calcium, vitamin C, essential oil; seed oil: fatty acids (including GLA and linoleic acid).
ACTIONS Leaf and flower: expectorant, diuretic, vulnerary, adrenal tonic, alterative, decongestant, demulcent, galactogogue, anti-inflammatory, antihypertensive, diaphoretic; seed oil: antiarthritic, anti-inflammatory, antihypertensive, hormone regulator.

Circulation • GLA in seed oil converts in the body to prostaglandin E1 (PGE1), which dilates blood vessels, reduces blood pressure and blood clots and lowers harmful cholesterol.
Mental and emotional • Relieves tension and anxiety, increases resilience to stress, supports adrenals, lifts spirits and improves mental energy.
Respiratory system • Decongestant and soothing expectorant for catarrh, coughs, bronchitis, pneumonia and pleurisy. • GLA reduces inflammation of the lungs and improves oxygenation; helpful in asthma, bronchitis and chronic airways obstruction.
Immune system • Increases sweat and urine production; clears heat and toxins. • GLA has anti-inflammatory properties; relieves eczema and other skin inflammation. • GLA is useful for diabetes, scleroderma, Sjögren's syndrome and to slow ageing • GLA is helpful in prostate cancer, allergies and inflammatory arthritis.
Urinary system • Cools and soothes irritation and inflammation; relieves cystitis, urinary tract infections and fluid retention.
Reproductive system • Increases milk flow in nursing mothers. • GLA is useful for PMS, menstrual problems and menopause.
Externally • Compress used for inflamed eyes and skin and bruises; gargle for sore throats.

Boswellia serrata
Frankincense

Native to North Africa and the Middle East, Frankincense is a small deciduous tree found growing in hot, dry places. The scored bark secretes a juice that hardens into a brown resin used for medicine and incense.

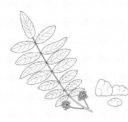

FAMILY Burseraceae
PARTS USED Gum resin from bark
CONSTITUENTS Triterpenes (boswellic acid A and B), sugars (arabinose), arabic acid, essential oils (bassorin, pinene, dipentene, uronic acids and sterols).
ACTIONS Anti-inflammatory, antiarthritic, antitumour, aphrodisiac, analgesic, hypocholesterolaemic, emmenagogue, antispasmodic.

Digestion • Anti-inflamatory, used for colitis, Crohn's disease and ulcerative colitis.
Circulation • Improves blood flow to the joints, prevents breakdown of tissues. • Reduces harmful cholesterol, clears ama from the blood[56]. • Traditionally used for relieving pain and arthritis, and for psoriasis. • Reduces inflammation and inhibits the formation of tumours.
Mental and emotional • Opens the mind; valued for its specific effect on the spiritual centre connected with the pituitary and hypothalamus gland.
Respiratory system • Clears catarrh, coughs, bronchitis and asthma[57].
Musculoskeletal system • Speeds the healing of broken bones. • Boswellic acid reduces the activity of pain- and inflammation-causing leukotrienes by inhibiting the production of 5-lipoxygenase enzyme[58]. • Inhibits the breakdown of connective tissue, increases blood supply to the joints and strengthens blood vessels[59].
Reproductive system • Used for uterine congestion, fibroids, cysts and painful periods with clots. • Brings blood to the penis and improves erectile function. • Reduces swelling, pain and morning stiffness in rheumatoid arthritis[60]. • Good alternative to non-steroidal anti-inflammatory drugs for rheumatoid arthritis, osteoarthritis, tendonitis, bursitis, MS and repetitive strain injuries[61].
Externally • Gum ointment for boils, wounds and sores[62], psoriasis and urticaria[63]. • Speeds healing of wounds and bruises, haemorrhoids and skin problems.

CAUTION Avoid during pregnancy. May cause mild gastric upset.

Calendula officinalis
Marigold

This popular garden annual, native to Europe and Asia, has been valued as a medicine since Roman times for digestive problems and infections, and the plague. Today it is prized as an excellent first-aid remedy.

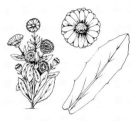

FAMILY Asteraceae
PARTS USED Flower
CONSTITUENTS Flavonoids (including rutin and isoquercetin), volatile oil, terpenoids (including lupeol), taraxerol, taraxasterol, saponins, polysaccharides, bitters, resin, mucilage, betacarotene.
ACTIONS Antiseptic, anti-inflammatory, diaphoretic, bitter tonic, digestive, antiulcer, antitumour, antioxidant, astringent, antiviral, detoxifying, antispasmodic, oestrogenic, diuretic.

Digestion • Reduces inflammation in gastritis and peptic ulcers. • Astringent for diarrhoea and bleeding. • Bitters stimulate liver and gall bladder function. • Improves digestion and absorption • Antimicrobial and anthelmintic for amoebic infections and worms, pelvic and bowel infections, dysentery, viral hepatitis and dysbiosis.
Circulation • Improves venous return; relieves varicose veins. • Enhances circulation and brings blood to the periphery, helping to throw off toxins.
Musculoskeletal system • Depurative and anti-inflammatory for rheumatism, arthritis and gout.
Immune system • Antioxidant and free-radical scavenging effects may account for its antibacterial and anti-inflammatory properties[64]. • Polysaccharides have immunostimulant properties[65], antibacterial[66] and antiviral activity[67] effective in flu and herpes viruses. • Reduces lymphatic congestion • Reputation as an anticancer remedy.
Urinary system • Antibacterial diuretic for infections and fluid retention.
Reproductive system • Hormone balancing, regulates menstruation and relieves menstrual cramps. • Relieves menopausal symptoms and reduces breast congestion. • Astringent for excessive menstrual bleeding and uterine congestion. • Reputation for treating tumours and cysts. • Promotes contractions in childbirth.
Externally • Stops bleeding, prevents infection and speeds healing of cuts and abrasions and ulcers.

CAUTION Avoid during pregnancy.

Capsicum minimum (also known as *C. frutescens*)
Cayenne pepper

Native to North and South America, this fiery plant excites the palate and enhances digestion. It is a great warming remedy for warding off coughs, colds and poor circulation.

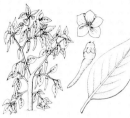

FAMILY Solanaceae
PARTS USED Fruit
CONSTITUENTS Alkaloid (capsaicin), carotenoids, vitamins A and C, flavonoids, volatile oil, steroidal saponins, salicylates.
ACTIONS Circulatory stimulant, vasodilator, hypotensive, rubefacient, analgesic, diaphoretic, digestive, carminative, depurative, antioxidant, antibacterial, expectorant.

Digestion • Enhances appetite, digestion and absorption.• Combats parasites and gastrointestinal infections. • Relieves wind, nausea, indigestion and symptoms of 'cold' such as diarrhoea and abdominal pain. • Clears toxins and reinforces immunity.
Circulation • Stimulates the heart, dilates arteries, improves blood flow and remedies chilblains.
• Antioxidant; protects arteries from damage. • Capsaicin stimulates the hypothalamus to lower blood temperature; aids tolerance of heat. • Reduces tendency to clots and the liver's production of cholesterol and triglycerides.
• Reduces blood pressure.
Mental and emotional • For lethargy, nervous debility and depression. • Stimulates secretion of endorphins that block pain and enhance wellbeing; eases pain of shingles, cluster headaches and migraine. • Improves memory.
Respiratory system • Diaphoretic and bactericidal properties and vitamin C enhance fight against infection.
• Thins and clears catarrh and prevents colds, coughs and chest infections; useful in emphysema. • Prevents cellular damage in the lungs; blocks irritation and constriction in bronchi from cigarette smoke and other pollutants.
Reproductive system • Relieves pain from poor circulation. • Rejuvenative for infertility and libido.
Externally • Topical analgesic, stimulates the release of substance P and reduces pain. • Component of salves for arthritic and postherpetic pain, trigeminal neuralgia, carpal tunnel syndrome, headaches and arthritis.

Carduus benedictus (also known as *Cnicus benedictus*)
Holy thistle

This prickly annual with its yellow flowers is native to the Mediterranean. It has an ancient reputation as a digestive and liver remedy with the power to fight off malaria, smallpox and even the plague.

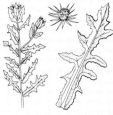

FAMILY Asteraceae
PARTS USED Root, aerial parts, seed
CONSTITUENTS Alkaloids, mucilage, tannin, bitter compound (cnicine) essential oil, flavonoids.
ACTIONS Galactogogue, diaphoretic, astringent, antimicrobial, digestive, nervine, carminative, decongestant, antispasmodic, stimulant, tonic, emmenagogue, expectorant.

Digestion • Bitters enhance appetite, digestion and absorption, stimulate liver function and the flow of bile; used for anorexia, indigestion, wind, colic and conditions associated with a sluggish liver such as skin problems, headaches, lethargy and irritability. • Good astringent for diarrhoea.
Circulation • Enhances the circulation and helpful for varicose veins.
Mental and emotional • Nerve tonic, improves memory and relieves nerve pain, backache, headaches, migraines and dizziness.
Respiratory system • Hot infusion is diaphoretic for fevers and expectorant for chest problems.
Immune system • Excellent tonic after illness, when tired and run-down. • Enhances immunity and has an antimicrobial and antitumour action. • Taken hot it reduces fevers and catarrh and improves circulation.
Urinary system • Diuretic; reduces fluid retention and cystitis.
Reproductive system • Increases milk production.
• Reduces heavy periods, menstrual headaches and period pain. • Emmenagogoue; brings on suppressed periods. • Helpful during menopause.
Externally • Antiseptic; staunches bleeding from cuts and speeds healing of wounds.

CAUTION Avoid during pregnancy.

Carduus marianus (also known as *Silybum marianum*)
Milk thistle

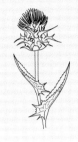

Native to the Mediterranean and naturalized in North America, Europe and Asia, milk thistle gets its name from the milky-white patterning on its toothed leaves, which resembles spilt milk. It has been used for centuries to treat liver and gall bladder problems.

FAMILY Asteraceae
PARTS USED Seed
CONSTITUENTS Flavonoids (silymarin), tyramine, histamine, gamma-linoleic acid (GLA), essential oil, mucilage, bitters.
ACTIONS Anti-inflammatory, antidepressant, antioxidant, appetite stimulant, astringent, bitter tonic, cholagogue, demulcent, diaphoretic, digestive, diuretic, emetic, emmanagogue, galactogogue, hepatoprotective, stomachic, tonic[68].

Digestion • Hepatoprotective for acute and chronic liver disease. Increases the resilience of healthy cells by preventing toxins entering liver cells and stimulates the repair of cells damaged by infection, alcohol and drug abuse, chemical exposure and drugs such as in chemotherapy. • Silymarin acts as an antioxidant, decreasing free radical damage in the liver. • Prevents fatal poisoning from liver damage from mushrooms such as death cap if administered intravenously within 48 hours[69]. • Indicated in acute and chronic viral hepatitis, bile duct inflammation and cirrhosis. • Traditionally used for gallstones and improving appetite and digestion in patients with liver disease. • Reduces cholesterol.
• Detoxifying; useful in skin problems such as psoriasis.
• Laxative; relieves haemorrhoids.
Immune system • Anti-inflammatory action. • Improves immunity by enhancing the function of neutrophils, T lymphocytes and leucocytes[70]. • May have anticancer actions in inhibiting the growth of breast, cervical and prostate cancer cells[71]. • Maintains gut flora; used to treat candida.
Urinary system • Protective action on the kidneys, reducing damage caused by toxins and drugs.
Reproductive system • Leaves traditionally used to enhance the flow of breast milk in lactating women.

Cassia senna (also known as *Senna alexandrina*)
Senna

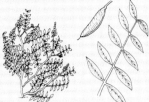

This perennial herb with spikes of yellow flowers is native to North Africa, parts of the Middle East and southern India. Senna has been popular in the Arab world since at least the ninth century and is now famous throughout the world as a powerful laxative.

FAMILY Caesalpiniaceae
PARTS USED Leaf, seed pod
CONSTITUENTS Calcium, sulphur, flavonoids, mannitol, anthraquinone glycosides (sennaosides and aloe-emodin), beta-sitosterol, chrysophanic acid, chrysophanol, tartaric acid, essential oil, mucilage, tannins, resin[72].
ACTIONS Cathartic, cholagogue, diuretic, febrifuge, laxative, purgative, stimulant, vermifuge.

Digestion • Laxative; for acute constipation, flatulence and haemorrhoids, to soften the stool in haemorrhoids and anal fissures[73]. Anthraquinones stimulate irritation and subsequent contraction of bowel muscle. It increases the flow of water and electrolytes into the large intestine and prevents fluid absorption, loosening and easing the passage of the stool. Best combined with aromatic herbs such as Ginger, Mint and Fennel, which relax intestinal muscles to prevent griping and improve bitter taste.
• Antimicrobial for bowel infections. • Clears heat from the liver; indicated for jandice and liver problems.
• Clears heat and toxins via the bowels; may be useful in fevers, arthritis and gout. • Anthelmintic action counteracts worms.
Circulation • Used in Traditional Chinese Medicine to combat the build-up of cholesterol in arteries, clear heat from the liver and to benefit the eyes. • Used in Ayurvedic medicine for anaemia.
Immune system • Contains emodin with antibacterial properties[74].
Skin • Clears heat and toxins; for skin problems such as acne, fungal infections, spots and boils.

CAUTION For short-term use only. Avoid in pregnancy and lactation, with IBS and gastrointestinal inflammation.
Drug interactions Avoid with cardiac glycosides such as digoxin.

Centella asiatica (also known as *Hydrocotyle asiatica*)
Gotu kola/Brahmi

This creeping annual native to Asia, Australia and the South Pacific is found in damp, marshy ground. Used traditionally to enhance memory and concentration, and promote intelligence.

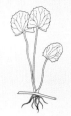

FAMILY Apiaceae
PARTS USED Aerial parts
CONSTITUENTS Essential oil, fatty oil, beta-sitosterol, tannins, resin, alkaloid (hydrocotylin), vellarine (bitter principle), pectic acid, polyphenols, saponins (braminoside and brahmoside), flavonoids.
ACTIONS Nerve tonic, cardiotonic, immunostimulant, febrifuge, alterative, diuretic, anthelmintic, vulnerary, rejuvenative, hair tonic, anticonvulsant, anxiolytic, analgesic, antibacterial, antiviral.

Digestion • Used for indigestion, acidity and ulcers.
• Antibacterial action contributes to its antiulcer properties.
Circulation • Relieves oedema, venous insufficiency and varicose veins[75]. • Excellent wound and scar healer. Stimulates synthesis of collagen and production of fibroblasts; protects skin against radiation. • Prevents bleeding; helpful for anaemia.
Mental and emotional • Famous brain tonic; protects against ageing effects and Alzheimer's disease.
• Improves memory and concentration; excellent for children with learning difficulties such as ADHD and mental problems[76], autism and Asperger syndrome.
• Used for depletion by stress and anxiety, insomnia and depression; calms mental turbulence. • Anticonvulsant for epilepsy.
Immune system • Antibacterial against *pseudomonas* and *Streptococcus* spp.; antiviral against *herpes simplex*.
• Clears toxins and allays inflammation; good for arthritis and gout.
Skin • Clears boils, acne and ulcers. • Keratinocyte antipoliferant for psoriasis[77]. • Increases synthesis of collagen and fibronectin; speeds wound healing[78].
Externally • Juice from fresh leaves mixed with Turmeric is applied to wounds to speed healing. • Prepared in coconut oil, it is applied to the head to calm the mind, promote sleep, relieve headaches and prevent hair loss; applied to the skin for eczema and herpes.

Drug interactions Can potentiate the action of anxiolytics.

Chamomilla recutita (also known as Chamomilla matricaria) and *Anthemis nobilis* (also known as *Chamaemelum nobile*)
German and Roman chamomile

German chamomile is native to Europe and northern Asia, while Roman chamomile is native to Europe. Both are renowned for their sedative effects.

FAMILY Asteraceae
PARTS USED Flowers
CONSTITUENTS Volatile oil (including chamazulene and bisabolol), flavonoids, coumarins, fatty acids, cyanogenic glycosides, choline, tannins.
ACTIONS Anti-inflammatory, antispasmodic, nervine, sedative, antiulcer, antihistamine, digestive, antimicrobial, diaphoretic, anodyne, diuretic, emmenagogue.

Digestion • Soothes stress-related digestive upsets; relieves spasm, colic (particularly in babies), wind, indigestion, heartburn and acidity. • Bisabolol speeds the healing of ulcers. • Antimicrobial; resolves infections such as gastroenteritis.
Mental and emotional • Calms anxiety and tension. Excellent relaxant for babies and children[79]. • Promotes sleep and relieves pain in headaches, migraine, neuralgia, flu, arthritis and gout.
Respiratory system • In warm tea it is used for fevers and infections such as sore throats, tonsillitis, colds and flu. • Reduces broncho-constriction in asthma.
Immune system • Enhances immunity • Active against bacteria including *Staphylococcus aureus* and fungal infections including candida[80]. • Antihistamine for allergies. • Reduces inflammation.
Urinary system • Antiseptic diuretic; soothes inflamed/irritable bladder and cystitis.
Reproductive system • Reduces period pain, PMS and premenstrual headaches. • Used for amenorrhea due to psychological problems. • For nausea and sickness in pregnancy. • Eases contractions and pain during childbirth. • Relieves mastitis. • Reduces menopausal symptoms.
Externally • Stimulates tissue repair, speeds healing of ulcers, sores, burns, varicose ulcers and skin disorders.
• Antiseptic wash for conjunctivitis; sitz bath for cystitis; and douche for vaginal infections.

CAUTION May cause contact dermatitis.

Cimicifuga racemosa (also known as *Actaea racemosa*)
Black cohosh

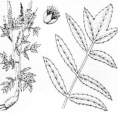

This attractive white-flowered perennial is native to North America and was renowned among Native Americans for easing mentrual problems and aiding childbirth.

FAMILY Ranunculaceae
PARTS USED Dried root, rhizome
CONSTITUENTS Triterpene glycosides (actein, 27-deoxyactein and cimicifugoside), flavonoids, isoferulic acid, tannin, volatile oil, resin, salicylates, ranunculin (which yields anemonin).
ACTIONS Antispasmodic, anti-inflammatory, anodyne, hypoglycaemic, hypotensive, sedative, uterine tonic, partus praeparator, diaphoretic, hormone balancing.

Circulation • Normalizes heart function. • Relaxes and dilates blood vessels; lowers blood pressure.
Mental and emotional • Anemonin depresses the central nervous system; excellent for nerve and muscle pain, rheumatoid and osteoarthritis and headaches.
• Eases cramps and muscle tension, ovarian and uterine pain, contractions during childbirth and breast pain.
• Sedative for insomnia. • Remedy for tinnitus and vertigo.
Respiratory system • Antispasmodic; useful in asthma, whooping cough, paroxysmal coughing and bronchitis.
Musculoskeletal system • Salicylates are anti-inflammatory, helpful in arthritis.
Reproductive system • Regulates the menstrual cycle. Relieves PMS, breast pain and swelling, menstrual cramps and painful contractions in childbirth. • Taken several weeks before childbirth for safe and easy delivery. It has amphoteric action, relaxing uterine muscles when tense and toning them when weak. • Reduces heavy bleeding; strengthens uterine muscles. • Hugely popular for easing menopausal symptoms including anxiety, depression, hot flushes, night sweats, headaches, palpitations, dizziness, vaginal atrophy and low libido.
• May normalize levels of luteinizing hormone and act on opiate receptors that affect mood, body temperature regulation and sex hormone levels.

CAUTION Avoid in pregnancy until last few weeks. It is an endangered species so only obtain from sustainable sources.
Drug interactions May interfere with oral contraceptives. Avoid with anticoagulant drugs.

Cinnamomum zeylanicum (also known as *C. cassia*)
Cinnamon

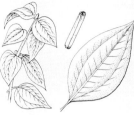

C. cassia is native to southern China; while *C. zeylanicum* grows in Sri Lanka. This sweet and aromatic spice, popular in cooking, is a warming remedy for warding off winter infections and improving digestion.

FAMILY Lauraceae
PARTS USED Inner bark
CONSTITUENTS Volatile oils (including eugenol), tannins, mucilage, gums, resin, coumarins.
ACTIONS Antibacterial, antiviral, antifungal, antioxidant, tonic, immunostimulant, nervine, adaptogen, circulatory stimulant, antispasmodic, astringent, digestive, anaesthetic, probiotic.

Digestion • Enhances digestion and absorption; used for indigestion, anorexia, colic, nausea and wind. • Protects gut lining against irritation and infection, prevents inflammation and ulcers. Good for gastroenteritis and dysentery. • Combats candida and other gut pathogens.
• Enhances effectiveness of insulin; helps prevent glucose intolerance that can predispose to diabetes.
Circulation • Lowers harmful cholesterol.
Mental and emotional • Improves resistance to stress.
• Lifts fatigue and low spirits, SAD and winter lethargy; used for chronic fatigue and ME. • Improves mental energy, concentration and motivation.
Respiratory system • Has a drying effect on mucosa.
• Expectorant for coughs and chest infections.
• Decongestant inhalations used for colds and catarrh.
Musculoskeletal system • Rich source of magnesium, essential for maintaining bone density. • Relieves arthritic pain, headaches and muscle stiffness.
Urinary system • Antiseptic for bladder problems.
Reproductive system • Rich in magnesium; helps maintain hormone balance. Good for PMS. • Uterine astringent, curbs heavy bleeding. • Aphrodisiac, used for low libido and impotence. • Used for painful periods.
Immune system • Antiviral and antibacterial, helps throw off fevers. • Essential oil powerfully antibacterial, antiviral and antifungal. Inhibits growth of *E. coli* and *Typhoid bacilli*. • Combats thrush and systemic candidiasis.
Externally • In massage oil relaxes aching muscles.

CAUTION Avoid large doses in pregnancy.

Codonopsis pilosula
Codonopsis

This perennial climbing herb
native to Asia has intricate
bell-like flowers. It is famous
as a tonic in Traditional
Chinese Medicine, with
properties similar to Ginseng.

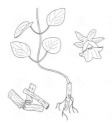

FAMILY Campanulaceae
PARTS USED Root
CONSTITUENTS Sterols, triterpenes, essential oil,
alkaloids, polysaccharides (inulin), phenylpropanoid
glycosides (tangshenosides), calcium, iron, zinc, proteins.
ACTIONS Blood tonic, adaptogen, aphrodisiac,
cardiotonic, demulcent, depurative, digestive,
emmenagogue, expectorant, styptic, immune tonic,
galactogogue, hypotensive, kidney tonic, stimulant.

Digestion • Improves digestion and assimilation.
Promotes appetite, improves metabolism and aids weight
loss. Used for anorexia, weak digestion and diarrhoea.
• Calms hyperacidity and dyspepsia[81]. Protects against
gastritis and ulcers. • May increase gastric motility.
• Reduces flatulence and nausea. • Protects the liver[82].
• Useful in diabetes.
Circulation • Dilates peripheral blood vessels, inhibits
adrenal cortex activity, calms palpitations and lowers
blood pressure[83]. • Reduces blood-clotting processes
and decreases risk of heart attacks and strokes. Useful
in angina. • Increases red blood cell and haemoglobin
count[84]; benefits anaemia. • Invigorates the spleen,
promotes the production of body fluid, improves the
condition of the blood and curbs excessive sweating.
Mental and emotional • Increases energy and enhances
resilience to stress; used for debility and chronic fatigue.
• Improves mental energy, memory and concentration.
Respiratory system • Used for asthma, chronic coughs,
shortness of breath, fevers and catarrh.
Musculoskeletal system • Relieves rheumatic and joint
pain[85]. • Used to treat 'tired limbs'[86], chronic fatigue
syndrome and fibromyalgia[87].
Immune system • Enhances the function of white blood
cells[88] and aids recovery from trauma, childbirth, surgery
and illness. • Used for chronic immune deficiency, HIV
and immune-suppressing effects of chemotherapy and
radiotherapy.
Reproductive system • Astringent properties reduce
excessive uterine bleeding[89]. • Strengthening to uterine
muscles; prevents prolapse.

Coleus forskohlii (also known as *Plectranthus barbatus*)
Forskohlii

This small perennial native
to India, Sri Lanka and Nepal
is used in Ayurveda as a
heart tonic and remedy for
the respiratory system and
eyes. Its active ingredient,
forskohlin, benefits the
heart, immune system and
fat metabolism.

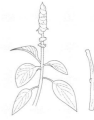

FAMILY Lamiaceae
PARTS USED Leaf, root
CONSTITUENTS Labdane diterpenes (including
forskolin), essential oil.
ACTIONS Hypotensive, antiplatelet, bronchodilator,
spasmolytic, cardiotonic, digestive stimulant, aromatic
digestive, antiobesity[90].

Digestion • Used for colic from muscular spasm.
• Enhances secretion of digestive enzymes.
Circulation • Inhibits platelet activity, decreasing risk of
blood clotting. • Increases force in heart muscle, improving
heart function. Useful in angina and congestive heart
failure. • Lowers blood pressure by dilating blood vessels[91].
Musculoskeletal system • Antispasmodic for muscle
tension and cramp, convulsions and bladder pain[92].
Immune system • Immunomodulatory effect, activating
macrophages and lymphocytes. • Useful in cancer
management by inhibiting tumour metastases[93].
• Reduces allergies and psoriasis associated with low
cyclic adenosine monophosphate and high platelet
activating factor (PAF) levels. Reduces histamine release
and inhibits inflammatory response. • Antihistamine and
bronchodilator and so excellent for asthma.
Endocrine system • Stimulates the release of thyroid
hormone, relieving hypothyroid symptoms such as
depression, fatigue, weight gain and dry skin[94].
• Increases fat metabolism and insulin production and
improves energy. Popular for the management of obesity
associated with low cyclic adenosine monophosphate.
Eyes • Applied topically for glaucoma. Decreases
intraocular pressure[95].

CAUTION Use with caution in hypotension and peptic
ulcers.
Drug interactions Possible interaction with hypotensive and
antiplatelet drugs.

Commiphora molmol (also known as *C. myrrha*)
Myrrh

This tree, native to North Africa, is famed as one of the gifts of the Magi. When the bark is scored it releases a yellow oil that hardens into a resin, which is used medicinally.

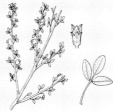

FAMILY Burseraceae
PARTS USED Oleogum resin[96], that is, air-hardened gum resin[97]
CONSTITUENTS Volatile oil: sesquiterpenes, heerabolene, dipentene, cinnamic aldehyde; resin: triterpenes, commiphoric acid, commiphorinic acid, commiferin; gum: arabinose, galactose.
ACTIONS Astringent, antibacterial, anti-inflammatory, vulnerary, anthelmintic, lymphatic, antioxidant.

Digestion • Protects the stomach lining from damage by drugs and alcohol[98]. Heals peptic ulcers. • Combats worms and parasites[99].
Circulation • Oleo-resins 'scrape' cholesterol out of the body. Used for congestive heart disorders, hypercholesterol and atherosclerosis[100]. • Stimulates lymphatic circulation; reduces lymphatic congestion, inflammation, lymphoedema and lymphatic swellings[101].
Respiratory system • Clears congestion[102]. Used for fevers, chronic bronchitis, colds and catarrh.
Musculoskeletal system • Anti-inflammatory for rheumatism and degenerative arthritis.
Immune system • Increases white blood cells and antimicrobial against *E. coli*, *Candida albicans* and *Staphylococcus aureus*[103]. • Sesquiterpenes are potent inhibitors of certain solid-tumour cancers[104].
Endocrine system • Antioxidant, thyroid-stimulating and prostaglandin-inducing properties[105].
Reproductive system • Stimulates circulation and moves stagnant blood; useful in amenorrhoea, endometriosis, fibroids, painful periods with clots, inflammation and congestion in the lower abdomen[106].
Externally • Astringent and antibacterial mouthwash and gargle used for gingivitis, sore throats, aphthous ulcers, pharyngitis, tonsillitis and halitosis. • Speeds repair in cuts, wounds and slow-healing skin sores[107], bruises and broken bones[108].

CAUTION Avoid in pregnancy, excessive uterine bleeding and kidney problems.

Commiphora mukul
Guggulu

This small tree is native to Asia and Africa. Its yellow resin is an honoured Ayurvedic remedy for 'scraping' toxins out of the body and lowering harmful cholesterol levels.

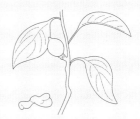

FAMILY Burseraceae
PARTS USED Gum resin
CONSTITUENTS Lignans, diterpenoids, sterols (guggulsterone, guggulsterol and beta-sitosterol), terpenes, essential oil, gum, calcium, iron, magnesium.
ACTIONS Anti-inflammatory, antiplatelet, hypocholesterolaemic, alterative, analgesic, antioxidant, antispasmodic, carminative, diaphoretic, expectorant, nervine, astringent, antiseptic, immunostimulant, rejuvenative, thyroid stimulant, emmenagogue.

Circulation • Increases breakdown of LDL cholesterol and reduces triglycerides. Increases HDL cholesterol. • Inhibits platelet aggregation, prevents formation of clots and reduces atherosclerosis[109]. Benefits ischaemic heart disease, angina and congestive heart failure. Reduces the risk of stroke and pulmonary embolism[110].
Respiratory system • Antimicrobial and antispasmodic for bronchitis and whooping cough.
Musculoskeletal system • Anti-inflammatory and detoxifying for gout and arthritis[111]. • Used for lumbago, rheumatism and sciatica. • Used for healing fractures.
Immune system • Increases white blood cell count, clears infections and promotes immunity[112]. • Used for growths and cancers[113].
Endocrine system • Specific for weight and obesity and hyperlipidemia[114], enhances thyroid function by improving iodine assimilation[115] and regulates fat metabolism[116]. • Can reduce blood sugar in diabetes.
Reproductive system • Reduces accumulations in the lower abdomen[117]. • Regulates the menstrual cycle. • Used for endometriosis and polycystic ovarian syndrome.
Skin • Reduces inflammation in chronic skin diease[118]. • Helps regenerate tissue granulation and enhances healing. • Clears tumours and reduces lipomas[119].

CAUTION Avoid in acute kidney infections, excessive uterine bleeding, thyroxicosis, pregnancy and breast-feeding.
Drug interactions Can reduce the effect of antihypertensives; care needed with hypoglycaemic medication.

Coriandrum sativum
Coriander

This highly aromatic
annual herb native to the
Mediterranean and Asia
is valued in Ayurvedic
medicine as a digestive and
for cooling heat in the body.

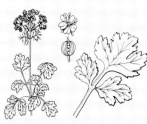

FAMILY Apiaceae
PARTS USED Seed, leaf
CONSTITUENTS Volatile oil (comprising coriandrol,
geraniol, borneol, camphor, carvone and anethole), resin,
malic acid, tannins, alkaloids, flavonoids.
ACTIONS Alterative, stimulant, carminative, diuretic,
antibacterial, antioxidant, nervine, decongestant,
antispasmodic, rejuvenative, aphrodisiac, digestive,
refrigerant, analgesic, diaphoretic.

Digestion • Enhances appetite, improves digestion and
absorption. Useful in anorexia nervosa. • Relaxant and
anti-inflammatory; relieves spasm, griping, wind,
bloating, nausea, gastritis, heartburn, indigestion,
nervous dyspepsia, halitosis, diarrhoea and dysentery.
• Seeds combined with laxatives used to prevent griping.
Circulation • Reduces harmful cholesterol.
Mental and emotional • Invigorating and
strengthening. • Clears the mind, improves memory,
reduces anxiety and tension and promotes sleep.
• Relieves headaches, migraine and other stress-related
problems, muscle pain, rheumatism and neuralgia.
Respiratory system • Seeds taken in hot teas for
colds, flu, fevers, coughs and to ward off infection.
• Decongestant for colds and catarrh, asthma and
bronchial congestion.
Immune system • Volatile oils in seeds are antibacterial
and antifungal. • Fresh leaves are rich in vitamins and
minerals used to chelate toxic metals from the body.
• Brings out rash in eruptive infections such as
chickenpox and measles[120].
Urinary system • Diuretic; cools hot burning symptoms
such as cystitis and urethritis. Reduces fluid retention.
Reproductive system • Antispasmodic for period pain
and uterine contractions during childbirth. • Aphrodisiac
and energizing for low libido. • Helpful for amenorrhoea,
PMS and hot flushes.
Externally • Leaf juice/tea used internally and externally
to soothe hot, itchy skin rashes such as eczema and
urticaria. • Seed decoction used as a gargle for sore
throats and oral thrush; eye lotion for conjuctivitis.

Crataegus monogyna
Hawthorn

This deciduous tree, bearing
clusters of white or pink
flowers in late spring, is native
to temperate climates. It
provides excellent medicines
for the heart and circulation.

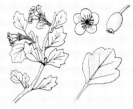

FAMILY Rosaceae
PARTS USED Flower, leaf, berry
CONSTITUENTS Saponins, glycosides, flavonoids
(rutin, vitexin and quercitrin), procyanidins, glycosides,
triterpenoids, tannins, pectin, vitamin C, B1 and B2,
choline, acetylcholine, calcium.
ACTIONS Antioxidant, hypotensive, vasodilator,
circulatory stimulant, cardiotonic, nutritive, rejuvenative,
adaptogen, nervine, sedative, antibacterial,
antispasmodic, astringent, digestive, antilithic.

Digestion • Used for diarrhoea, dysentery and
dyspepsia. • Regulates metabolism.
Circulation • Best remedy for heart and circulation,
regulating blood pressure and preventing the build-up of
atherosclerosis. Lowers harmful cholesterol. Strengthens
heart muscle and regulates heart rhythm. • Prescribed in
coronary insufficiency, palpitations, arrhythmias, angina
and degenerative heart disease. • Protects heart muscle,
reduces inflammation in blood vessels and helps prevent
clots and heart attacks. • Peripheral vasodilator for poor
circulation, Raynaud's disease and Buerger's disease,
intermittent claudication and varicose veins. • Used for
anaemia and altitude sickness.
Mental and emotional • Relieves anxiety and stress;
promotes sleep. • Recommended in ADD and ADHD.
• Used for emotional heartache.
Musculoskeletal system • Benefits joint linings,
synovial fluid, collagen, ligaments and vertebral discs.
• Antioxidant for inflammatory connective tissue
disorders[121]. Useful in arthritis, gout and tendonitis[122].
Urinary system • Diuretic; helps reduce fluid retention.
• Dissolves stones and gravel.
Reproductive system • Regulates blood flow; used
for amenorrhoea. • Promotes libido and fertility.
• Recommended in threatened miscarriage. • Used
for menopausal night sweats and hot flushes.
Eyes • Used for macular degeneration.

CAUTION Drug interactions May potentiate effects of
heart drugs such as digoxin amd beta-blockers.

Curcuma longa
Turmeric

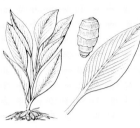

This perennial native to South Asia has a long orange root that produces a yellow spice popular in Indian cooking. Turmeric is a great aid to digestion and an effective anti-inflammatory remedy.

FAMILY Zingiberaceae
PARTS USED Rhizome
CONSTITUENTS Curcumin, tumerone, zingiberone, carotene equivalent to 50 IU of vitamin A per 100 g[123].
ACTIONS Antioxidant, antibiotic, anti-inflammatory, digestive, analgesic, antiobesity, anticarcinogenic.

Digestion • Aids digestion, absorption and metabolism. Aids weight loss. • Stimulates bile flow from liver, aids detoxification and protects the liver against damage. • Regulates intestinal flora; good after antibiotics. • Used for worms, heartburn, wind, bloating, colic and diarrhoea. • Soothes gut mucosa; boosts stomach defences against the effects of stress, excess acid, drugs and other irritants, reducing the risk of gastritis and ulcers. • Lowers blood sugar in diabetics.
Circulation • Lowers harmful cholesterol and inhibits blood clotting by blocking prostaglandin production[124]. • Helps prevent and remedy atherosclerosis.
Respiratory system • Immune enhancing and antimicrobial; wards off colds, sore throats and fevers.
Immune system • Enhances immunity. • Powerful antioxidant; protects against damage by free radicals. • Protects against cancer, especially of colon and breast. Enhances production of important cancer-fighting[125] cells. In China it is used to treat the early stages of cervical cancer[126]. • Curcumin is a powerful anti-inflammatory, excellent for arthritis, liver and gall bladder problems.
Reproductive system • Relieves pain and minor breast problems.
Externally • Antibiotic and anti-inflammatory. Mixed with Aloe vera gel for inflamed and infected skin problems such as eczema, acne, psoriasis, scabies, fungal infestations and skin cancer.

CAUTION Avoid large doses in pregnancy and with peptic ulcers, obstruction of the biliary tract and gallstones.
Drug interactions Avoid large doses with anticoagulant and non-steroidal anti-inflammatory drugs.

Cynara scolymus
Globe artichoke

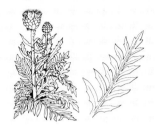

The hardy perennial, indigenous to the Mediterranean region, is one of the oldest cultivated vegetables, valued by the ancient Greeks and Romans. It was used as a medicine by medieval Arab physicians mainly to treat the liver and sluggish digestion.

FAMILY Asteraceae
PARTS USED Leaf
CONSTITUENTS Sesquiterpene lactones (including cynaropicrin, dehydrocynaropicrin, cynaratriol and grossheimin), caffeic acid derivatives (including cynarin), flavonoids, alpha-selinene, caryophyllene, eugenol.
ACTIONS Cholagogue, diuretic, antispasmodic, antioxidant, hepatoprotective, antioxidant, hypocholesterolaemic, astringent, cardiotonic, detoxifier, digestive stimulant, diuretic, hypotensive.

Digestion • Enhances digestion and absorption; stimulates metabolism. • Protective liver tonic, acts as an antioxidant, promotes regeneration of damaged liver cells and protects liver from damage from drugs, alcohol or chemicals. Often combined with Milk thistle, Turmeric or Schisandra for this and for hepatitis B and C[127]. • Increases bile secretion and lowers harmful cholesterol. Indicated in liver and gall bladder disorders. • Anti-inflammatory and digestive action in the gut is useful in the treatment of Crohn's disease, IBS, dyspepisa, poor appetite, inability to digest fats, constipation and flatulence.
Circulation • Protects the heart and arteries by lowering harmful cholesterol and lipid levels. Inhibits cholesterol synthesis.
Immune system • Antioxidant; protects against free radical damage in cardiovascular system, immune system and liver. • 3,5 dicaffeoylquinic acid and 4,5 dicaffeoylquinic acid have demonstrated anti-inflammatory activity[128].
Urinary system • Diuretic; relieves fluid retention. Aids elimination of toxins via the kidneys.

CAUTION Avoid in cases of obstruction in the biliary tract and gallstones[129].

Daucus carota
Wild carrot

This attractive biennial, also
known as Queen Anne's
Lace, is the ancestor of the
domestic carrot. Native to
Europe and parts of Asia, it
is found in hedgerows and
stony or sandy ground near
the sea.

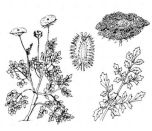

FAMILY Apiaceae
PARTS USED Aerial parts, seed, root
CONSTITUENTS Seed: volatile oil (including asarone,
carotol, pinene and limonene), alkaloids; root: vitamins C,
B and B2, flavonoids, carotene, asparagine, sugars,
pectin, minerals; leaf: porphyrins.
ACTIONS All parts: anthelmintic, astringent,
carminative, antilithic, galactogogue, diuretic, ophthalmic;
seed: emmenagogue, abortifaecient, contraceptive,
antitumour, spasmolytic, hepatoprotective, antifertility;
root: antibacterial, liver tonic, urinary antiseptic.

Digestion All parts: improve appetite, digestion and
absorption and expel worms from the intestines. • They
relax the gut and relieve wind, bloating, colic and
indigestion. • Stimulate the bile flow from the liver. Used
for gallstones, sluggish liver and hangovers and to clear
toxins. • May prevent damage to the liver from toxins,
drugs and alcohol.
Immune system • Cultivated carrots are rich in
betacarotene, boosting immunity, helping to prevent
degenerative disease and reducing the risk of cancer and
heart disease.
Urinary system • Seeds are particularly diuretic and
dissolve stones and gravel. Used for fluid retention,
cystitis, urethritis, prostatitis and bladder problems.
• They aid elimination of toxins via the kidneys; helpful in
gout and arthritis. • Root is more antiseptic for urinary
tract infections.
Reproductive system • Seeds traditionally used as a
contraceptive. Research shows that they interfere with
the implantation of fertilized eggs in the lining of the
uterus and oil from the seeds may block synthesis of
progesterone[130]. • Root contains porphyrins, which
stimulate pituitary gland and increase the secretion of
female sex hormones[131].
Eyes • Betacarotene enhances eyesight and night vision.

CAUTION Avoid seeds during pregnancy.

Dioscorea villosa
Wild yam

Wild yam is a creeping plant
native to North and Central
America. Until 1970 it was the sole
source of the hormone material
diosgenin, used in the
contraceptive pill and other
steroid hormones.

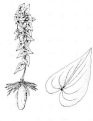

FAMILY Dioscoreaceae
PARTS USED Root, rhizome
CONSTITUENTS Steroidal saponins (yielding
diosgenin), tannins, starch, alkaloids (dioscorin).
ACTIONS Antispasmodic, anti-inflammatory, nutritive,
rejuvenative, reproductive tonic, analgesic,
antirheumatic, aphrodisiac, oestrogen-modulating,
diuretic, cholagogue, relaxant, peripheral vasodilator.

Digestion • Antispasmodic throughout the gut; relieves
colic, spasms, IBS, biliary colic, painful wind and
bloating. • Indicated in inflammatory conditions of the
bowel such as colitis and diverticulitis.
Mental and emotional • Calms anxiety, lifts depression
and relaxes muscle tension.• Combats tiredness.
• Relieves mood swings in PMS and menopause.
Musculoskeletal system • Relieves muscular spasm
and pain, muscle twitches, restless legs and leg cramps.
• Reduces inflammation; useful in arthritis and gout.
Immune system • Anti-inflammatory, can be helpful in
autoimmune disease such as rheumatoid arthritis and
lupus.• Enhances immunity; may stimulate interferon
production.
Reproductive system • Regulates levels of oestrogen
and progesterone; steroidal saponins are converted to
diosgenin in the body, a precursor of progesterone.
• Relieves tension and cramps in the uterus and ovaries;
used for spasmodic dysmenorrhoea with nausea[132] and
ovarian pain. • Recommended to balance hormones and
as a nourishing tonic in low libido, infertility, erectile
dysfunction, low sperm count and PMS. • Used for
nausea and cramping in pregnancy, especially when
related to stress and tension, and for threatened
miscarriage. • Can be helpful for menopausal symptoms
such as hot flushes, insomnia and night sweats.
Externally • Used in creams to balance hormones and
reduce menopausal symptoms.

CAUTION An excess may cause nausea, vomiting,
diarrhoea and headache[133].

Echinacea angustifolia, E. purpurea and E. pallida
Echinacea

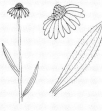

This beautiful plant has deep pink flowers and is native to North America. It was traditionally valued as a blood cleanser for wounds, burns, insect bites and joint pains. Research has demonstrated its efficacy in combating infections.

FAMILY Asteraceae
PARTS USED Whole herb, root
CONSTITUENTS Echinacosides, chlorogenic acid, alkylamides, echinacein, isobutylamides, polyacetylenes, D-acidic arabinogalactan polysaccharide.
ACTIONS Alterative, antibiotic, diaphoretic, antioxidant, anti-inflammatory, immunostimulant, antimicrobial, decongestant, antitumour, diaphoretic, vulnerary.

Respiratory system • Wards off infections especially when taken at the onset of sore throats, colds, chest infections, tonsillitis and glandular fever. • Relieves chronic respiratory tract infections and whooping cough. • Traditionally used for TB.
Immune system • Immune-stimulating; increases the activity of white blood cells[134]. • Antibiotic, antifungal, antiviral[135] and antiallergenic action. • Recommended for candida and post-viral fatigue syndrome. • Particularly useful for lowered immunity that causes repeated infections and antibiotic resistance. • Helps support immunity in cancer and after chemotherapy and radiotherapy. • The anti-inflammatory effect[136] of Echinacea helps relieve arthritis and gout, skin conditions and pelvic inflammatory disease. • Taken in hot infusion it stimulates circulation and sweating, reducing fevers. • Traditionally used for malaria and typhus.
Reproductive system • Indicated for gynaecological infections, pelvic inflammatory disease, urinary infections and post-partum infection.
Skin • Blood cleanser for septic conditions; clears skin of infections, boils and abscesses. • Relieves allergies such as urticaria and eczema.
Externally • Anti-inflammatory and antiseptic for skin problems. • Gargle and mouthwash used for sore throats and infected gums; douche for vaginal infections.

CAUTION Occasional sensitivity may cause anaphylaxis, asthma or urticaria[137].

Eclipta alba
Bhringaraj

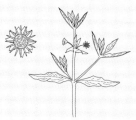

This herb has a white daisy-like flower and is native to India where it is traditionally used to enhance memory and as an anti-ageing remedy. Its bitter taste indicates its cooling, anti-inflammatory effect.

FAMILY Asteraceae
PARTS USED Aerial parts, root, seed
CONSTITUENTS Saponins, alkaloids (ecliptine), wedelic acid, luteolin, triterpene glycosides, flavonoids, isoflavonoids.
ACTIONS Antioxidant, liver deobstruent and tonic, alterative, purgative, antiseptic, antimicrobial, antiviral, rejuvenative, febrifuge, anti-inflammatory, haemostatic, anthelmintic.

Digestion • Improves appetite, stimulates digestion and absorption. • Aids elimination of toxins by stimulating the bowels; indicated in constipation. • Excellent for liver problems including cirrhosis and infective hepatitis[138]. • Protects liver against damage from drugs, chemicals and alcohol. • Acts as a deobstruent to promote bile flow. • Protects parenchymal liver tissue in viral hepatitis and other conditions involving liver enlargement.
Circulation • Reduces blood pressure and nervous palpitations. • Used for anaemia.
Mental and emotional • Valued in Ayurveda as a rejuvenative. Antioxidant properties reduce oxidative and ischaemic damage to the brain and improve brain function, memory and concentration. Prevents onset of age-related mental decline and Alzheimer' disease. • Calms nervous tension and anxiety; helpful in insomnia, mental agitation and anger. • Traditionally used for vertigo, dizziness, declining eyesight and hearing problems.
Respiratory system • Combats upper respiratory infections and clears catarrhal congestion.
Skin • Aids liver in its cleansing work. It is beneficial for skin problems including urticaria, eczema, psoriasis and vitiligo. • Reduces itching and inflammation; traditionally reputed to promote a lustrous complexion.
Externally • Combined with coconut oil, it is a popular remedy for balding and premature hair greying by nourishing the roots.

Elettaria cardamomum
Cardamom

Native to India, aromatic and spicy Cardamom has long been esteemed for its ability to lift the spirits and induce a calm, meditative state of mind. It can neutralize the overstimulating effects of caffeine and reduce the mucous-forming properties of milk by aiding its digestion.

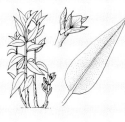

FAMILY Zingiberaceae

PARTS USED Seed

CONSTITUENTS Essential oils (including limonene), cineol, terpineol, terpinene, capricylic acid, potassium mucilage resin.

ACTIONS Carminative, antispasmodic, decongestant, expectorant, diaphoretic, digestive, circulatory stimulant, nervine, antibacterial, aphrodisiac.

Digestion • Warming and invigorating, cardamom improves appetite, digestion and absorption and sweetens breath. • Seeds chewed or in teas are used for relaxing stress-related problems, indigestion, colic, wind, nausea, vomiting (including that related to chemotherapy) and travel sickness. Often combined with Fennel.
• Counteracts excess acidity in the stomach • Prevents post-prandial drowsiness and hangovers from alcohol.
• It has a mild laxative effect.

Circulation • Enhances circulation and increases energy; good when run-down and tired in the winter.

Mental and emotional • For tension and anxiety, lethargy and nervous exhaustion. • Lifts the spirits, calms the mind. • Improves memory and concentration.

Respiratory system • Seeds chewed soothe sore throats and dry coughs. • Stimulating expectorant action clears phlegm from the nose, sinuses and chest in colds, coughs, asthma and chest infections.

Musculoskeletal system • Essential oil is anti-inflammatory and analgesic for joint pain.
• Antispasmodic for muscle pain and spasm.

Urinary system • Strengthening for a weak bladder, involuntary urination and bed-wetting in children.
• Antibacterial for urinary tract infections[139].

Reproductive system • Traditionally used as an aphrodisiac and added to love potions.

CAUTION Avoid large amounts in cases of gastro-oesophageal reflux and gallstones.

Eleutherococcus senticosus
Siberian ginseng

A famed tonic that grows in Siberia, China, Korea and Japan and long used for increasing vitality, improving mental and physical performance and protecting against stress. Used in China for more than 2,000 years, it was extensive Russian research in the 1960s that put it in the spotlight.

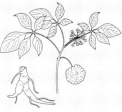

FAMILY Araliaceae

PARTS USED Root

CONSTITUENTS Triterpenoid saponins: eleutherosides A to G, polysaccharides, glycans.

ACTIONS Adaptogen, antioxidant, immunostimulant, hypocholesterolaemic, anti-inflammatory, rejuvenative.

Digestion • Improves digestion and absorption of nutrients, increasing strength and relieving lethargy, diarrhoea and bloating from weak digestion. • Protects the liver; enhances its ability to break down toxins.
• Regulates blood sugar levels.

Circulation • Reduces harmful cholesterol and triglycerides. • Relieves angina. • Relaxes arteries; reduces stress-related blood pressure. • Normalizes body temperature; helpful in hypothermia.

Mental and emotional • Increases blood flow through the arteries to the brain; improves memory and concentration and increases mental stamina. Used for ADHD and failing memory in the elderly. • Supports optimum adrenal function; useful for adrenal fatigue.

Musculoskeletal system • Excellent for athletes. Powerful anti-fatigue effect; increases endurance and ability of the mitochondria in the cells to produce energy.
• Increases cells' ability to dispose of lactic acid causing sore muscles after a workout.

Immune system • Wide research in Russia on athletes and workers demonstrated its ability to help cope with and recover from adverse conditions and physical performance. • Enhances immunity against infections including coughs and colds, protects against carcinogens including environmental pollutants and radiation and inhibits tumour formation. • Speeds recovery after physical exertion; prevents immuno-depletion from excessive work[140].

CAUTION **Drug interactions** Avoid with digoxin.

Emblica officinalis (also known as *Phyllanthus emblica*)
Amalaki/Indian gooseberry

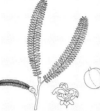

Native to India, this fruit is one of the richest natural sources of vitamin C, containing approximately 20 times the vitamin C content of an orange. It is one of the most valued rejuvenative tonics in Ayurvedic medicine.

FAMILY Euphorbiaceae
PARTS USED Mainly fruit, to a lesser extent seed, leaf, root, bark, flower
CONSTITUENTS Ascorbic acid, fatty acids, bioflavonoids, polyphenols, cytokinins, B vitamins, calcium, potassium, iron, tannins, pectin.
ACTIONS Rejuvenative, antioxidant, hepatoprotective, hypocholesterolaemic, anti-inflammatory, laxative, hypoglycaemic, stomachic, tonic, diuretic, antifungal.

Digestion • Enhances appetite, digestion and absorption. • Antibacterial and anti-inflammatory properties helpful for peptic ulcers, acidity, nausea, vomiting, gastritis, hepatitis, colitis and haemorrhoids. • An ingredient of the cleansing formula Triphala. A bowel tonic for IBS and chronic constipation. • Antioxidant properties protect the liver.
Circulation • Decreases LDH cholesterol levels; reduces atherosclerosis. • Reduces the risk of blood clots.
Mental and emotional • Famous rejuvenative for debility following illness, stress or in old age. Main ingredient of tonic Chayawanprash to improve mental and physical wellbeing. • Improves memory and concentration and resilience to stress. Calms anger and irritability.
Respiratory system • Antibiotic activity against a wide range of bacteria; used for coughs, colds, flu, chest infections and asthma.
Immune system • Shown to slow the growth of cancer cells, probably through its ability to enhance natural cell mediated cytotoxicity. • Antifungal; useful for candida. • Antiviral for colds and flu. • Active against a range of organisms including *Staphylococcus aureus*, *E. coli*, *L. albicans*, *Mycobacterium tuberculosis* and *Staphylococcus typhos*. • Antioxidant and immunomodulating.
Urinary system • Antiseptic diuretic; resolves cystitis.
Externally • Ingredient of hair oils to prevent hair loss. Lotion used for inflammatory eye problems.

CAUTION Avoid in diarrhoea and dysentery.

Equisetum arvense
Horsetail

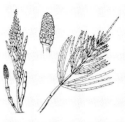

Horsetail is a prehistoric-looking perennial and is one of the oldest plants on the planet. Native to Europe, Asia, Africa and North America, it is found growing wild in damp ground. It is highly valued as a rich source of minerals and trace elements.

FAMILY Equisetaceae
PARTS USED Aerial parts
CONSTITUENTS Saponins, silica, manganese, potassium, sulphur, magnesium, tannins, alkaloids (including nicotine, palustrine and palustrinine), flavonoids (including apigenin, kaempferol, luteolin and quercetin), glycosides, sterols (including cholesterol).
ACTIONS Diuretic, styptic, antihaemorrhagic, alterative, anodyne, antibacterial, antifungal, anti-inflammatory, antiseptic, astringent, diaphoretic, kidney tonic, lithotriptic, nutritive, rejuvenative, tonic, vulnerary.

Digestion • Astringent and toning useful for treating diarrhoea, rectal prolapse and haemorrhoids[141].
Circulation • Stops bleeding of wounds, nosebleeds and in the respiratory and urinary tract. • Good tonic in anaemia. • Protects arteries from atherosclerosis.
Musculoskeletal system • Rich in soluble silica, which is readily absorbed. Supports regeneration of bones, cartilage and other connective tissue; increases strength and elasticity[142]. • Ability to increase bone density in post-menopausal women with osteoporosis. • Strengthening for teeth and brittle nails. • Used for rheumatic and arthritic problems.
Urinary system • Used for cystitis, urethritis and urinary stones. • Beneficial in prostate problems, acute and chronic prostatitis and benign prostatic hyperplasia. • Astringent tannins stem bleeding and are toning for prolapse, urinary incontinence and bed-wetting in children.
Other • For signs of nutritional deficiency such as white spots on nails, dull hair, hair loss and brittle nails. Silica encourages absorption and uptake of calcium.
Externally • Stops bleeding and speeds healing of cuts and wounds. • Antiseptic and anti-inflammatory for skin problems.

CAUTION Horsetail breaks down vitamin B1. Take alongside B complex supplementation. Avoid in oedema[143].

Eschscholzia californica
California poppy

This vibrant yellow-orange flower is the state flower of California and native to western North America. It was first introduced to Europe as an ornamental and medicinal plant, but now has a reputation as a non-addictive alternative 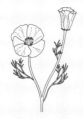 to the opium poppy for aiding sleep and reducing pain. It was used for colicky pains and toothache by the Native American tribes and settlers in America.

FAMILY Papaveraceae
PARTS USED Whole fresh plant including root and seed pod.
CONSTITUENTS Morphine alkaloids (including protopine, sanguinarine and chelerythrine), eschscholtzione, glycosides.
ACTIONS Sedative, hypnotic, antispasmodic, anodyne, nervine, febrifuge.

Digestion • Antispasmodic, relaxes the muscles in the gut; relieves colic in the stomach and gall bladder.
Circulation • By calming the nervous system it influences the heart and circulation; slows rapid heart, relieves palpitations and reduces blood pressure.
Mental and emotional • Cousin to the opium poppy, but far less powerful. It is a safe sedative to calm excitability, restlessness, anxiety, tension and relieve insomnia; suitable for calming children. • Painkilling and relaxing for migraine, headaches, neuralgia, back and muscle pain, arthritis, sciatica and shingles. • Balances emotions and reduces stress. • Helpful in withdrawal from addiction to alcohol, drugs or tobacco. Helps to maintain mental stability. • Used for stress-related bed-wetting in children. • Beneficial for treating behavioural problems in children such as ADD and ADHD, improves memory and concentration.
Externally • Applied to areas of pain such as toothache and headaches.

CAUTION Avoid in pregnancy and breastfeeding.

Eupatorium perfoliatum
Boneset

Boneset is native to eastern North America, found in meadows and marshland. It was renowned among the Native American tribes, who used it for flu and fevers. In fact, the plant was so named because it can relieve the 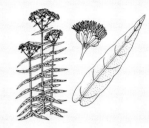 aching that accompanies flu, which feels as though it is penetrating to the bones.

FAMILY Asteraceae
PARTS USED Aerial parts
CONSTITUENTS Sesquiterpene lactones (eupaflin and euperfolitin), polysaccharides, flavonoids (kaempferol, quercitin, hyperoside and rutin), glucoside (eupatorin), diterpenes, gallic acid, sterols, essential oil[144].
ACTIONS Aperient, antispasmodic, astringent, bitter, carminative, diaphoretic, emetic, expectorant, febrifuge, immunostimulant, laxative, stimulant, tonic, antibacterial analgesic and nervine.

Digestion • Clears toxins by its action on the liver and laxative effects. Useful in arthritis, skin conditions and worms[145]. • Used for indigestion and traditionally for weak digestion in the elderly.
Respiratory system • In hot infusion it clears congestion in allergic rhinitis, bronchitis, catarrh, colds and coughs[146].
Immune system • Famous as a flu remedy; promotes sweating, reduces fevers, and clears heat and toxins.
• Polysaccharides and sesquiterpene lactones increase white blood cell production and phagocytosis, boosting immunity to bacterial and viral infections, including herpes simplex type 1 and 11[147]. • It has been shown to have anti-inflammatory and antitumour actions[148]. Sesquiterpene lactones and eupatorin have cytotoxic action[149].
Externally • Tea made from Boneset can be used as a wash to reduce fevers[150].

CAUTION Large doses can cause vomiting and diarrhoea[151].

Eupatorium purpureum
Gravel root/Joe Pye weed

This handsome perennial with
a mass of pink-purple flowers
is native to Europe and North
America and is found in moist
woodland and by streams. Its
common name is after Joe Pye,
a New England medicine man
who cured fevers and typhus
with this plant.

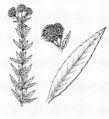

FAMILY Asteraceae
PARTS USED Rhizome, root
CONSTITUENTS Protein, carbohydrates
(polysaccharides), flavonoids (quercitin and euparin),
oleoresin (eupatorin), sesquiterpene lactones, essential
oil, resin, tannins.
ACTIONS Antirheumatic, astringent, carminative,
diaphoretic, diuretic, emmenagogue, immunostimulant,
nervine, tonic, alterative, antilithic.

Immune system • Used by Native American tribes as
a diaphoretic to induce perspiration and reduce fevers.
Urinary system • Diuretic, stimulant and astringent
tonic to the urinary tract. • Reduces fluid retention. • Tea
made from the roots and leaves drunk lukewarm to cool
is used to prevent and treat kidney and bladder stones.
• Reduces inflammation and soothes dysuria in cystitis,
urethritis and prostatitis. • Helpful in treating arthritis
and gout by increasing the elimination of uric acid and
toxins via the kidneys. • Astringent action is helpful in
treatment of urinary incontinence, bed-wetting in
children and haematuria[152].
Reproductive system • Tones and strengthens
uterine muscles; stimulates contractions in childbirth.
Recommended for threatened miscarriage and
uterine prolapse[153]. • Relieves menstrual pain. • Anti-
inflammatory and astringent for pelvic inflammatory
disease. • Indicated in benign prostatic hypertrophy
and erectile dysfunction.

CAUTION Large doses may cause vomiting. Avoid during
pregnancy. Contains pyrrolizidine alkaloids; do not take for
more than 6 weeks[154].

Euphrasia officinalis
Eyebright

This delicate flowering
annual is partially parasitic,
taking nourishment from
nearby grass roots. It is a
member of the foxglove
family, originally from
Europe and Asia, but grows
happily throughout the USA.

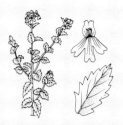

FAMILY Scrophulariaceae
PARTS USED Aerial parts
CONSTITUENTS Iridoid glycosides (including aucubin),
saponins, tannins, resin, flavonoids (including quercitrin),
volatile oil.
ACTIONS Astringent, digestive, liver tonic, alterative,
demulcent, anti-inflammatory, expectorant, antibacterial,
antiviral, antifungal, decongestant.

Digestion • Bitters improve digestion and absorption
and enhance bile flow, aiding the liver's detoxifying work
and benefiting the eyes.
Mental and emotional • Traditionally used to lift the
spirits, for 'troubles of the mind' and to improve memory
and concentration. • Regarded as a 'visionary herb',
enhancing insight.
Respiratory system • Astringent action relieves
irritation and catarrh in nose, throat, sinuses, ears and
chest. Used for sore throats, post-nasal drip, otitis media,
sinusitis, sinus headaches and coughs. • Helps relieve
allergic rhinitis/hay fever.
Eyes • Used for centuries to improve and preserve
eyesight. • Antimicrobial astringent for inflammatory eye
infections such as conjunctivitis, styes, blepharitis and
watery eye conditions. • Clears mucous, keeps eye
mucosa clear and healthy. • Particularly used for red,
itchy eyes with discharge, as in hay fever or measles. For
oversensitive eyes that run in cold and wind and irritation
from smoky/stuffy atmospheres. • Reduces inflammation
in tired, strained eyes and puffiness. • Enhances
circulation to the eyes; improves eyesight in the elderly.
Externally • Gargles used for sore and catarrhal throats;
mouthwashes for mouth ulcers. • To treat eye conditions
it is best taken internally and used topically in sterile
saline solutions as drops or compresses. • A few drops of
dilute tincture or infusion in the nostrils used for clearing
catarrhal congestion.

Filipendula ulmaria
Meadowsweet

These elegant flowers grow in damp meadows and by rivers and streams. When crushed they give off the characteristic smell of salicylicates, which offer similar benefits to aspirin.

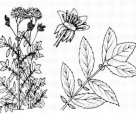

FAMILY Rosaceae
PARTS USED Aerial parts
CONSTITUENTS Essential oils (salicyladehyde and methylsalicylate), salicylic acid, spireine, gaultherine, flavonoids, (quercetin, rutin and spiraeoside), vanillin, coumarin, glycoside, mucilage, tannins.
ACTIONS Analgesic, anodyne, antacid, antibacterial, antiemetic, anti-inflammatory, antispasmodic, astringent, cholagogue, diaphoretic, diuretic, relaxant, stomachic, urinary antiseptic.

Digestion • Excellent antacid and anti-inflammatory for acid indigestion, heartburn, gastritis, peptic ulcers, gastro-oesophageal reflux[155] and other inflammatory conditions. • Astringent tannins protect and heal the gut lining. • Antiseptic and antispasmodic; useful for enteritis and diarrhoea, IBS, colic, flatulence and distension.
Mental and emotional • Analgesic for headaches and neuralgia. • Relaxant; eases spasm and induces sleep.
Musculoskeletal system • Rich in vitamin C, iron, calcium, magnesium and silica. Speeds the healing of connective tissue. • Anti-inflammatory and analgesic; relieves pain and swelling in arthritis and gout.
Immune system • Anti-inflammatory, analgesic and antipyretic activity[156]; useful in acute infections, fevers, colds and flu. • Brings out rashes in eruptive infections such as measles and chickenpox.
Urinary system • Mild antiseptic diuretic for cystitis and urethritis, fluid retention and kidney problems. • Helps eliminate toxins and uric acid, which contribute to arthritis, gout and skin problems.
Externally • Promotes tissue repair and staunches bleeding of cuts, wounds, ulcers and skin irritations.

CAUTION Salicylate sensitivity[157].
Drug interactions Possible interaction with anticoagulants[158]. Do not take simultaneously with mineral supplements, thiamine or alkaloids[159].

Foeniculum vulgare
Fennel

This feathery perennial has large umbels of flowers that bear aniseed-tasting seeds. The Greeks used Fennel to overcome obesity and for stimulating milk flow in nursing mothers.

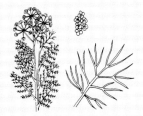

FAMILY Apiaceae
PARTS USED Seed, leaf, root
CONSTITUENTS Vitamins, minerals, essential oil, fixed oil, phenolic acids, flavonoids, coumarins, furanocoumarins.
ACTIONS Anaesthetic, antibacterial, antiemetic, antifungal, anti-inflammatory, antispasmodic, antitussive, aperient, carminative, digestive, diuretic, expectorant, galactogogue, mucolytic, hormone balancing, stimulant.

Digestion • Improves energy by enhancing appetite, digestion and absorption. Aids digestion of fatty foods. • Added to laxative blends to ease griping. • Stabilizes blood sugar levels and reduces sugar craving[160]. • May aid weight loss by increasing metabolism and elimination. • Settles the stomach; relieves hiccups, colic, bloating, wind, nausea, vomiting, halitosis, indigestion, heartburn, diarrhoea and IBS. • Decongests the liver; clears stagnation[161]. Volatile oil increases liver regeneration[162].
Respiratory system • Decongestant and expectorant in hot tea. • Relaxes the bronchi; useful in asthma and coughs.
Musculoskeletal system • Diuretic action aids the elimination of toxins. This supports its anti-inflammatory effects in arthritis and gout.
Urinary system • Aids elimination of toxins via the kidneys; used for cellulite, cystitis, fluid retention and urinary infections. • Helps dissolve stones[163].
Reproductive system • Antispasmodic; relieves period pains. • Slightly oestrogenic[164]. Regulates the menstrual cycle; used in amenorrhea, endometriosis, low libido and PMS. • Helpful during menopause. • Stimulates milk production in nursing mothers.
Externally • Decoction of seeds makes an anti-inflammatory eyewash for sore eyes and conjunctivitis, and a gargle for sore throats.

CAUTION Seeds are potentially toxic; do not exceed the recommended dose[165]. In excess they can overstimulate the nervous system. Avoid therapeutic doses during pregnancy[166].

Fucus vesiculosus
Bladderwrack

A seaweed growing in
offshore waters and temperate
coastal parts of Europe and
North America. Rich in iodine,
it stimulates the thyroid gland.

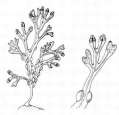

FAMILY Fucaceae
PARTS USED Whole plant
CONSTITUENTS Alginic acid, fucoidan, fucoxanthin,
carrageenan, minerals, mucopolysaccharides, mannitol,
zeaxanthin, protein, betacarotene, vitamins C, D and E.
ACTIONS Antiobesity, thyroid stimulant, alterative,
antimicrobial, anthelmintic, antioxidant, antitumour,
demulcent, diuretic, emollient, laxative, nutritive.

Digestion • Enhances energy as rich in nutrients.
• Enhances digestion, mild laxative. • Probiotic for
candida and intestinal worms[167]. • Binds radioactive
strontium, barium and cadmium in the gastrointestinal
tract. • Relieves heartburn, gastritis and peptic ulcers.
Circulation • Reduces harmful cholesterol levels
through inhibition of bile acid absorption. • Reduces risk
of heart disease, atherosclerosis, hypotension,
hypertension and anaemia[168].
Musculoskeletal system • Detoxifying, nourishing and
anti-inflammatory for arthritic conditions.
Immune system • Enhances immunity. • Contains the
highest antioxidant activity of edible seaweeds, possibly
due to fucoxanthin[169]; helps reduce cellular damage.
• Antibacterial and antifungal properties. Polyphenols
and polysaccharides have anti-viral and anti-
inflammatory action; useful in herpes simplex and HIV
activity[170]. • May inhibit cancer.
Urinary system • Diuretic; aids elimination of toxins.
• Soothes inflammation in cystitis and urethritis.
Reproductive system • Helps regulate the menstrual
cycle. • Used to prevent breast cancer in Japan and can
be helpful in fibrocystic breast disease.
Thyroid • Used for low thyroid function and goitre.
• Increases metabolism[171], demonstrating potential for
controlling weight and cellulite.
Skin • Clears toxins; useful in chronic skin complaints
including boils, eczema, psoriasis and herpes.

CAUTION Avoid in hyperthyroidism, pregnancy and
lactation[172].
Drug interactions Avoid with anticoagulants. Use with
caution with insulin and antidiabetic drugs[173].

Galega officinalis
Goat's rue

This bushy plant with lilac
blue flowers is an attractive
perennial member of the pea
family and is native to
Europe, Russia and Iran. It
was once important for
treating the plague, fevers
and infectious diseases and
for treating diabetes mellitus.

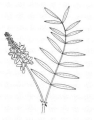

FAMILY Fabaceae
PARTS USED Aerial parts
CONSTITUENTS Alkaloid (galegine), flavonoids,
saponins, traces of chromium, glycosides, tannins.
ACTIONS Hypoglycaemic, antidiabetic, galactogogue,
diaphoretic, diuretic, digestive, antibacterial, febrifuge.

Digestion • Galegine lowers blood sugar levels[174] and
helps manage late-onset diabetes. It contains guanidine,
which reduces blood sugar by decreasing insulin
resistance, helping cells to use insulin to metabolize
glucose more efficiently. • Decreases absorption of
glucose from the gut and reduces glucose formation in
the liver; increases uptake and utilization of glucose in fat
and muscle cells (metformin is a chemical derived from
Goat's rue used to treat diabetes). • Helps non-insulin-
dependent diabetics to regulate blood sugar levels and
insulin-dependent diabetics to stabilize blood sugar levels
and decrease insulin dosage. • Reduces appetite and
increases weight loss; useful in metabolic syndrome X[175].
• Enhances digestion and pancreatic function. Used for
digestive problems caused by lack of digestive enzymes[176]
including constipation and indigestion.
Immune system • Exhibits significant antibacterial
activity against certain types of bacteria and inhibits
blood clotting[177]. • Diaphoretic; reduces fevers.
Urinary system • Diuretic; reduces fluid retention and
aids elimination of toxins via the kidneys.
Reproductive system • Stimulates milk production in
nursing mothers.
Externally • Ointments are used to hasten healing after
surgery[178].

Drug interactions Use with caution in patients on
antidiabetic drugs or insulin[179].

Galium aparine
Cleavers

This common hedgerow perennial native to Europe has long, sticky stems and seeds that cling to anything they touch. It is a member of the bedstraw family, so called because it was used as a strewing herb in less hygienic times, giving off a smell of newly mown hay.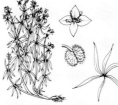

FAMILY Rubiaceae
PARTS USED Aerial parts
CONSTITUENTS Iridoids (including asperuloside), polyphenolic acids, alkanes, flavonoids, tannins, citric acid, saponins, coumarins, scopoletin.
ACTIONS Depurative, lymphatic, diuretic, aperient, tonic, astringent, anti-inflammatory, diaphoretic, vulnerary, cholagogue.

Digestion • Improves digestion. • Stimulates bile flow from the liver. • May be helpful in hepatitis.
Circulation • Lowers blood pressure, perhaps through its diuretic action. • Asperuloside may have hypotensive action.
Immune system • Lymphatic tonic enhancing lymphatic circulation, aiding the body in its cleansing and immune work and purifying the blood. Recommended for lymphatic congestion, swollen lymph glands, glandular fever, ME and tonsillitis. • May have antitumour activity. • Clears heat and resolves inflammation; helpful in arthritis and gout. • Promotes immune function and reduces fevers.
Urinary system • Diuretic; aids elimination of fluid toxins via the kidneys. Used for losing weight. • Traditionally used as tea or a vegetable as a cleansing 'spring tonic', cooling heat and clearing toxins. • Used for stones, urinary infections such as cystitis and irritable bladder.
Skin • Cleansing for chronic skin disorders such as eczema, acne, boils, psoriasis and rosacea. • Helps resolve eruptive infections such as measles and chickenpox.
Externally • Skin wash used for skin disorders, cuts and scrapes. • As a hair rinse for dandruff.

Ganoderma lucidum
Reishi

This mushroom grows on hardwoods in China, Japan, Russia and the USA. Known as the 'mushroom of immortality', Reishi was used for centuries as a longevity tonic. It supports homeostasis, regulating blood sugar and enhancing immunity.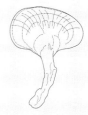

FAMILY Polyporaceae
PARTS USED Mushroom
CONSTITUENTS Polysaccharides, beta-glucans, adenosine, triterpenes, protein, phytosterols, lipids, ganesterone, vitamins C and B2.
ACTIONS Tonic, immunostimulant, hypoglycaemic, antitumour, anti-inflammatory, antioxidant, expectorant, adrenal stimulant, radiation protective, cardio tonic, hypocholesterolaemic, antihistamine.

Circulation • Enhances heart function and improves coronary artery circulation, protecting against heart attacks. • Relieves palpitations and arrhythmias, prevents clotting, normalizes blood pressure and prevents atherosclerosis[180]. • Lowers cholesterol levels[181]. • Increases oxygen level in the blood; used to combat altitude sickness[182].
Mental and emotional • Reduces stress and anxiety. • Improves adrenal function and sleep quality.
Respiratory system • Antihistamine action helps in allergic asthma and rhinitis. • Expectorant for chronic bronchitis[183], pneumonia and respiratory problems.
Immune system • Beta-glucans enhance immunity and T-cell activity and increase production of leucocytes and macrophage activity; they protect against cancer[184]. • Antibacterial to *Staphylococci* and *Streptococci* bacteria. • Antifungal; combats candida. • Used for HIV, herpes, hepatitis B and C, chronic fatigue syndrome, acute myeloid leukaemia and nasopharyngeal carcinomas[185]. • Protects against the harmful effects of chemotherapy or radiotherapy[186]. • Helpful in allergies; sulphur compounds inhibit histamine release from mast cells[187]. • Gandosterone is hepatoprotective; beneficial for cirrhosis and hepatitis. • Excellent rejuvenative for the elderly and during convalescence[188].

CAUTION Avoid with mushroom allergies. May cause diarrhoea in large doses[189].

Gentiana lutea
Gentian

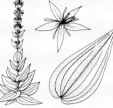

This beautiful perennial with
yellow star-shaped blooms is
found growing wild in lime-
rich soil in the high altitudes
of the European mountains.
It has long been valued as a
panacea for all ills and a vital
ingredient of elixirs of life. It
was used for stomach and bowel
disorders, liver and heart problems,
to neutralize poisons and to prolong life.

FAMILY Gentianaceae
PARTS USED Root, rhizome
CONSTITUENTS Bitter glycosides (amarogentin and
gentiopicrin), alkaloids, quinic acid, inulin, xanthones,
triterpenes, iron, volatile oils.
ACTIONS Digestive, bitter tonic, anthelmintic,
antiseptic, anti-inflammatory, antibiliary, emmenagogue,
febrifuge, sialogogue.

Digestion • The root contains the bitter glycoside
amarogentin. Bitters stimulate the flow of digestive
enzymes and stimulate appetite and digestion,
particularly of protein and fats. • Aids absorption of
essential minerals and vitamins and improves the
elimination of wastes. • Stimulates bile flow from the
liver. • Promotes peristalsis and movement of food and
wastes through the gut. • Helpful in poor appetite,
nausea, indigestion and wind. • Anti-inflammatory and
cooling in gastritis and colitis. • Anthelmintic and
antiseptic for clearing worms and infections.
Immune system • Strengthening tonic due to its
beneficial effect on digestion and absorption, which
increases energy and immunity. • Traditionally used as
a 'spring bitter' to purify the blood. • Anti-inflammatory,
nourishing and cleansing. Relieves rheumatism, arthritis
and gout. • Reduces fevers. • Gentiopicrin is highly
poisonous to *Plasmodium*, accounting for its traditional
use in treating malaria.
Reproductive system • Emmenagogue; brings on
periods and regulates menstruation. • Nerve tonic for
PMS and menopausal mood swings.

Ginkgo biloba
Ginkgo

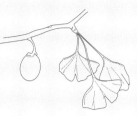

Native to China, this tree is
thought to be the oldest on
the planet, reputedly
growing 190 million years
ago. It is popular for slowing
the effects of ageing, such as
poor memory, hearing loss
and risk of stroke.

FAMILY Ginkgoaceae
PARTS USED Leaf
CONSTITUENTS Terpenesditerpene ginkgolides,
sesquiterpenes (bilobalides), proanthocyanidins, vitamin
C, flavonoids (quercetin, kaempferol and rutin), organic
acids, essential oils, tannins.
ACTIONS Antioxidant, circulatory stimulant,
neuroprotective, antibacterial, anticoagulant, antifungal,
anti-inflammatory, brain tonic, cardiotonic, decongestant,
kidney tonic, rejuvenative, vasodilator.

Circulation • Improves blood flow and specifically
cerebral circulation; protects against and treats altitude
sickness, Alzheimer's disease, senile dementia and age-
related poor memory, diminishing eyesight and hearing
loss. • Indicated in impaired peripheral circulation,
gangrene, Raynaud's syndrome and peripheral
neuropathies. • Improves coronary circulation and
relieves angina, arteriosclerosis and varicose veins.
• Decreases blood viscosity; prevents clots. • Improves
recovery in heart attacks, strokes and injury to the head.
Mental and emotional • Relieves anxiety and depression.
Respiratory system • Inhibits the activity of platelet-
activating factors and inflammatory compounds
associated with respiratory allergies such as asthma and
chronic obstructive airways disease[190]. • Enhances
immunity to infections; helps prevent colds and coughs
and chest infections.
Immune system • Reported to have antitumour
activity[191].
Eyes • Protects the eye from damage by reducing free-
radical damage to the retina[192]. • Used for macular
degeneration and impaired retinal blood flow[193].
• Slows or prevents glaucoma, cataracts and diabetic
retinopathy[194].

CAUTION Can cause headaches. Avoid a week before
surgery and in haemophilia.
Drug interactions Avoid with anticoagulant drugs.

Glechoma hederacea (also known as *Nepeta hederacea*)
Ground ivy

Ground ivy is a creeping perennial with purple-blue flowers growing in profusion on grassland and in hedgerows and woods. Popular as a medicine since at least 2nd-century CE Greece, it 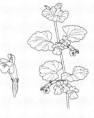 has been used for treating inflamed eyes, chronic bronchitis and nervous headaches. It is a gentle herb, perfect for children with catarrhal problems of the ear, nose and throat.

FAMILY Lamiaceae
PARTS USED Aerial parts
CONSTITUENTS Volatile oils, tannins, bitters, resin.
ACTIONS Anodyne, anti-inflammatory, appetizer, astringent, decongestant, digestive, diuretic, stimulant, tonic, expectorant, anthelmintic.

Digestion • A pleasant-tasting digestive, enhancing appetite, digestion and the absorption of nutrients. • Protects the gut lining from irritation and inflammation and can be used for indigestion, wind, bloating, nausea and diarrhoea. • Traditionally used for expelling worms.
Respiratory system • Astringent, antiseptic and decongestant; dries excess mucous in the nose, throat and chest. • Taken hot it makes a good decongestant for colds, catarrh, congestive headaches, coughs and bronchial phlegm, and helps to relieve fevers. • Safe and effective, it can be given to children to clear chronic catarrh and treat chronic conditions such as glue ear and sinusitis. • Traditional remedy for catarrhal deafness and tinnitus.
Urinary system • Antiseptic diuretic; helps reduce fluid retention and clear toxins from the system. • Used for cystitis, urinary frequency and urinary tract infections.
Externally • Used as a gargle for sore throats. • Makes a good lotion to bathe inflamed eyes and speed the healing of bruises, cuts and abrasions.

Glycyrrhiza glabra
Liquorice

This vetch-like perennial is native to Europe, Asia and North and South America. It has an affinity with the endocrine system. In Traditional Chinese Medicine it is said to harmonize the effects of other herbs.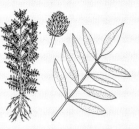

FAMILY Papilionaceae
PARTS USED Peeled root, runner
CONSTITUENTS Glycyrrhizin, triterpenoid saponins, polyphenols, flavonoids (isoflavones), bitter principle (glycymarin), phytoestrogens, asparagin, volatile oil, coumarins, tannins.
ACTIONS Demulcent, expectorant, tonic, laxative, anti-inflammatory, antipyretic, diuretic, adaptogen, antacid, antitussive, adrenal tonic, antiviral, antiallergenic, hypocholesterolaemic.

Digestion • Lowers stomach acid and relieves heartburn and indigestion. • Excellent for healing ulcers[195]. • Mild laxative. • Increases bile flow from the liver. Useful in chronic hepatitis and cirrhosis[196].
Circulation • Isoflavones reduce harmful cholesterol and atherosclerosis[197].
Mental and emotional • Adaptogenic strengthening tonic. Improves resistance to physical and mental stress, possibly by its action on the adrenal glands.
Respiratory system • Anti-inflammatory; soothes sore throats and dry coughs. • Expectorant for irritating coughs, asthma and chest infections. • Antiallergenic for hay fever, rhinitis, conjunctivitis and bronchial asthma.
Immune system • Glycyrrhizin resembles adrenal hormones with anti-inflammatory and antiallergic effects similar (but without the side effects) to cortisone. Useful when coming off steroid drugs. • Antiviral; used for cytomegalovirus[198] and herpes simplex[199]. • Anti-inflammatory for arthritis, skin problems such as eczema and psoriasis. • Classed as a desmutagen; binds to toxic chemicals and carcinogens.
Reproductive system • Mild oestrogenic properties; used for menstrual and menopausal problems.

CAUTION Avoid prolonged use and large doses. May increase blood pressure. Avoid during pregnancy.
Drug interactions May cause potassium loss if combined with diuretics/laxatives. May potentiate prednisolone.

Gymnema sylvestre
Gymnema

This climbing vine, native to India and Australia, has been used for thousands of years in Ayurvedic medicine for balancing blood sugar. Its Sanskrit name *gurmar* means 'sweet destroyer' because eating fresh leaves numbs bitter and sweet receptors on the tongue.

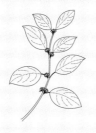

FAMILY Asclepiadaceae
PARTS USED Leaf
CONSTITUENTS Saponins (gymnemic acids and gymnemasaponins), gurmarin (polypeptide of 35 amino acids), tartaric acid, stigmasterol, betaine, choline.
ACTIONS Antidiabetic, astringent, diuretic, laxative, refrigerant, hypocholesterolaemic, hypolipidaemic, antiobesity.

Digestion • Reduces sweet cravings and excessive appetite. Gymnemic acid binds to sugar receptors on the tongue for 1–2 hours, blocking the taste of sugar and reducing the desire for sweet foods[200]. Helpful for weight loss. • Used in management of diabetes types 1 and 2, and blood sugar disorders[201]. Increases production of insulin by the pancreas, helps to regulate blood glucose levels, helps the regeneration of beta cells in the pancreas that release insulin and stops adrenaline from stimulating the liver to produce glucose.
Circulation • Saponins lower cholesterol[202] and triglycerides[203].

CAUTION Saponins may cause or aggravate gastro-oesophageal reflux[204]. Not to be used by patients with hypoglycaemia[205]. Use with caution in heart conditions, as it can stimulate the heart[206].
Drug interactions In patients taking hyperglycaemic drugs and insulin, monitor blood sugar levels carefully so that the dosage of drugs can be adjusted[207].

Hamamelis virginiana
Witch hazel

This deciduous shrub, native to North America, has distinctive yellow flowers that appear before the leaves in early spring. Native Americans used it as snuff for nosebleeds and mixed it with flax seed for painful swellings and tumours. It is a household remedy for scalds and burns, to stop bleeding and bruising.

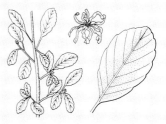

FAMILY Hamamelidaceae
PARTS USED Leaf, bark, twig
CONSTITUENTS Tannins, saponins, choline, resins, flavonoids.
ACTIONS Astringent, haemostatic, styptic, vulnerary, slightly sedative, anodyne, antibacterial, anti-inflammatory, antioxidant.

Digestion • Traditionally used for diarrhoea, dysentery, colitis and respiratory catarrh.
Reproductive system • Astringent for uterine prolapse and a debilitated state after miscarriage and childbirth, as it tones up the uterine muscles.
Externally • Tannins stop bleeding, speed healing, reduce pain, inflammation and swelling and provide a protective coating on cuts and wounds to inhibit the development of infection. It can be used in decoction, tincture or distilled form. As a douche for vaginal discharge and irritation; a gargle for sore throats, tonsillitis and laryngitis; and a mouthwash for mouth ulcers and bleeding gums. • Lotion can be applied to varicose veins, ulcers and phlebitis, insect bites and stings, aching muscles and broken capillaries. • Used as a poultice or compress for burns, inflammatory skin problems such as boils, swollen engorged breasts, bedsores, bruises, sprains and strains.• It makes a refreshing eyebath mixed with rosewater; relieves sore, tired or inflamed eyes such as conjunctivitis. • Potent antioxidant, used in antiageing skin preparations[208].

CAUTION Take internally only for short periods. Avoid in pregnancy and breast-feeding.
Drug interactions May impair the absorption of ephedrine, codeine, theophylline, atropine or pseudoephedrine taken internally.

Harpagophytum procumbens
Devil's claw

This shrubby evergreen vine is native to the desert sands of Africa. It has been used by African tribes for hundreds of years to ease the pain of inflamed joints and clear toxins from the body.

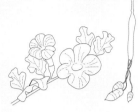

FAMILY Pedaliaceae
PARTS USED Root (secondary tuber)
CONSTITUENTS Essential oil (mainly ligustilide and n-butylidene phthalide), ferulic acid, coumarins, phytosterols.
ACTIONS Anti-inflammatory, antirheumatic, analgesic, alterative, antibacterial, febrifuge, hypotensive, laxative, antispasmodic, bitter tonic, digestive.

Digestion • Enhances appetite, improves digestion and absorption and eases stomach upsets[209]. Useful in anorexia[210]. • Bitter tonic for indigestion, flatulence, bloating and constipation.
Circulation • May help lower both blood pressure and heart rate[211].
Musculoskeletal system • Anti-inflammatory for arthritis[212], bursitis and tendonitis. • Used for degenerative disorders[213], osteoarthritis, rheumatoid arthritis, myalgia, lower back pain and gout[214]. • Anodyne properties aid pain relief.
Externally • Poultice can be applied to ulcers, boils and other skin lesions[215].

CAUTION Not advised in peptic ulcers, pregnancy and breast-feeding.
Drug interactions May interact with antiarrhythmic medications[216].

Humulus lupulus
Hops

A trailing plant that grows in Europe, Asia, North America and Australia. Hops used to be smoked for their narcotic effect, put in pillows for insomnia and used by monks to kerb sexual desire.

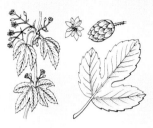

FAMILY Cannabaceae
PARTS USED Female flowers (strobiles)
CONSTITUENTS Bitter resin lupulin (including valerianic acid, humulone and lupulone), essential oil (including sesquiterpenes) humulene, tannins, flavonoids, asparagin, choline, oestrogenic chalcone.
ACTIONS Sedative, anaphrodisiac (male), bitter tonic, phytoestrogenic, antispasmodic, digestive, antiseptic, astringent, diuretic, anodyne, anti-inflammatory, antihistamine, expectorant, anthelmintic, febrifuge.

Digestion • Bitters enhance appetite and digestion. • Eases muscle tension, spasm and inflammation; used for colic, IBS, diverticulitis, indigestion and stress-related problems including peptic ulcers, Crohn's disease and ulcerative colitis. • Tannins aid healing of irritated and inflammatory conditions and stem diarrhoea. • Lupulon and humulon are antiseptic[217] and combat infections such as gastroenteritis.
Mental and emotional • Sedative and antispasmodic; relieves tension and anxiety as well as pain.
Respiratory system • Antispasmodic, antimicrobial and expectorant; relieves coughs, chest infections, bronchitis and asthma.
Musculoskeletal system • Anti-inflammatory and pain relieving for joint and muscle pain.
Urinary system • Asparagin is a soothing diuretic • Aids elimination of toxins and helps clear skin problems such as eczema and acne.
Reproductive system • Calms sexual desire in men and enhances it in women. • Reduces menstrual cramps. • Helps regulate periods and menopausal symptoms. • Enhances milk supply in nursing mothers.
Externally • Add to a night-time bath to ease aching muscles and use in pillows to promote sleep.

CAUTION Avoid in depression. May cause contact dermatitis and stimulate oestrogen-positive tumours[218].
Drug interactions Avoid with central nervous system depressant drugs.

Hydrastis canadensis
Golden seal

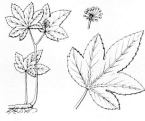

This perennial woodland plant is native to North America and was a favourite of Native American tribes, including the Cherokees, Comanches and Iroquois. A powerful antimicrobial and anti-inflammatory, it has been used for ulcers, wounds and acute infections, including cholera, *Giardia* and amoebic dysentery.

FAMILY Ranunculaceae
PARTS USED Rhizome, root
CONSTITUENTS Alkaloids (hydrastine and berberine).
ACTIONS Bitter tonic, anti-inflammatory, laxative, stomachic, anticancer, astringent, mucosal tonic, antimicrobial, antiseptic, antifungal, antispasmodic.

Digestion • Improves appetite, digestion and absorption. • Relieves stomach upsets and indigestion. • Antimicrobial for gastroenteritis, diarrhoea and dysentery. • Probiotic; helps re-establish gut flora and combats candida. • Stimulates bile flow from the liver and helps the liver in its detoxifying work.
Circulation • Enhances heart function and circulation; used in heart problems.
Immune system • Stimulates the production of white blood cells to ward off infection. • Berberine has been found to be active against a wide range of bacteria, including *Staphylococcus* spp., *Giardia* and tapeworms[219]. • Toxic to certain types of cancer cells[220]. • Reduces fevers. • Used for sore throats, coughs, colds, catarrh, flu, chest infections and whooping cough.
Externally • Drops used for inflamed eyes and earache. • Gargle used for sore throats; mouthwash for ulcers and inflamed gums.

CAUTION Avoid in pregnancy and with high blood pressure. This is an endgangered species, so only obtain it from sustainable sources.

Hypericum perforatum
St John's wort

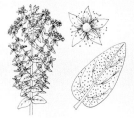

This perennial blooms at midsummer. Its yellow flowers contain a red pigment believed to indicate its power to heal wounds and staunch bleeding.

FAMILY Clusiaceae
PARTS USED Flowering top
CONSTITUENTS Glycosides (including red pigment hypericin), hyperforin, flavonoids, tannins, resin, volatile oil.
ACTIONS Antidepressant, anxiolytic, antimicrobial, antiviral, vulnerary, antineoplastic, antioxidant, anti-inflammatory, sedative, astringent, expectorant, diuretic.

Digestion • Astringent and antimicrobial for gastroenteritis, diarrhoea and dysentery. • Heals peptic ulcers and gastritis. • Protects liver against toxins.
Circulation • Reduces blood pressure and capillary fragility.
Mental and emotional • Nervine for nervous exhaustion, tension, anxiety and depression. • Increases sensitivity to sunlight; reduces SAD during winter and jet lag. • Improves sleep and concentration. • Mood-elevating properties can take 2–3 months to produce a lasting effect. • Reduces nerve pain and neuralgia such as trigeminal neuralgia, sciatica, back pain, headaches, shingles and rheumatic pain. • Useful after surgery and laceration of nerve tissue.
Respiratory system • Expectorant action clears phlegm from chest; relieves coughs and chest infections.
Immune system • Anti-inflammatory for gout and arthritis. • Hypericin has shown antitumour activity[221]. • Antiviral; active against TB and influenza A, herpes, HIV and hepatitis B and C[222].
Urinary system • Diuretic and astringent. • Used for bed-wetting in children and incontinence.
Reproductive system • For painful, heavy and irregular periods, PMS and menopausal emotional problems.
Externally • Oil eases pain and speeds healing in nerve pain such as sciatica and shingles, burns, cuts, varicose veins, ulcers, sunburn and inflammatory conditions.

CAUTION Can cause photosensitivity. Avoid during pregnancy.
Drug interactions Avoid with theophylline beta-2 agonists, SSRIs, protease inhibitors and cyclosporin.

Hyssopus officinalis
Hyssop

This attractive evergreen member of the mint family is native to Europe and Asia. It was valued by the Romans as an effective antimicrobial remedy to protect against sickness, including the plague, and was used in the Middle Ages to clean churches and the houses of the sick.

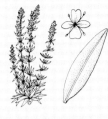

FAMILY Lamiaceae
PARTS USED Flower, leaf
CONSTITUENTS Volatile oils, resin, gums, silica, bitters, tannins, flavonoid glycosides, sulphur.
ACTIONS Expectorant, diaphoretic, diuretic, digestive, anthelmintic, antiviral, astringent, cholagogue, circulatory stimulant, decongestant, vasodilator, nervine, antiseptic, carminative, emmenagogue.

Digestion • Increases appetite and digestion. • Relieves indigestion, constipation and flatulence. • Antispasmodic; reduces spasm, colic and IBS.
Circulation • Pungent and warming; stimulates circulation, causes sweating, reduces fevers and increases the elimination of toxins via the skin.
Mental and emotional • Traditionally used in epilepsy and as a cordial for the heart and to lift the spirits.
• Nerve tonic to relieve anxiety, tension, exhaustion and depression, and give support during times of stress.
Respiratory system • Stimulating decongestant and expectorant for colds, flu, catarrh, sinus problems, hay fever, coughs, asthma and pleurisy. • Volatile oils are antiseptic and expectorant; used for bronchitis, TB and viruses such as colds, flu and herpes simplex.
Immune system • Excellent for warding off infection and enhancing immunity.
Externally • Used as oils and liniments for bruises, sprains, cuts and wounds, aching joints and muscles, to relieve swelling and speed healing. • Oil in a vaporizer is used to purify the atmosphere, dispel infection, enhance clarity and concentration and steady the nerves when studying for exams. • Gargle used for tonsillitis and sore throats; inhalation for catarrh and hay fever.

CAUTION To be avoided by epileptics.

Inula helenium
Elecampane

This perennial with yellow daisy-like flowers is native to Europe and northern Asia. The bitter, aromatic root was traditionally used for children's coughs and catarrh.

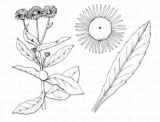

FAMILY Asteraceae
PARTS USED Root, rhizome (flower in Traditional Chinese Medicine)
CONSTITUENTS Volatile oils (including alantolactone, azulene and helenin), polysaccharide inulin, sterols, resin, pectin, mucilage, calcium, magnesium.
ACTIONS Antimicrobial, expectorant, anti-inflammatory, analgesic, bitter, aromatic digestive, antispasmodic, bronchodilator, carminative, decongestant, anthelmintic, antibacterial, antifungal, emmenagogue, rejuvenative, vulnerary, diuretic.

Digestion • Enhances appetite, digestion and absorption. • Relaxes tension and spasm and combats infection. • Calms nausea, indigestion, flatulence, colic, IBS, diarrhoea and gastroenteritis. • Stimulates bile flow from the liver. • Helps maintain healthy gut flora.
• Alantolactone is active against roundworm, threadworm and hookworm infection[223].
Respiratory system • A warming decongestant and expectorant, excellent for catarrh, colds, hay fever and bronchitis. Inulin is an expectorant. • Antispasmodic and antibacterial; used for sore throats, tonsilitis, laryngitis, whooping cough, asthma, emphysema, chest infections, pneumonia and pleurisy. Alantolactone has been found to be active against TB[224].
Immune system • Enhances immunity and reduces inflammation; helpful in arthritis and autoimmune disease. • Antibacterial and antifungal; combats candida and dysbiosis. • Taken hot it helps to reduce fevers and increases circulation.
Urinary system • Antiseptic diuretic; relieves fluid retention and urinary tract infections. • Antispasmodic for irritable bladder.
Externally • Good antiseptic wash for cuts, wounds and skin infections such as scabies and herpes. • Traditionally used for facial neuralgia and sciatica[225].

CAUTION Avoid during pregnancy. Large doses may cause diarrhoea, vomiting and allergic hypersensitivity[226].

Iris versicolor
Blue flag

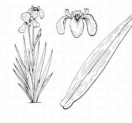

This beautiful perennial bog plant with purple-blue flowers is found growing wild in wet, peaty areas in North America and is the provincial flower of Quebec, Canada. It was popular among Native Americans as a remedy for skin diseases such as boils, abscesses and acne.

FAMILY Iridiaceae
PARTS USED Dried rhizome
CONSTITUENTS Acrid resin (irisin), volatile oil, starch, salicylates, alkaloid, tannin.
ACTIONS Alterative, digestive, bitter tonic, diuretic, anti-inflammatory, cholagogue, diaphoretic, sialogogue, laxative.

Digestion • Laxative, improves digestion and absorption, relieving flatulence, constipation, heartburn, indigestion and nausea. • Relieves headaches, skin problems and lethargy associated with poor digestion. • Improves liver and gall bladder function, aids the digestion of fats and enhances the detoxifying work of the liver.
Respiratory system • Clears congestion in the chest, throat and nose. • Relieves swollen glands and sore throats. • Traditionally used in thyroid and pancreatic disorders.
Immune system • Enhances lymphatic circulation and immunity. Used for swollen glands, chronic tonsillitis and lowered immunity. • Traditionally used to clear heat and toxins, as a cleansing and anti-inflammatory remedy for skin disease such as boils, abscesses, psoriasis, herpes and acne.
Urinary system • Diuretic; aids the elimination of toxins and excess fluid via the urine.
Externally • Root was used in poultices by Native Americans to relieve pain and swelling of sores, wounds, bruises and arthritic joints.

CAUTION The fresh root is poisonous. Only use the dried root in small amounts. Avoid during pregnancy and lactation. Emetic in large doses.

Juglans regia
Walnut

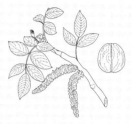

This handsome tree, a native of Iran, grows happily throughout Asia and Europe. Walnut trees live a long time, some as much as 1,000 years. Many of the large trees seen in Europe and Britain were planted by monastic orders and in the grounds of convents for their nutritious nuts and the medicinal values of their leaves and green outer shell of the nuts.

FAMILY Juglandaceae
PARTS USED Leaf, nut, bark, husks
CONSTITUENTS Napthaquinones (juglone), tannins, flavonoids, ellagic acid, gallic acid, volatile oils.
ACTIONS Alterative, astringent, anthelmintic, laxative, tonic, restorative, disinfectant.

Digestion • Astringent action combats irritation and inflammation of the gut lining. Relieves indigestion, gastroenteritis, nausea and diarrhoea. • Traditionally used for worms and lowering blood sugar.
Respiratory system • Clears catarrh and catarrhal coughs.
Immune system • Walnuts are a good source of omega-3 essential fatty acids and linolenic acid, which benefits immunity and protects heart and circulation from degenerative disease. • Reduces harmful cholesterol.
• Bark is detoxifying and enhances the function of the lymphatic system. Clears skin problems such as acne, lymphatic congestion and swollen glands.
Urinary system • Diuretic and depurative action; aids elimination of toxins via the urine.
Externally • Infusion/decoction of the leaves is used as a lotion for cold sores, shingles, chilblains, excessive perspiration of the hands and feet, piles, varicose veins and ulcers, inflammatory eye problems such as styes and sore throats. • Used as a douche for vaginal discharges. • Husks boiled in water are used as a hair dye (to cover up grey hair) and to thicken the hair. • The vinegar from pickled young walnuts can be used as a gargle for sore throats.

Lactuca virosa
Wild lettuce

This is the more bitter wild ancestor of the cultivated lettuce, native to North America, Europe and Asia. Its Latin name derives from *lac*, meaning 'milk', because of the white latex that exudes from the fresh stem, which has narcotic and euphoric properties. Dried leaves were traditionally smoked for relaxation and to relieve pain.

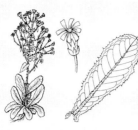

FAMILY Asteraceae
PARTS USED Leaf, latex
CONSTITUENTS Sesquiterpene alkaloids (lactucine, lactucopicrin and lactucic acid), mannitol, flavonoids (quercitrin), coumarins, phenylamine[227].
ACTIONS Sedative, antispasmodic, anodyne, narcotic, antitussive, diuretic, febrifuge, galactogogue, anaphrodisiac, bitter, digestive, cholagogue, hypoglycaemic.

Digestion • Bitters stimulate bile flow from the liver; aid the elimination of toxins and the digestion of fats. • Used for nausea, indigestion, colic, pain and stress-related digestive problems.
Mental and emotional • Alkaloids have a narcotic and euphoric effect similar to opium in large amounts, but not addictive. Calming for anxiety, panic attacks, hyperactivity, restlessness and agitation. Great sedative for inducing sleep. • Antispasmodic and analgesic; relieves pain and tension in tight muscles.
Respiratory system • Antispasmodic and sedative to the cough reflex; calms dry, irritating coughs, particularly those that disturb sleep. • Used for bronchitis and whooping cough.
Externally • Cooling wash used for inflammatory skin problems such as acne, spots and rash from poison ivy[228]. • Latex is used to treat warts, applied daily.

CAUTION Can cause drowsiness if used during the day or in large doses. Latex from the fresh plant can cause eye irritation and rashes[229].

Lavandula spp.
Lavender

This perennial shrub with its spikes of scented mauve flowers is native to the Mediterranean. It was popular during the Middle Ages as a strewing herb to perfume and sanitize houses and churches, and to ward off the plague.

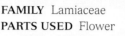

FAMILY Lamiaceae
PARTS USED Flower
CONSTITUENTS Volatile oils (including linalool, geraniol, cineole and linionene), tannins, coumarins, flavonoids, antioxidant (rosmarinic acid), triterpenoids.
ACTIONS Carminative, diuretic, antispasmodic, nerve tonic, analgesic, stimulant, digestive, sedative, antimicrobial, antiseptic, diaphoretic, expectorant, antidepressant, antioxidant.

Digestion • Releases spasm and colic and combats wind and bowel problems related to tension and anxiety. • Volatile oils active against bacteria and fungi[230]. Used for infections causing vomiting and diarrhoea.
Mental and emotional • Excellent for anxiety and stress-related symptoms such as headaches, migraines, neuralgia, palpitations, insomnia. • Helpful in agitated behaviour in dementia[231]. • Lifts the spirits. • Restores energy in tiredness and nervous exhaustion.
Respiratory system • Antimicrobial; increases resistance to colds, coughs, chest infections, flu, tonsillitis and laryngitis. • Decongesting and expectorant; clears phlegm and relieves asthma. • Antispasmodic for asthma and croup.
Immune system • Volatile oils are antibacterial, antifungal and antiseptic[232]. • Rosmarinic acid has antioxidant and anti-inflammatory action. • Taken as hot tea it reduces fevers and increases the elimination of toxins via the skin and urine.
Reproductive system • Analgesic and antiseptic; used in baths to speed healing and reduce pain after childbirth[233].
Externally • Antiseptic for inflammatory and infective skin problems such as eczema, acne, varicose ulcers and nappy rash. • Stimulates tissue repair; minimizes scar formation when oil is applied neat to burns, cuts and wounds, sores and ulcers. • Oil repels insects and relieves bites and stings, soothes pain of bruises, sprains, gout, arthritis and muscle tension.

Lentinula edodes
Shiitake mushroom

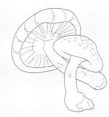

This delicious edible mushroom is native to China. Known as the 'mushroom of immortality', it has been used to prevent premature ageing for thousands of years[234].

FAMILY Polyporaceae
PARTS USED Mushroom
CONSTITUENTS Amino acids (lysine and arginine), polysaccharide (lentinan), eritadenin, vitamin C, D, B2 and B12, calcium, potassium, purines[235].
ACTIONS Immunostimulant, rejuvenative, antitumour, antioxidant, antiviral, aphrodisiac, hepatoprotective, hypocholesterolaemic, hypotensive.

Digestion • Protects the liver against damage from toxins, chemicals, alcohol, drugs and infection[236]. Can reduce elevated liver enzymes[237]. • Regulates blood sugar.
Circulation • Reduces cholesterol, blood pressure and atherosclerosis. Prevents clots. • Antioxidant action helps prevent cardiovascular disease, strokes and heart attacks. • Strengthening tonic for anaemia.
Respiratory system • Boosts interferon production, which fights flu viruses[238]. Enhances immunity; prevents frequent colds and coughs and bronchitis. • Antiallergenic for hay fever and asthma.
Immune system • Powerful natural immunostimulant and restorative. Strengthens immunity of patients with cancer, HIV and TB[239], autoimmune disease, chronic fatigue syndrome and fibromyalgia[240]. • Used for allergies, arthritis, environmental illness, fatigue and hepatitis[241]. • Compound in cooked Shiitake (thiazolidine-4-carboxylic acid) can inhibit the formation of potentially carcinogenic nitrites in the stomach[242]. • Lentinan can improve survival times of cancer patients when used concurrently with chemotherapy[243]. • Stimulates stem cells in bone marrow to produce B and T cells; inhibits blood platelet aggregation[244] and boosts production of interferon and natural killer cells, which help suppress tumours[245]. • Antiviral action used for herpes simplex 1 and 11.

CAUTION Avoid in extreme weakness or with diarrhoea[246]. Rarely causes mild gastric upset and rashes[247].
Drug interactions Thyroxin and hydrocortisone inhibit the antitumour activity of lentinan[248]. Water-soluble extracts may reduce platelet coagulation; use cautiously with blood thinners[249].

Leonurus cardiaca
Motherwort

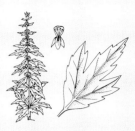

This perennial is found growing in hedgerows in many parts of Europe. It has been praised since the days of the ancient Greeks as a relaxing remedy for expectant mothers, hence its name.

FAMILY Lamiaceae
PARTS USED Aerial parts
CONSTITUENTS Triterpenes (including ursolic acid), iridoid glycosides (leonuride), alkaloids, leonurine, tannins, resins, vitamin A.
ACTIONS Antispasmodic, anxiolytic, cardiotonic, hypotensive, diaphoretic, astringent, bitter, partus praeparator, parturient, emmenagogue, nervine, thymoleptic, immunostimulant, antiviral, antibacterial.

Digestion • Bitter and cooling for acidity and heartburn. • Antispasmodic for stress-related digestive problems.
Circulation • Benefits the heart; reduces palpitations and blood pressure. • Reduces blood clotting, harmful cholesterol and atherosclerosis.
Mental and emotional • Calms anxiety and aids sleep. • May help heartbreak. • Reduces nervous palpitations and irregular heart rates, particularly useful during menopause. • Relieves headaches and muscular twitches and spasms.
Immune system • Active against viruses such as Epstein Barr[250], herpes and bacterial and fungal infection. • Ursolic acid has been found to inhibit cancers including leukaemia and lung, breast and colon cancer[251].
Reproductive system • Antispasmodic and tonic; for painful or delayed periods, cramps, back pain and vaginismus. • Enhances fertility, increases libido. • Helps prepare for childbirth, taken in the last few weeks; eases tension or anxiety about birth. • Eases childbirth. • Helps prevent post-partum infection. • Helps prevent post-natal depression. • Stimulates menstruation; may be helpful in amenorrhoea and scanty flow. • Soothes anxiety, anger and irritability; good for PMS and menopausal mood swings. • Helpful in menstrual headaches. • Cooling for hot flushes.
Other • May have hypothyroid activity.
Externally • Used as a douche/lotion for leucorrhoea and vaginal infection such as candida.

CAUTION May increase menstrual flow. Use only in the last few weeks of pregnancy.

Lonicera japonica
Honeysuckle

This woody, deciduous twining shrub is loved for its honey-sweet scent. So named because the sweet nectar can be sucked from the flowers. A syrup of the flowers is a traditional remedy for croup, cramps and asthma, and for speedy delivery in childbirth.

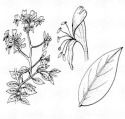

FAMILY Caprifoliaceae
PARTS USED Aerial parts
CONSTITUENTS Essential oils (including borneol), mucilage, glucoside, salicylic acid, invertin.
ACTIONS Antimicrobial, antiseptic, rejuvenative, alterative, laxative, expectorant, astringent, diaphoretic, diuretic, hypotensive, antispasmodic, anti-inflammatory, vulnerary, decongestant.

Digestion • Gentle laxative. • Anti-inflammatory and antiseptic; useful for diarrhoea, dysentery, food poisoning and Crohn's disease.
Respiratory system • Anti-inflammatory, expectorant, decongestant, antibiotic and antispasmodic properties; useful for spasm and phlegm in asthma, croup, whooping cough, bronchitis and chest infections. • Active against several bacteria including TB[252]. Used with *Forsythia suspensa* in Traditional Chinese Medicine for infections including tonsillitis, pneumonia, TB and middle ear infection. • The Japanese use flowers for sore throats, colds, flu, tonsillitis, bronchitis and pneumonia. • In hot infusion used for colds, catarrh, sinusitis and bronchial congestion.
Immune system • Traditionally used in China to clear damp heat and toxins. • Enhances immunity; promotes longevity. • Essential oils are antimicrobial; active against several bacteria and enhance the system's fight against infection. • Salicylic acid has an aspirin-like action, relieving aches and pains, headaches, flu, fevers, arthritis and rheumatism. • May protect against breast cancer[253].
Urinary system • Diuretic; soothing in cystitis and irritable bladder. • Aids elimination of toxins.
Skin • Detoxifying and anti-inflammatory; clears spots, boils, acne, psoriasis and eczema.
Externally • Lotion soothes rashes and sore eyes. • Gargle used for sore throats; mouthwash for mouth ulcers.

CAUTION The berries are poisonous.

Marrubium vulgare
White horehound

A perennial native to Europe, Asia and North Africa, with woolly, silvery-green leaves and a musky aroma loved by bees. Popular in brewing, White horehound used to be made into sweets for catarrh and coughs as well as medicines for snake bites and poisoning.

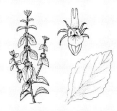

FAMILY Lamiaceae
PARTS USED Aerial parts
CONSTITUENTS Flavonoids (luteolin), saponins, tannins, volatile oils (pinene, limonene and campene), mucilage, bitter lactone, alkaloids (betonicine and stachydrine), sterols, diterpene alcohol (marrubiol), bitters, vitamin C, iron.
ACTIONS Expectorant, decongestant, diaphoretic, bitter tonic, anthelmintic, antibacterial, cholagogue, digestive, antispasmodic, diuretic, emmenagogue, laxative.

Digestion • Its bitter taste stimulates appetite and digestion; promotes flow of digestive juices and bile from the liver. • Laxative. • Antibacterial and anthelmintic. • Indicated in indigestion, wind, colic, gastroenteritis, diarrhoea and worms.
Circulation • Used for calming palpitations, dilating the arteries and normalizing the circulation. Essential oils have a vasodilatory action. • Contains iron; used for anaemia.
Respiratory system • Renowned as an antibacterial, antispasmodic and expectorant remedy for coughs, colds, catarrh, flu, croup, asthma, bronchitis, chest infections, emphysema and bronchial catarrh. • Traditionally used for laryngitis, tonsillitis, pneumonia, TB and whooping cough. • Taken hot it increases perspiration and relieves fevers and catarrhal congestion.
Reproductive system • Stimulates the uterus; brings on menstruation in delayed periods and amenorrhoea. • Traditionally used to expel the placenta after childbirth.

CAUTION Avoid in pregnancy. Fresh juice may cause skin irritation.

Melissa officinalis
Lemon balm

This perennial herb, native to the Mediterranean, was introduced to Britain by the Romans, who valued it to improve memory and lift the spirits. It was a favourite of the Arab world in the Middle Ages to promote longevity, now explained by the presence of the antioxidant rosmarinic acid.

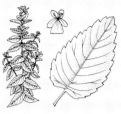

FAMILY Lamiaceae
PARTS USED Aerial parts
CONSTITUENTS Volatile oils (including citronellal, geraniol and linalool), polyphenols, tannins, flavonoids (including isoquercetrin), rosmarinic acid, triterpenoids.
ACTIONS Diaphoretic, carminative, nervine, antispasmodic, antihistamine, antimicrobial, sedative, antiviral, partus praeparator, antioxidant, decongestant.

Digestion • Reduces pain and spasm. • Soothes stress-related problems. • Stimulates the liver and gall bladder.
Circulation • Calms nervous palpitations and arrhythmias. • Reduces hypertension.
Mental and emotional • Sedative and analgesic; reduces tension, anxiety and agitation. Useful in dementia[254] and insomnia. • Relieves headaches, migraine, vertigo and tinnitus. • Mood elevating. • Improves memory and concentration.
Respiratory system • Relaxant, antimicrobial and decongestant; helps resolve colds, flu, catarrh, chest infections, coughs and asthma.
Immune system • Antiviral against herpes simplex, mumps, possibly HIV[255]. • Volatile oils are antibacterial, antifungal and antihistamine; helpful in hay fever and allergic rhinitis. • Rosmarinic acid is antioxidant and anti-inflammatory and influences complement activity[256].
Urinary system • Antispasmodic and diuretic.
Reproductive system • Helpful in irregular and painful periods, PMS and menopausal depression. • Eases and speeds childbirth when taken prior to and during the birth.
Other • Thyroid-inhibitory effect; used in the management of hyperthyroidism.
Externally • Antiseptic for cuts and wounds. • Dilute oils used in massage for period pains, neuralgia, joint and muscle pain and cold sores. • Eardrops used for infections.

Drug interactions Avoid with thyroid drugs.

Mentha piperita
Peppermint

With its refreshing taste and stimulating action, Peppermint is traditionally used as a digestive, analgesic and decongestant for headaches and colds.

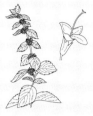

FAMILY Lamiaceae
PARTS USED Aerial parts
CONSTITUENTS Volatile oil menthol and derivatives, flavonoids, phytol, carotenoids, rosmarinic acid, tannins.
ACTIONS Diaphoretic, carminative, nervine, antispasmodic, antiemetic, antiseptic, digestive, circulatory stimulant, analgesic, antimicrobial.

Digestion • Relieves pain and spasm in stomachaches, colic, flatulence, heartburn, indigestion, hiccups, constipation, IBS and diarrhoea. • Enhances appetite and digestion. • Relieves nausea and travel sickness. • Tannins protect gut lining from irritation and infection; useful in Crohn's disease and ulcerative colitis. • Bitters stimulate liver and gall bladder function.
Circulation • In warm infusion it improves circulation, dispersing blood to the periphery and causes sweating.
Mental and emotional • Used as a brain tonic to clear the mind and improve concentration. • Calms anxiety and tension. • Analgesic and antispasmodic; relieves tension headaches, joint and muscle pain.
Respiratory system • Decongestant in hot infusion. • Clears airways and reduces spasm in asthma.• Enhances resistance to infections. Relieves colds, flu and fevers.
Immune system • Increases energy and immunity by enhancing digestion and absorption. • Volatile oils are antibacterial, antiparasitic, antiviral and antifungal. • Active against a wide range of bacteria including *Helicobacter pylori*, *Salmonella enteritidis* and *E. coli*[257] and fungi including candida. • Flavonoid luteolin-7-O-rutinoside has antihistamine action[258].
Reproductive system • Relaxes smooth muscle in the uterus; reduces menstrual pain and cramps.
Externally • Oils/lotion are useful for herpes simplex and ringworm. • Oil used as an inhalant for colds, catarrh and sinusitis; added to lotions for muscular pains and aching feet. • Tea/tincture used as a gargle for sore throats; mouthwash for gum infections and mouth ulcers.

CAUTION Oil should always be used diluted, and avoided in pregnancy. Do not use on babies or small children.

Myrica cerifera
Bayberry

This perennial shrub is native to eastern North America. The greenish berries are edible and produce wax that has long been used to make candles and soap. Powerfully astringent, it is excellent for toning lax muscles.

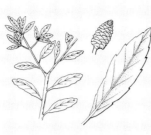

FAMILY Myricaceae
PARTS USED Bark, root bark
CONSTITUENTS Tannins, triterpenes (taraxerol, taraxerone and myricadol), flavonoids (myricitrin), vitamin C, phenols, fatty acids (palmitic, stearic and myristic acids), gum.
ACTIONS Astringent, alterative, anti-inflammatory, antibacterial, antioxidant, circulatory stimulant, diuretic, diaphoretic, expectorant, hepatoprotective, styptic.

Digestion • Astringent tannins protect the gut lining from irritation and inflammation. • Antibacterial actions also help combat infections. • Useful in gastritis, heartburn, acid indigestion, gastroenteritis, diarrhoea, dysentery, colitis and IBS.
Circulation • Stimulates the flow of blood and lymph, clearing lymphatic congestion and supporting the detoxification work of the lymphatic system. • Used for varicose veins.
Respiratory system • Astringes mucous membranes, protecting against irritation and infection and reducing excess mucous. • It has expectorant properties and brings down fevers. • Useful in colds, nasal congestion, catarrhal coughs, flu, sinusitis, sore throats and tonsillitis.
Urinary system • Astringent diuretic, reducing fluid retention; recommended in urinary incontinence and bed-wetting.
Reproductive system • Reduces blood flow; used for heavy periods. • Tones pelvic muscles; excellent for prolapse.
Externally • Mouthwash used for bleeding gums and mouth ulcers, gargle for sore throats, and lotion for varicose veins. • Decoction used as a douche for vaginal discharge and combating infection. • Used in tooth powders for bleeding gums.

CAUTION Avoid during pregnancy. Large doses can be emetic.

Myristica fragrans
Nutmeg

Nutmeg is the dried kernel of the seeds of an evergreen tree native to the Indonesian Molucca Islands. In large amounts it has euphoric effects and has long been used in love potions as well as perfumes and incense.

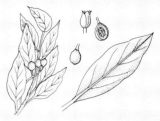

FAMILY Myristicaceae
PARTS USED Kernel
CONSTITUENTS Essential oil myristicin (borneol, camphene, pinene, linalool and eugenol), oleic, palmitic and linoleic acids, saponins.
ACTIONS Sedative, euphoric, stimulant, anti-inflammatory, antimicrobial, antispasmodic, digestive, carminative, aphrodisiac, circulatory stimulant, astringent.

Digestion • Relaxes muscles throughout the gut, stimulates the flow of digestive enzymes and promotes appetite, digestion and absorption. Relieves halitosis, indigestion, hiccups, colic, wind, bloating and nervous digestive problems. • Anti-inflammatory and antiseptic for Crohn's disease, colitis, infections, diarrhoea, dysentery, gastroenteritis, nausea and vomiting.
• Traditionally used with coconut water in India for dehydration caused by vomiting and diarrhoea, particularly in cholera.
Circulation • Protective effect on the cardiovascular system. Lowers harmful cholesterol. Prevents clotting.
Mental and emotional • Powerful brain stimulant yet promotes sleep. • Relaxes muscles; eases muscle spasm and pain.
Respiratory system • Decongestant for catarrh.
Reproductive system • Traditionally used to prolong lovemaking and heighten sensitivity.
Externally • Ground nutmeg mixed with water is applied to skin problems such as ringworm and eczema. • Essential oil can be applied to numb toothache while awaiting dental help. • The oil is anti-inflammatory and pain relieving used in rubs for arthritis, nerve and muscle pain.

CAUTION No more than 3 g should be taken daily. Large amounts can produce toxic symptoms such as nausea, vomiting, convulsions, tachycardia, restlessness, dizziness and hallucinations.

Ocimum sanctum
Holy basil/Tulsi

Tulsi is one of the most sacred
plants in India, dedicated to
Vishnu and Krishna. It has an
uplifting and strengthening
effect on mind and body. Its
aroma is traditionally used to
purify the atmosphere.

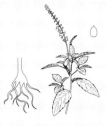

FAMILY Lamiaceae
PARTS USED Leaf, seed, root
CONSTITUENTS Essential oils (including eugenol,
carvacrol, linalool and camphor), triterpenes, sterols,
polyphenols, flavonoids, fatty acids (myristic, stearic,
palmitic, oleic, linoleic and linolenic).
ACTIONS Demulcent, antibacterial, antifungal,
expectorant, anticatarrhal, antispasmodic, anthelmintic,
febrifuge, nervine, adaptogen, immunostimulant,
digestive, laxative, mood elevating.

Digestion • Antispasmodic and warming; relieves spasm,
wind and bloating. • Appetizing and digestive and
improves absorption. • Used for anorexia, nausea,
constipation, vomiting, abdominal pain, ulcers and
worms. • Increases the production of protective stomach
mucous, preventing irritation from acidity drugs and
toxins.
Mental and emotional • Uplifting and strengthening.
Clears lethargy and congestion that dampen the spirits
and fog the mind. • Reduces anxiety, mild depression,
insomnia, and stress-related problems such as headaches
and IBS. • Increases resilience to stress.
Respiratory system • Decongestant, expectorant and
antispasmodic. • Protects against histamine-induced
bronchospasm; helpful in asthma and rhinitis. • Active
against micro-organisms including *E. coli*, *Staphylococcus
aureus* and *Mycoplasma tuberculosis* and fungi such as
Aspergillus spp. • Used for coughs, colds, fevers, sore
throats and flu.
Immune system • Anti-inflammatory; inhibits
prostaglandin production. • Protects healthy cells from
the toxicity of radiation and chemotherapy. • Used for
allergies such as hay fever and rhinitis. • Anthelmintic;
active against enteric pathogens and candida.
Urinary system • Relieves dysuria, cystitis and urinary
tract infections. Clears toxins through diuretic effect.
Endocrine system • Lowers blood sugar, harmful
cholesterol and triglyceride levels.

Oenothera biennis
Evening primrose

This biennial has sweet-
scented pale-yellow flowers.
It was originally brought to
Europe from America. The
oil is a good source of
omega-6 fatty acids, vital for
the healthy functioning of
the immune, nervous
and hormonal systems.

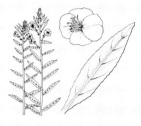

FAMILY Onagraceae
PARTS USED Oil from seeds
CONSTITUENTS Omega-6 essential fatty acids
(including gamma-linoleic acid/GLA, linoleic, oleic,
palmitic and stearic acid).
ACTIONS Antispasmodic, nervine, sedative, antioxidant,
antiallergenic, hormone regulator, hypotensive.

Digestion • Counteracts the effects of alcoholic
poisoning • Encourages regeneration of damaged liver.
Helps withdrawal from alcohol and alcoholic depression.
Circulation • Reduces high blood pressure and harmful
cholesterol levels; helps prevent blood clots and coronary
artery disease.
Mental and emotional • Mildly sedative, helpful in
nervous indigestion, colic and hyperactivity in children.
• Well known for its beneficial use in MS.
Respiratory system • Antispasmodic effects help
to relieve asthma and paroxysmal coughing, as in
whooping cough.
Immune system • Fatty acids are helpful in the
treatment of allergies such as eczema, hyperactivity,
ADHD, asthma, migraine, metabolic disorders, diabetes,
high cholesterol, viral infections and arthritis. • GLA
reduces inflammation by reducing prostaglandin E.
• May inhibit the production of free radicals and slow
tumour growth.
Reproductive system • Fatty acids help maintain
hormone balance. Indicated in PMS, menstrual
irregularities, breast problems, menopausal problems
and acne. • Increases fat content of breast milk in
lactating[259] women.
Skin • Provides GLA, which cannot be produced by the
body; excellent when breakdown in GLA production from
linoleic acid is related to eczema or acne.

CAUTION Avoid in epilepsy. Supplement with omega-3 oils
simultaneously at ratio of 3:1.

Olea europaea
Olive

The Olive is one of the
oldest cultivated plants of
the Mediterranean, thought
to have been grown at least
5,000 years ago in Egypt
and Crete for its oil.
Olympic athletes would rub
olive oil into their skin to
keep their muscles and joints supple.

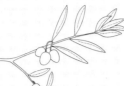

FAMILY Oleaceae
PARTS USED Fruit, oil, leaf
CONSTITUENTS Oil: antioxidants, olein, palmetin,
aracluin, stearin, cholesterin, cyclorarthanol, benzoic
acid; leaf and unripe fruit: mannite.
ACTIONS Nutritious, demulcent, emollient, antiseptic,
astringent, febrifuge, antioxidant, cholagogue, hypotensive,
hypocholesterolaemic.

Digestion • Soothes irritated and inflamed conditions
such as indigestion, heartburn, gastritis, colitis and peptic
ulcers. • Warm enemas help to relieve constipation.
• Traditionally used as a gastric lavage for poisoning by
alkalis/corrosives to soothe irritated mucosae and hasten
elimination. • Stimulates bile flow; used for liver and gall
bladder problems. Alternated with lemon juice to dissolve
and encourage the passing of gallstones. • Leaves lower
blood sugar; helpful in diabetes.
Circulation • Cold-pressed oil is high in oleic acid; can
lower harmful cholesterol, blood pressure and reduce
risk of atherosclerosis, clots, heart attacks and strokes.
• Leaves relax blood vessels and lower blood pressure;
used for hypertension, angina and other circulatory
problems. • Hot infusion of leaves increases sweating and
reduces fevers.
Respiratory system • Soothes harsh, dry coughs,
laryngitis and croup. • Reduces catarrh.
Immune system • Antioxidants make cell membranes
less susceptible to destruction by free radicals. May
reduce development of cancer and retard ageing.
Externally • Applied to boils, eczema, cold sores, dry
skin, brittle nails, insect bites and stings and minor burns
to speed healing. • Warm oil dropped into the ear softens
wax; used with essential oils such as garlic or lavender to
relieve earache. • Massaged over kidneys for bed-
wetting. • Infusion of leaves used as a mouthwash for
bleeding/infected gums; and gargle for sore throats.

Origanum majorana
Sweet marjoram

With its white flowers and
grey-green leaves Marjoram
is a half-hardy annual in cool
temperate areas and a
perennial found growing
wild in warmer areas of
Europe and the USA. The
ancient Greeks used it to
nourish the brain and remedy
the digestion.

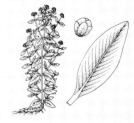

FAMILY Lamiaceae
PARTS USED Flower, leaf
CONSTITUENTS Essential oil (including camphor,
borneol, terpinene and sabinene), mucilage, bitters,
tannins, antioxidants.
ACTIONS Digestive, carminative, tonic, stimulant,
diaphoretic, antispasmodic, diuretic, antiviral,
antioxidant, expectorant.

Digestion • Antispasmodic and warming; used for
indigestion, poor appetite, wind and colic, nausea,
diarrhoea and constipation.
Circulation • Stimulates blood flow and taken hot clears
toxins via the skin; used for poor circulation, chilblains,
arthritis and gout.
Mental and emotional • Traditionally used to calm
unwanted sexual desire and to ease loneliness,
bereavement and heartbreak. • Relaxes mental and
physical tension; relieves insomnia, restlessness, anxiety,
depression, aching muscles and stress-related symptoms
such as indigestion, colic, headaches, migraine, period
pains, PMS, poor concentration and memory.
Immune system • Antioxidants minimize damage from
free radicals and retard ageing. • Enhances immunity and
increases circulation. • Essential oils are antimicrobial
against bacteria such as TB, viruses such as herpes
simplex and fungal infections such as candida; protect
against winter infections such as coughs and colds.
• Clears phlegm, soothes coughs and relieves sinusitis
and fevers. • Probiotic.
Urinary system • Antiseptic diuretic for infections and
fluid retention. Clears toxins via urine.
Externally • Diluted essential oils can be massaged into
painful joints, aching muscles, sprains and strains.

Paeonia lactiflora, P. officinalis and *P. suffrcticosa*
Peony

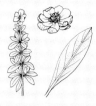

There are 33 species of Peony native to Europe, China and North America. *P. lactiflora,* with red, white or pink-scented flowers, was cultivated in China from 900 BCE.

FAMILY Paeoniaceae
PARTS USED Root, seed, flower
CONSTITUENTS Benzoic acid, asparagin, essential oil, alkaloid.
ACTIONS *P. officinalis*: diuretic, emmenagogue, bitter tonic, alterative, nervine, astringent; *P. lactiflora* cultivated root (bai-shao): liver tonic, astringent, antispasmodic, sedative, antiseptic, diuretic, nourishing; wild harvested root (chi-shao): anodyne, cooling, febrifuge; *P. suffruticosa* bark of the root (mu-dan-pi): antiseptic, diuretic, nourishing.

Digestion • Liver and gall bladder remedy; dissolves gallstones. • Root reduces pain and spasm in the stomach and intestines, use for diarrhoea, dysentery and stress-related gastric ulcers.
Circulation • Improves venous return; benefits varicose veins and haemorrhoids. • Bai-shao used in Traditional Chinese Medicine for hypertension, hypertensive headaches, fevers, dizziness due to poor circulation and blood deficiency with liver heat.
Mental and emotional • Bai-shao is calming; relaxes spasm in the chest, gut and uterus and has anticonvulsive properties. • Traditional remedy for spasms, epilepsy, nervous twitches and St Vitus's dance.
Immune system • Root is anti-inflammatory, antibacterial and antiviral. Clears signs of heat such as boils. • Used for stiff joints.
Urinary system • Diuretic; helps dissolve stones.
Reproductive system • Stimulates uterine muscles; aids contractions in childbirth and expulsion of the placenta.
• Bai-shao reduces painful periods and night sweats.
Externally • A knife wound with bleeding and pain is commonly treated with bai-shao in Chinese Traditional Medicine.

CAUTION Avoid in early pregnancy.

Panax ginseng
Korean ginseng

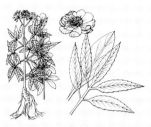

For centuries in the East, top-grade Ginseng roots have been valued more highly than gold. There are many different grades of Ginseng – Wild ginseng, particularly that from Manchuria, being considered the best.

FAMILY Araliaceae
PARTS USED Root
CONSTITUENTS About 30 hormone-like saponins (ginsenosides), volatile oil, sterols, starch, pectin, vitamins B1, B2 and B12, choline, minerals (including zinc, copper, magnesium, calcium, iron).
ACTIONS Tonic, nervine, adaptogen, alterative, stimulant, immunostimulant, rejuvenative.

Digestion • Reduces blood sugar; useful for diabetics.
• Improves the appetite and digestion and lowers harmful cholesterol.
Mental and emotional • Chinese 'qi' tonic. Adaptogen; increases energy and resilience to stress. • Optimizes pituitary and adrenal function when stressed. • Increases efficiency of nerve impulses, enhancing overall mental and physical performance, memory, stamina and muscular strength. • Excellent when undergoing harsh physical training, recovering from illness or surgery, studying for exams or taking on a large project at work. • Rejuvenating tonic; reduces the impact of the ageing process.
• Quietens the spirit and imparts wisdom.
Respiratory system • Acts as a tonic to the lungs, reducing wheezing and shortness of breath.
Immune system • Immune enhancer. Some 3,000 scientific studies confirm its ability to increase resistance to stress caused by extremes of temperature, excessive exertion, illness, hunger, mental strain and emotional problems. • Increases white blood cell action. • Improves liver function, aiding resistance to hepatotoxins and radiation. • Reduces depression of bone marrow when on anticancer drugs. • Decreases allergic responses.
Reproductive system • Saponins stimulate sexual function in men and women; increase sperm production.
• Reduces menopausal symptoms such as depression.

CAUTION Avoid in acute inflammatory conditions such as bronchitis.

Passiflora incarnata
Passion flower

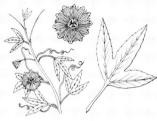

This perennial climber indigenous to South America has stunningly beautiful, intricate flowers. It derives its name from the resemblance of the centre of the flower to the cross and crown of thorns, symbolizing the Passion of Christ. This prompted its Spanish discoverers in Peru to send it to Pope Paul V in 1605.

FAMILY Passifloraceae
PARTS USED Vine, flower
CONSTITUENTS Alkaloids, sugar, gum, sterols, flavonoids, coumarin derivatives, essential oil.
ACTIONS Anodyne, anticonvulsive, nervine, sedative, antispasmodic, anxiolytic, hypotensive.

Digestion • For stress-related digestive problems including wind, colic and indigestion.
Circulation • Relaxes tension through the arterial system; reduces blood pressure and nervous palpitations.
Mental and emotional • An excellent relaxant and sedative for stress-related and painful conditions.
• Improves circulation and nutrition to the nerves.
• Calms nervous anxiety, restlessness and agitation.
• Improves concentration and combats exam nerves.
• Soothes pain in headaches, neuralgia, shingles, muscular aches, backache and period pains. • Cooling in conditions of excess heat, inflammation, anger, intolerance and irritability. • Non-addictive tranquillizer for chronic insomnia. For best results, take during the day as well as before retiring. • Antispasmodic for Parkinson's disease, muscle twitching and cramps, high blood pressure and colic.
Respiratory system • Antispasmodic; relieves irritating and nervous coughs, croup and asthma.

Drug interactions Avoid with monoamine oxidase-inhibiting antidepressants.

Phytolacca decandra
Poke root

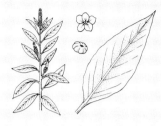

This striking herb, native to North America, has reddish-purple berries, which are poisonous when raw. It is a potent remedy for the immune system and is being researched for its potential in treating cancer, HIV, bilharzia and arthritis.

FAMILY Phytolaccaceae
PARTS USED Root
CONSTITUENTS Triterpenoid saponins, resin, sugars[260], phytolaccosides, alkaloid (phytolaccine), phyolaccic acid, formic acid, lectins, tannin, proteins, histamines, fatty oil.
ACTIONS Alterative, anodyne, anti-inflammatory, antirheumatic, antitumour, antiviral, laxative, expectorant, hypnotic, immunostimulant, lymphatic decongestant, narcotic, purgative, spermicide[261].

Respiratory system • Strengthens immunity and combats acute and chronic infections; used for sore throats, throat infections, colds and flu viruses.
Musculoskeletal system • Phytolaccosides have potent anti-inflammatory action[262]. Detoxifying and anti-inflammatory for rheumatic and arthritic conditions[263].
Immune system • Immune enhancing and cleansing. Supports the lymphatic system in its detoxifying and immune work. Used in swollen lymph nodes, tonsillitis, mumps, swollen breast and mastitis. • The proteins are antiviral; they can inhibit the replication of the influenza and herpes simplex viruses and poliovirus[264]. • Used in HIV and cancers including leukaemia and liver cancer[265].
• The peptide PAFP-s has antifungal activity[266].
Externally • Antifungal, antiseptic and anti-inflammatory wash used for athlete's foot, spots, acne, boils, abscesses, psoriasis, eczema, herpes, shingles, chickenpox, measles, tumours, impetigo and scabies, swelling sprains and strains.

CAUTION Only use in small doses. Avoid internal use during pregnancy, lactation and gastrointestinal irritation. Do not apply to broken skin.
Drug interactions Do not use with immunosuppressive drugs[267].

Piper longum
Long pepper

Native to tropical India, and a close relative of black pepper. It has warming and energizing properties and acts as a stimulant and a tonic for those feeling cold and run-down.

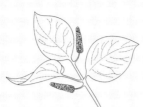

FAMILY Piperaceae
PARTS USED Root, seed
CONSTITUENTS Volatile oils, alkaloids (piperine and piplartine), lignans, resin, esters.
ACTIONS Stimulant, carminative, laxative, diuretic, febrifuge, tonic, expectorant, anthelmintic, digestive, antiseptic, emmenagogue, rejuvenative, analgesic, cardiac stimulant, hypocholesterolaemic.

Digestion • Enhances appetite, digestion and absorption up to 30 per cent[268]. Piperine stimulates an enzyme that enhances the uptake of amino acids from the gastrointestinal tract. Used for anorexia, dyspepsia, flatulence, constipation, colic and weak digestion.
• Antimicrobial for amoebae, worms and candida.
• Hepatoprotective, enhancing the liver's ability to break down toxins; reduces liver damage.
Circulation • Vasodilatory. • Stimulates circulation and reduces harmful cholesterol. • Used for anaemia.
Mental and emotional • Promotes energy and vitality.
• Reduces tension, anxiety and insomnia.
Respiratory system • Decongestant for colds, catarrh, bronchial congestion and bronchitis. • Traditionally used in milk to reduce bronchospasm in asthma.
Immune system • Anti-inflammatory for gout, arthritis and muscle and back pain. • Enhances immunity; activates macrophages and phagocytosis. • Found to be helpful in the treatment of hepatitis. • Broad spectrum antibiotic activity against gram+ and gram- bacteria[269], including *Staphylococcus aureus*[270]. • Reduces allergic conditions including hay fever and eczema. • Antioxidant and rejuvenative. • Reduces fevers; traditionally used for typhoid and chronic fevers[271].
Reproductive system • May have a contraceptive effect; reduces sperm count. • Reputed to be an aphrodisiac.
• Antispasmodic for dysmenorrhoea.
Externally • Rubefacient ingredient of liniments for pain and swelling.

CAUTION May increase drug absorption. Use cautiously in acidity. Avoid in pregnancy and lactation.

Plantago major
Greater plantain
Also *P. minor* (Lesser plantain); *P. lanceolata* (Ribwort plantain); *P. psyllium* (Psyllium)

This common perennial with cylindrical spikes of seeds grows in lawns and on cultivated and waste ground. It is historically famous as a wound healer and an antidote to poisons.

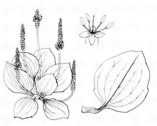

FAMILY Plantaginaceae
PARTS USED Leaf, seed of *P. psyllium*
CONSTITUENTS Leaf: iridoid glycosides, triterpenoids, caffeic acid, polysaccharides, tannins, flavonoids, silica; seed: mucilage, monoterpene alkaloids, glycosides, fixed oil, fatty acids, tannins, sugars.
ACTIONS Leaf: astringent, alterative, diuretic, vulnerary, demulcent, refrigerant, detoxifying, decongestant, expectorant, antiseptic, antispasmodic. Seed: bulk laxative, demulient.

Digestion • Leaf: astringent and soothing. Counters irritation and inflammation in the stomach and bowels; used for gastritis, diarrhoea, colitis and stomach and bowel infections. • Reduces spasm and colic. • Seeds are used as a bulk laxative.
Respiratory system • Leaf depresses mucous secretion in colds, catarrh, sinusitis, bronchial congestion and allergies such as hay fever and asthma. Helps prevent glue ear and ear infections. • Mucilage protects mucosae from irritation; soothes cough reflex. • Expectorant and antispasmodic for coughs and asthma. • Antiseptic for colds, tonsillitis and chest infections.
Immune system • Leaf: polysaccharides have an immunomodulating effect[272]. • Tannins reduce swelling and inflammation, staunch bleeding and promote healing. • Clears heat and toxins; reduces fevers, infections and skin problems. • Antiviral against herpes viruses and adenoviruses[273], and urinary tract infections.
Reproductive system • Astringent for excessive menstrual bleeding. • Useful for prostatitis enlargement.
Externally • Used for cuts, stings and insect bites.

CAUTION Take seeds with plenty of fluid to prevent bowel obstruction.
Drug interactions Care needed with patients on insulin, as seeds can lower blood sugar. Separate by 2 hours from other drugs. May inhibit absorption.

Polygonum multiflorum
Polygonum

A perennial vine, native
to Japan, Vietnam and China,
where it is highly valued as
an adaptogen. In Chinese
Medicine it is used as a
rejuvenating kidney tonic and
to prevent hair from greying.

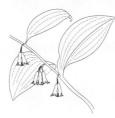

FAMILY Polygonaceae
PARTS USED Processed root
CONSTITUENTS Phenolic glucosides,
tetrahydroxystilbene, tannins, anthraquinones,
phospholipids (including lecithin), allantoin, minerals.
ACTIONS Adaptogen, immune tonic, rejuvenative,
hypocholesterolaemic, nervine, bitter, alterative,
antibacterial, antioxidant, aphrodisiac, demulcent,
cholagogue, laxative, astringent, blood tonic, cardiotonic,
hypoglycaemic, kidney tonic, sedative.

Digestion • Protects liver against damage from toxins,
chemicals, alcohol and drugs. • Enhances liver and gall
bladder function. • Reduces gut irritation. • Useful in
constipation from dryness. Best combined with digestive
herbs such as Ginger. • Lowers blood sugar.
Circulation • Reduces blood pressure and harmful
cholesterol; prevents atherosclerosis. • Increases cerebral
circulation; used for dizziness with tinnitus and anaemia.
Mental and emotional • Increases energy and resilience
to stress. • Used for nervous exhaustion and insomnia.
Excellent tonic for the elderly and during convalescence.
• Improves memory. May protect against Alzheimer's
disease and be useful in Parkinson's disease[274].
Musculoskeletal system • Strengthens bones, muscles
and tendons[275].
Immune system • Adaptogenic and antioxidant; enhances
immunity and protects against cancer. • Antiageing
through the inhibition of brain monoamine oxidase[276].
• Increases secretion of adrenal and thyroid hormones;
enhances T lymphocyte and macrophage activity[277].
Reproductive system • Strengthening tonic and
aphrodisiac for impotence, low sperm count, infertility
and menopausal problems. • For signs of kidney
weakness including low libido, poor vision, weak knees
and grey hair.

CAUTION May cause diarrhoea.
Drug interactions Avoid with tetracycline, statins and
acetaminophen[278].

Prunella vulgaris
Selfheal

A small perennial, with
purple flowers, growing wild
in Europe, North America
and China. It was historically
used for throat complaints,
since its corolla resembles a
throat with swollen glands.

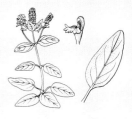

FAMILY Lamiaceae
PARTS USED Aerial parts
CONSTITUENTS Volatile oils (including camphor and
fenchone), bitters, saponins, tannins, sugar, glycoside
(aucubin), urosolic acid, flavonoids, antioxidants
(including rosmarinic acid).
ACTIONS Astringent, styptic, vulnerary, tonic, anti-
inflammatory, relaxant, antibiotic, diuretic, digestive, liver
tonic, antiallergenic, antioxidant, restorative.

Digestion • Astringent for diarrhoea and inflammatory
bowel problems such as colitis. • Bitters stimulate the
liver and gall bladder.
Mental and emotional • Used for headaches,
particularly when related to tension, vertigo,
oversensitivity to light and high blood pressure. • Used
in China for hyperactivity in children.
Immune system • Enhances immunity. Research
indicates a potent antiviral action, including activity
against HIV[279], and the polysaccharides have an
immunomodulatory effect[280]. • Rosmarinic acid
contributes to its antioxidant effects[281]. • Research
indicates antimutagenic effects, indicating possible
anticancer use[282]. • Recommended in lowered immunity,
HIV, chronic fatigue syndrome and allergies. • Effective
antibiotic against a range of bacteria. • Used for swollen
glands, mumps, glandular fever and mastitis.
• Detoxifying; clears inflammatory skin problems.
• Reduces fevers.
Urinary system • Urosolic acid is a diuretic that has
anticancer properties[283]; clears toxins and excess uric acid
via the kidneys. Recommended for gout.
Reproductive system • Astringent; curbs heavy
menstrual bleeding.
Externally • Traditional wound remedy. • Gargle used
for sore throats; mouthwash for mouth ulcers and
bleeding gums. • Tea/fresh plant used to stop bleeding,
reduce swelling from minor injuries, burns, bites and
stings, piles, varicose veins and ulcers. • Drops used for
inflammatory eye problems such as conjunctivitis.

Rehmannia glutinosa
Rehmannia

Native to China, where it is famous as a yin and blood tonic, increasing energy and immunity, and a strengthening tonic for children.

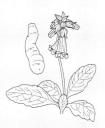

FAMILY Scrophulariaceae
PARTS USED Root; uncured (sheng di) or cured (shu di huang)
CONSTITUENTS Iridoid compounds, polysaccharides (astragalans), glucuronic acid, glycosides (jionosides), flavones, iso-flavones, saponins, b-sitosterol, arginine, manitol, stimasterol, tannins.
ACTIONS Haemostatic, adaptogen, antioxidant, antibacterial, hepatoprotective, immune tonic, antipyretic, demulcent, alterative, laxative, anti-inflammatory.

Digestion • Astringent for diarrhoea. • Increases appetite. • Regulates blood sugar.
Circulation • Improves coronary blood flow; helps prevent cardiovascular disease.
Respiratory system • Strengthens lung energy; prevents colds, flu, fevers, coughs, bronchitis, pneumonia, asthma and TB. • Reduces phlegm.
Musculoskeletal system • Strengthens bones, muscles and tendons; prevents muscle weakness and prolapse.
Immune system • Protects against infections such as glandular fever, Coxsackie B virus and post-viral fatigue. • Inhibits formation of tumours and prevents immunosuppression by chemotherapy[284]. • Used for inflammatory conditions associated with depletion, including TB. • Uncured root useful in autoimmune disease such as rheumatoid arthritis, and allergies[285]. • Protects and supports the liver and adrenal glands. Enhances production of corticosteroids[286].
Urinary system • Strengthens kidneys, stems bleeding and reduces urinary frequency and incontinence. • Prevents damage from toxins, drugs and infection.
Reproductive system • Prepared root used in Chinese Medicine for low kidney energy and yin deficiency, night sweats, vertigo, tinnitus, lower back pain; regulates menstrual flow. • Curbs bleeding in heavy periods. • Reduces menopausal night sweats and hot flushes.

CAUTION Best prepared with Cardamom or Ginger to prevent indigestion.
Drug interactions Use cautiously with immunosuppressant drugs.

Rhodiola rosea
Rhodiola

A perennial plant with red, pink or yellowish flowers, native to the Himalayas and found growing at high elevations in Asia, Europe and North America. It has long been considered a tonic to increase physical and mental endurance and strength.

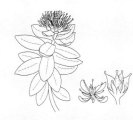

FAMILY Crassulaceae
PARTS USED Root, stem, leaf, flower, seed
CONSTITUENTS Phenylpropanoids (collectively known as rosavins, including rosavin, rosarin and rosin), salidroside, rosiridin, flavonoids, tannins, essential oil[287].
ACTIONS Adaptogen, tonic, antioxidant, antitumour[288], cardiotonic, brain tonic, thymoleptic, immunostimulant.

Circulation • Cardioprotective; normalizes heart rate after intense exercise. • Protects against altitude sickness. • Used in anaemia and cardiovascular disorder[289]. • Combats the effects of excess adrenaline, which causes raised blood pressure and blood lipids.
Mental and emotional • Reputed to be more powerful than other adaptogens. Increases ability to deal with stress. • Increases blood supply to the brain and muscles. • Improves memory and concentration and increases attention span[290]. • Recommended for elevating mood in depression[291]. • Useful sedative for insomnia in higher doses.
Musculoskeletal system • Energy tonic; increases protein synthesis, useful in increasing strength and endurance in athletes and the elderly[292]. Recommended for combating fatigue, physical stress, chronic fatigue syndrome and fibromyalgia[293].
Immune system • Stimulates immunity directly by increasing natural killer cells, improving T-cell immunity and increasing resilience to stress. • Helps combat infections, including TB. • Helps prevent cancer as it has antitumour, antimetastatic and antimutagenic properties, which increase resistance to toxins and chemicals that could be potentially harmful. • Supportive during chemotherapy or radiotherapy[294]; shortens recovery time of suppressed white blood cells following chemotherapy or radiation therapy.

CAUTION Do not take simultaneously with mineral supplements.

Rosa spp.
Rose

Roses have long been praised
for their beauty as well as their
medicinal benefits, valued for
their cooling properties, for
strengthening the heart and
refreshing the spirit.

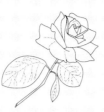

FAMILY Rosaceae
PARTS USED Hip, leaf, flower
CONSTITUENTS Tannins, pectin, carotene, fruit acids,
fatty oil, nicotinamide, vitamins C, B, E and K.
ACTIONS Diaphoretic, carminative, stimulant,
emmenagogue, laxative, decongestant, febrifuge,
nervine, anti-inflammatory, astringent, antimicrobial,
thymoleptic, analgesic.

Digestion • Combats infection and helps re-establish
normal gut flora. • Tannins reduce hyperacidity and
stomach overactivity causing excessive hunger and
mouth ulcers. Useful for diarrhoea and enteritis. • Rose
hip syrup or decoction of empty seed cases relieves
diarrhoea, stomach cramps, constipation and nausea.
Mental and emotional • Flowers are uplifting and
calming. Used for insomnia, depression, irritability, anger
and mental and physical fatigue.
Respiratory system • Stimulates action of the
mucociliary escalator, antimicrobial and decongestant;
helps to prevent and relieve colds, flu, sore throats,
catarrh, coughs and bronchitis.
Immune system • Combats infection and clears heat and
toxins. Hips are famous for an immune-enhancing syrup;
a rich source of vitamin C, A, B and K. • Hips have anti-
inflammatory effects[295]; reduce pain and increase flexibility
in osteoarthritis[296]. • Leaves and flowers reduce fevers.
Urinary system • Flowers and seeds relieve infections
and fluid retention; hasten the elimination of toxins.
• Reduces inflammation and dissolves stones.
Reproductive system • Flowers relieve uterine
congestion that causes pain, heavy and irregular periods.
• Antispasmodic and relaxing for menstrual cramps and
PMS. • Cooling for menopausal hot flushes, night sweats
and mood swings.
Externally • Rosewater cleanses and tones skin; clears
infection and inflammation in acne, spots, boils, and sore
eyes, minor cuts and wounds. • Reduces swelling of
bruises and sprains.

CAUTION Avoid in pregnancy.

Rosmarinus officinalis
Rosemary

Native to the Mediterranean,
this perennial shrub has been
recognized as a rejuvenating
brain tonic since the ancient
Egyptians, perhaps because it
is rich in antioxidants.

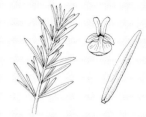

FAMILY Lamiaceae
PARTS USED Aerial parts
CONSTITUENTS Volatile oils, flavonoids, phenolic acids,
tannins, bitters, resins.
ACTIONS Diaphoretic, carminative, emmenagogue,
nervine, antioxidant, cholagogue, thymoleptic,
decongestant, antispasmodic, antimicrobial, circulatory
stimulant, febrifuge.

Digestion • Tannins protect the gut lining from irritation
and inflammation, reducing bleeding and diarrhoea.
• Antimicrobial for infections. • Stimulates appetite,
digestion and absorption, relieves flatulence and
distension. • Enhances elimination. • Bitters stimulate bile
flow from the liver and gall bladder, aid digestion of fats
and clear toxins. • Traditional remedy for hangovers,
jaundice, gallstones, gout, arthritis and skin problems.
Circulation • Stimulates blood flow to the head, reduces
inflammation and muscle tension. Specific for migraines
and headaches. • Stimulates general circulation,
improving peripheral blood flow. • Used for varicose
veins, chilblains and arteriosclerosis.
Mental and emotional • Excellent brain tonic, improves
concentration and memory[297]. • Calms anxiety and lifts
depression, relieves exhaustion and insomnia.
Respiratory system • Volatile oils dispel infection. • Hot
tea used for fevers, catarrh, sore throats, colds, flu and
chest infections. • Antispasmodic[298]; helpful in asthma.
Immune system • Volatile oils are antibacterial, antifungal
and antiviral[299], and enhance immunity. • Antioxidant; may
have potential as an anticancer remedy[300]. Stimulates liver
enzymes that detoxify poisons including carcinogens. •
Anti-inflammatory; relieves arthritis and gout.
Urinary system • Diuretic; enhances elimination of
wastes.
Reproductive system • Reduces heavy menstrual
bleeding and relieves dysmenorrhoea.
Externally • Diluted essential oil is rubbed onto the skin
for joint pain, headaches and poor concentration.

CAUTION Avoid in pregnancy.

Rubus idaeus
Raspberry

Native to Europe and temperate Asia, Raspberry is well known for its delicious fruit, while the leaves have traditionally been valued for their astringent properties. They were given to relieve diarrhoea and were best known as a parturient, to prepare women for childbirth.

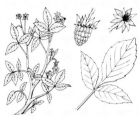

FAMILY Rosaceae
PARTS USED Leaf, fruit
CONSTITUENTS Fragarine, tannins, volatile oil, pectin, vitamin C, niacin, manganese and other minerals and trace elements.
ACTIONS Anti-inflammatory, astringent, birthing aid, decongestant, oxytocic, antiemetic, ophthalmic, antioxidant, antiseptic, antidiarrhoeal, diaphoretic, diuretic, choleretic, partus praeparator, hypoglycaemic.

Digestion • Astringent. Protects gut lining from irritation and inflammation; relieves nausea and diarrhoea. • Helps normalize blood sugar levels. Manganese may effect glucose regulation.
Respiratory system • Antiseptic astringent. Taken in hot tea for sore throats, colds, flu and catarrh.
Reproductive system • Uterine astringent used for frequent or excessive menstruation, painful periods and other menstrual disorders. • Relieves nausea in pregnancy and helps prevent miscarriage. • Infusion of leaves in last 3 months of pregnancy tones uterine and pelvic muscles to prepare for childbirth. By relaxing over-tense muscles and toning over-relaxed muscles, the leaves enable the uterus to contract effectively during childbirth, easing and speeding the birth. • Taken afterwards, they stimulate the flow of breast milk and speed healing. • Raspberries are nutritious; useful in pregnancy to combat anaemia.
Externally • Used as a gargle and mouthwash for sore throats, tonsillitis, mouth ulcers and inflamed gums.
• Poultice/lotion used for sores, conjunctivitis, minor cuts and wounds, burns and varicose ulcers.

Rumex crispus
Yellow dock

A common inhabitant of hedgerows, meadows, ditches and roadsides in temperate areas. The leaves are well known for relieving nettle stings, while the whole plant has been valued since the ancient Greeks, for cleansing toxins and aiding digestion.

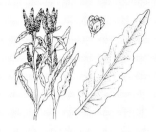

FAMILY Polygonaceae
PARTS USED Root
CONSTITUENTS Anthraquinone glycosides, tannins, iron, bitters, chrysarobin, rumicin.
ACTIONS Alterative, antiscorbutic, astringent, antitumour, cholagogue, depurative, laxative, tonic.

Digestion • Famous for its detoxifying properties. Gentle laxative properties due to anthraquinones, which stimulate peristalsis and cleanse the bowel. • Astringent tannins check irritation and inflammation, and curb diarrhoea. • Bitters stimulate the liver and benefit digestion. Used for liver and gall bladder complaints, headaches and lethargy.
Circulation • Affinity with blood, enriching it with iron and clearing impurities. Traditionally used for anaemia, bleeding of the lungs and bleeding haemorrhoids.
• Stimulates lymphatic circulation; reduces chronic lymphatic congestion and glandular swellings.
Immune system • Invigorating tonic; cleansing and nutritive. • Traditionally used as an anticancer remedy.
• Anti-inflammatory; useful in arthritis.
Urinary system • Diuretic properties increase the elimination of toxins via the kidneys; useful for fluid retention, cystitis, gout and arthritis.
Skin • Cleansing and anti-inflammatory as it aids elimination of toxins through the bowels and kidneys. For chronic skin diseases such as acne, eczema and psoriasis.
Externally • Lotion used for swellings, skin rashes, cuts, sores, ulcers and infections. • Crushed leaves are applied to burns, scalds and nettle stings.

CAUTION Excess doses can cause gastric disturbance, nausea and dermatitis.

Salix alba and *S. nigra*
White and Black willow

White willow is a large, elegant tree that grows by riverbanks and in damp places throughout Europe, North Africa and Central Asia, while Black willow is native to eastern North America.

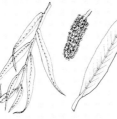

FAMILY Salicaceae
PARTS USED Bark
CONSTITUENTS Salicylic glycosides (including salicin, salicortin and fragilin), tannins.
ACTIONS Febrifuge, analgesic, anti-inflammatory, astringent, tonic, stomachic, diuretic, anodyne, antiseptic, sedative.

Digestion • Astringent tannins protect the gut lining from irritation and inflammation. Relieves diarrhoea and dysentery and stems bleeding. • Indicated in weak digestion, dyspepsia, heartburn acidity and worms.
Respiratory system • Decongestant for head colds, flu and fevers. • Tonic to restore strength after illness.
Musculoskeletal system • Pain reliever and anti-inflammatory for rheumatism, arthritis, gout, aching muscles, inflammatory stages of autoimmune diseases, backache, tendonitis, bursitis and sprains.
Immune system • The original source of salicylic acid; used like aspirin for fevers, muscular aches and pains accompanying flu, headaches, inflammation and arthritic pain without side effects. • Traditionally used for intermittent fevers as in malaria.
Urinary system • Diuretic; reduces fluid retention and helps to eliminate toxins from the body via the urinary system.
Reproductive system • Astringent for heavy periods.
Externally • Lotion used for cuts and wounds; gargles for sore throats; mouthwashes for mouth ulcers and bleeding gums; and poultices for inflamed joints.

CAUTION Avoid in bleeding problems and if allergic to salicylates. Children and teenagers with chickenpox, flu or any undiagnosed illness should not take it without first consulting a practitioner due to theoretical risk of Reye's syndrome.
Drug interactions Use with caution with non-steroidal anti-inflammatory drugs such as ibuprofen or naproxen.

Salvia officinalis
Sage

An evergreen perennial shrub, native to southern Europe and the Mediterranean. It was regarded as the 'immortality herb' by the ancient Greeks and was vital to medieval prescriptions for longevity and 'elixirs of life'.

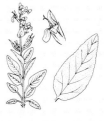

FAMILY Lamiaceae
PARTS USED Leaves
CONSTITUENTS Volatile oils, tannins, phenolic acids, bitters, flavonoids, resins, phytoestrogens.
ACTIONS Antimicrobial, astringent, antiseptic, bitter tonic, digestive, antioxidant, rejuvenative, diuretic, phytoestrogenic, antihydrotic, carminative, cholagogue, vasodilator.

Digestion • Improves appetite, digestion and absorption, particularly of fats. • Relaxes tension and colic. • Relieves bloating and wind. • Beneficial effect on the liver and pancreatic function. Lowers blood sugar.
Mental and emotional • Reduces anxiety, lifts depression and decreases excessive salivation, as in Parkinson's disease.
Respiratory system • Decongestant, antimicrobial and expectorant; excellent for catarrh, colds and chest infections.
Immune system • Antibacterial, antiviral and antifungal for colds, flu, fevers, sore throats and chest infections. Effective against candida, herpes simplex type 2 and influenza virus II. • Traditionally used for TB and profuse perspiration. • Antioxidant actions explain its rejuvenative effects.
Urinary system • Aids elimination of toxins via the kidneys; useful for arthritis and gout.
Reproductive system • Hormone balancing and antispasmodic for irregular, scanty and painful periods. • Used for menopausal problems such as night sweats and insomnia. • Reduces excessive lactation.
Externally • Antiseptic lotion for cuts, burns, insect bites, skin problems, ulcers and sunburn; gargle for sore throats; mouthwash for inflamed gums and ulcers. • Applied leaves relieve toothache. • Poultice used for sprains, swellings and ulcers.

CAUTION May be toxic in large dosages or over a prolonged period. Avoid in pregnancy and breast-feeding and with epilepsy.

Sambucus nigra
Elder

The fragrant, deciduous
Elder tree with its abundance
of white flowers has been
called the 'medicine chest of
the country people', as it has
so many health benefits.

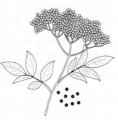

FAMILY Caprifoliaceae
PARTS USED Flower, berry
CONSTITUENTS Flower: tannins, flavonoids, essential
oil, mucilage, triterpenes; berry: sugar, cytokinins,
vitamin C, bioflavonoids, anthocyanins, fruit acids.
ACTIONS Relaxant, antioxidant, adaptogen,
decongestant, diuretic, immune enhancing, alterative,
astringent, anti-inflammatory, antimicrobial, febrifuge.

Digestion • Flowers are antispasmodic and astringent to
the gut, protecting it against irritation and inflammation;
useful for heartburn, indigestion, gastritis, diarrhoea,
gastroenteritis, colic and wind.
Circulation • Anthocyanins in berries protect blood
vessel walls against oxidative stress, preventing vascular
disease. • Berries reduce harmful cholesterol and help
prevent atherosclerosis.
Mental and emotional • Flowers are calming and
soothing for tension, anxiety and depression. • Induces
sleep. • Berries increase resilience to stress.
Respiratory system • Hot infusion of flowers is
beneficial at the onset of colds, fevers, flu, tonsillitis and
laryngitis. • Decongestant and relaxant effects relieve
catarrh, bronchial congestion, asthma and tight coughs.
Immune system • Flowers and berries are antimicrobial
and decongestant. • Berries activate immunity by
increasing cytokine production[301] and prevent damage
caused by free radicals. Their proteins help regulate the
immune response. • Berries have antiviral action,
inhibiting colds and influenza A and B[302] and herpes
virus; may be helpful in HIV. • Berries have collagen-
stabilizing action, useful for varicose veins, haemorrhoids,
sprains and arthritis.
Urinary system • Flowers enhance kidney function,
relieve fluid retention and eliminate toxins and heat.
Externally • Used as a gargle for sore throats;
mouthwash for mouth ulcers and inflamed gums;
eyewash for conjunctivitis and sore, tired eyes.

CAUTION Leaves may cause a reaction in sensitive skins.
Avoid use of the root and bark.

Schisandra chinensis
Schisandra

Native to China, the red berries with their
five tastes are considered to balance all
bodily systems in Traditional Chinese
Medicine. Schisandra is famous as a tonic
to increase kidney 'jing', preserving
youth and beauty and enhancing energy
and immunity.

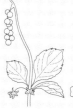

FAMILY Schisandraceae
PARTS USED Fruit, seed
CONSTITUENTS Dibenzo cycloactadiene lignans
(including gomisins and schizandrol), volatile oils,
vitamins A,C and E, organic acids (oleic, linoleic, linolenic
and palmitic).
ACTIONS Adaptogen, antibacterial, antidepressant,
antitussive, aphrodisiac, antioxidant, anti-inflammatory,
astringent, antiasthmatic, hepatotonic, immune tonic,
rejuvenative, hypoglycaemic, nervine, sedative.

Digestion • Lignans in the seeds have liver-protective
properties against chemical toxins. • Besides hepatitis
and other liver ailments, Schisandra is also helpful in
intestinal infections including chronic gastritis.
Circulation • Reduces nervous palpitations, improves
blood flow through coronary arteries and protects the
heart from ischaemic damage[303].
Mental and emotional • Increases energy, endurance
and resilience to stress. • Prevents altitude sickness.
• Used for depletion from stress, chronic fatigue
syndrome, anxiety, depression, irritability, dizziness and
Ménière's disease. • Anticonvulsive; may help in
Parkinson's disease. • Improves memory and
concentration. • Helpful in neuralgia, insomnia and
nervous palpitations.
Respiratory system • Boosts immunity, reduces
allergies and moistens lungs; used in chronic coughs and
allergic asthma.
Immune system • Prevents damage from free radicals.
• Improves liver regeneration and recovery after
hepatitis. Enhances glutathione protection in the liver,
stimulates glycogen and protein synthesis and may
protect against liver cancer[304]. • Stimulates production
of interferon and lymphocytes[305]. • Anti-inflammatory.
Reproductive system • Relieves night sweats, frequent
urination, low libido, spermatorrhoea, premature
ejaculation and low sperm count. • Enhances fertility.

CAUTION Avoid in pregnancy and epilepsy.

Scutellaria baicalensis
Baikal skullcap

A small perennial, native
to Siberia, Russia, North China,
Mongolia and Japan, it is used in
Traditional Chinese and Tibetan
medicine to clear 'damp heat', and
as a strengthening nerve and
immune tonic.

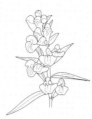

FAMILY Lamiaceae
PARTS USED Root
CONSTITUENTS Flavones, flavone glycosides (including
baicalein, wogonin and scutellarein).
ACTIONS Antihistamine, antioxidant, anti-inflammatory,
sedative, antitumour, anticlotting agent, vasodilator,
antibacterial, diuretic, febrifuge, choleretic, nervine.

Digestion • Clears heat from the gut in bowel infections,
diarrhoea and dysentery, and is indicated in chronic
hepatitis and other liver problems.
Urinary system • Antiseptic diuretic for urinary tract
infections, dysuria and haematuria.
Circulation • Protective effect on the heart and
circulation. Dilates peripheral arteries, reduces blood
pressure and prevents clots.
Mental and emotional • Energizing nerve tonic and
sedative for depletion from stress, anxiety, convulsions,
cramps and nervous heart conditions.
Immune system • Antihistamine for allergies including
eczema, asthma, hay fever, urticaria and rhinitis. Inhibits
release of histamine from mast cells. • Useful for
autoimmune problems such as rheumatoid arthritis and
lupus. • Antibacterial against a wide range of infecting
organisms including *Staphylococcus aureus*,
Pseudomonas aeruginosa and *Streptococcus pneumoniae*.
Has an affinity with the respiratory, urinary and digestive
tracts. • Reduces fevers.
Reproductive system • Traditionally used to prevent
miscarriage.
Eyes • Clears soreness and inflammation associated with
'liver heat'[306].

Scutellaria laterifolia
Skullcap

An attractive perennial
with a pretty blue flower
indigenous to North
America, and found
growing in damp places
and meadows. It was
traditionally used to treat
nervous disorders and
infertility, and to dampen
down unwanted sexual desires.

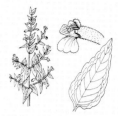

FAMILY Lamiaceae
PARTS USED Aerial parts
CONSTITUENTS Flavonoid glycosides (including
scutellarin), volatile oil, diterpenoids, bitters, tannins,
linoleic, oleic and palmitic acids, phenols, B vitamins,
minerals (iron, silica, calcium, potassium, magnesium).
ACTIONS Antispasmodic, nervine, anticonvulsant,
anaphrodisiac, anodyne, astringent, brain tonic, diuretic,
emmenagogue, febrifuge.

Digestion • Bitter tonic. Enhances appetite and digestion
and stimulates liver function. • Reduces spasm and colic;
relieves wind and bloating and nervous stomachaches.
Mental and emotional • Rich in nutrients essential to
a healthy nervous system. • Helpful in anxiety, tension,
muscle pain, obsessive compulsive disorder and panic
attacks. • Scutellarin enhances the production of
endorphins; lifts depression, dispels tiredness and
nervous exhaustion and promotes sleep. • May help
rebuild myelin sheath and benefit MS[307]. • Recommended
for addiction, when withdrawing from orthodox
tranquillizers and antidepressants. • Relieves pain in
tension headaches, neuralgia, period pain and arthritis.
• Improves memory and concentration; useful in ADD.
• Antispasmodic; used for twitching muscles, facial tics,
tremors, Parkinson's disease, restless leg syndrome,
epilepsy (petit and grand mal), cramps and palpitations.
Urinary system • Diuretic; aids elimination of excess
fluid and toxins via the kidneys. Useful in cystitis and
irritable bladder where there is a nervous component.
Reproductive system • Antispasmodic for period pain.
• Combined with hormone-balancing herbs such as Wild
yam and Vitex, useful for PMS and menopausal irritability,
depression and mood swings. • Traditionally used for
excess libido.

Serenoa repens
Saw palmetto

A small plant bearing dark blue-black berries native to North America. Its benefits were first discovered by farmers who observed that animals that fed on the berries looked healthy despite the summer drought. In humans it increases strength and energy.

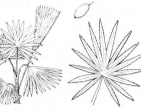

FAMILY Arecaceae
PARTS USED Berry
CONSTITUENTS Fatty acids (including caprylic, oleic, linoleic, linolenic and palmitic), polysaccharides, phytosterols (beta-sitosterol and campesterol), resins.
ACTIONS Anti-inflammatory, adaptogen, rejuvenative, anabolic, antiandrogenic, decongestant, diuretic, nutritive, digestive, demulcent, antitumour, antibacterial, immunostimulant, hypocholesterolaemic, aphrodisiac.

Digestion • Enhances appetite and digestion. Used for anorexia, diarrhoea and gall bladder problems.
Mental and emotional • Reduces tension; increases resilience to stress and induces sleep.
Respiratory system • Soothes irritation and resolves infection. • Expectorant, clears catarrh. • Used in whooping cough, laryngitis, chronic coughs, TB, bronchitis and asthma[308].
Immune system • A tonic to increase strength and weight. • Adaptogenic; enhances immunity and endurance. Used for frequent infections and allergies.
Urinary system • Soothing diuretic; relieves cystitis, irritable bladder, infections and incontinence. • Clears toxins and helps resolve skin problems.
Reproductive system • Tonic for low libido, low sperm count and erectile dysfunction. • Inhibits prolactin; may suppress milk flow in nursing mothers. • Specific for benign prostatic hypertrophy; improves the flow of urine, relieves pain, reduces swelling and inhibits further growth of the prostate by increasing breakdown of dihydrotestosterone (DHT) without affecting prostate-specific antigen (PSA) readings[309]. Reduces inflammation in prostatitis, orchitis and epididymitis. • Used with Vitex for polycystic ovaries, hirsutism, acne and in fertility problems related to excess androgens.

CAUTION Avoid when breast-feeding.

Smilax ornata
Sarsaparilla

A climbing vine native to South and Central America, the Caribbean and parts of Asia. It was famous among pirates as an antimicrobial and cleansing remedy for venereal disease.

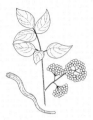

FAMILY Smilacaceae
PARTS USED Rhizome
CONSTITUENTS Steroidal saponins, phytosterols (including beta- and e-sitosterol), starch, resin, sarsapic acid, minerals.
ACTIONS Alterative, antimicrobial, anti-inflammatory, antiseptic, antitumour, aphrodisiac, astringent, carminative, cholagogue, demulcent, diaphoretic, diuretic, hepatoprotective, rejuvenative, stimulant, digestive, tonic, antirheumatic.

Digestion • Supports and protects the liver. • Reduces oxidative load in the bowel[310]. • Nutritive; increases the body's metabolic processes.
Mental and emotional • Strengthening tonic for debility and depression, especially in menopause.
Musculoskeletal system • Increases muscle mass and improves strength and athletic performance. • Diuretic properties help clear excess uric acid helpful in gout and arthritis.
Immune system • Antimicrobial, anti-inflammatory and detoxifying. • Steroidal saponins bind to toxins in the gut and inhibit their absorption. Beneficial in autoimmune problems such as psoriasis, rheumatoid arthritis and ulcerative colitis, which can be associated with toxicity[311]. • Saponins have antibiotic activity[312]. May help leptospirosis and syphilis[313].
Urinary system • Diuretic; clears toxins via the kidneys. Recommended for infections, stones, renal colic, bed-wetting and urinary incontinence.
Reproductive system • Tonic and aphrodisiac for low libido, impotence and erectile dysfunction[314]. • Regulates menstrual cycle. Used for menorrhagia, menstrual cramps, ovarian cysts, pelvic inflammatory disease, PMS and infertility. • Helpful during menopause for hot flushes and night sweats.
Skin • Anti-inflammatory and detoxifying. Useful in eczema and psoriasis; relieves itching and dryness.

CAUTION Avoid during pregnancy.
Drug interactions Avoid with warfarin[315].

Solidago virgaurea
Goldenrod

A perennial with bright
yellow flowers native to
North America. It was
traditionally used to stop
bleeding and heal wounds.

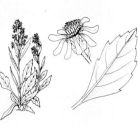

FAMILY Asteraceae
PARTS USED Aerial parts
CONSTITUENTS Flavonoids (quercitin, rutin,
isoquercitrin and astragalin), saponins, diterpenes,
phenolic glycosides, inulin, leiocarposide, salicylic acid,
essential oil, tannins.
ACTIONS Analgesic, anthelmintic, anticatarrhal,
antifungal, anti-inflammatory, antioxidant, antiseptic,
astringent, carminative, decongestant, diaphoretic,
diuretic, expectorant, haemostatic, hepatic, hypotensive,
alterative, stimulant, vulnerary.

Digestion • Astringent, antispasmodic and antiseptic;
useful for maintaining gut flora and treating candida,
wind, colic, indigestion, diarrhoea, gastroenteritis,
nausea, peptic ulcers and worms. • Stimulates bile flow
from the liver; used for liver problems and gallstones.
Circulation • Reduces blood pressure.
Respiratory system • Decongestant, expectorant and
antimicrobial; helps combat infection in throat infections,
colds, flu, catarrh, sinusitis, middle ear infections,
catarrhal deafness, hay fever[316], coughs and bronchitis.
Also used in asthma.
Immune system • Astringent and antimicrobial;
combats infection in the digestive, respiratory and
urinary tracts. • Anti-inflammatory and analgesic; can be
helpful in rheumatoid and osteoarthritis[317].
Urinary system • Antiseptic diuretic; aids elimination of
toxins; useful in gout, inflammatory problems, cystitis,
acute and chronic urinary tract infections, bed-wetting,
bladder weakness and incontinence. • Helps dissolve
kidney and bladder stones[318].
Reproductive system • Used for benign prostate
enlargement. • Regulates the menstrual cycle, relieves
menstrual cramps and heavy and irregular periods[319].
Externally • Poultice/compress/lotion used for arthritis,
boils, burns, fungal infections, eczema, swellings and
wounds. • Gargle used for sore throat, laryngitis and
candida; and mouthwash for toothache.

CAUTION Avoid in oedema from heart or kidney failure and
in known allergy.

Stachys betonica (also known as *Betonica officinalis*)
Wood betony

Native to Europe, Wood betony
grows wild in hedgerows and
meadows and is a specific for
headaches. Traditionally, it was
taken internally, smoked and
powdered for snuff and mixed
with Eyebright to clear congestion from colds.

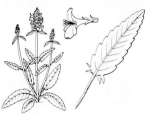

FAMILY Lamiaceae
PARTS USED Aerial parts
CONSTITUENTS Tannins, saponins, alkaloids
(betonicine, stachydrine and trigonelline), betonicine,
stachydrine, trigonellin, betaine, choline, tannins.
ACTIONS Digestive, circulatory stimulant, nerve tonic,
sedative, vulnerary, astringent, liver tonic, anthelmintic,
antiseptic, carminative, cholagogue, diuretic,
emmenagogue, expectorant.

Digestion • Enhances appetite and digestion. • Astringent
tannins protect the gut lining from inflammation and
infection. • Used for indigestion, colic, wind, heartburn,
diarrhoea and parasites. • Reduces liver and gall bladder
problems. • Trigonellin lowers blood sugar; useful for
diabetes.
Mental and emotional • Tonic and sedative to nerves.
Relieves pain, particularly in trigeminal neuralgia and
sciatica. • Reduces tension and anxiety; lifts depression.
• Improves circulation to the head, stimulates liver
function and reduces tension; specific for headaches
whether from poor circulation, a sluggish liver or tension.
• Improves memory and concentration. • Traditionally
used for convulsions and nervous palpitations.
Respiratory system • Astringent and antiseptic. • In hot
tea it stimulates the circulation and helps throw off colds,
catarrh, sinusitis and coughs.
Urinary system • Diuretic; aids elimination of toxins and
excess uric acid, helpful in gout and arthritis.
Reproductive system • Relieves period pain and PMS.
• Stimulates uterine muscle, brings on delayed periods.
• Relaxing for menopausal flushes, insomnia and depression.
Externally • Stems bleeding, speeds repair and inhibits
infection of cuts and wounds, ulcers, varicose veins and
haemorrhoids. • Lotions/creams used for bruises, sprains
and strains. • Draws splinters and thorns. • Traditionally
taken as snuff for nosebleeds and headaches.

CAUTION Avoid during pregnancy.

Stellaria media
Chickweed

Native to Eurasia, Chickweed is highly nutritious and considered a delicacy in Europe. Eaten in salads and cooked like spinach it acts as a blood tonic for the spring and during convalescence. It is thought to improve eyesight, as it is rich in vitamin A.

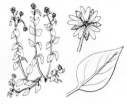

FAMILY Caryophyllaceae
PARTS USED Aerial parts
CONSTITUENTS Saponins, mucilage, copper, tin, potash salts, iron, vitamins A, C, thiamine, riboflavin, niacin, minerals (calcium, phosphorus, iron, magnesium, sodium, potassium and zinc).
ACTIONS Demulcent, refrigerant, anti-inflammatory, diuretic, astringent, carminative, depurative, emmenagogue, expectorant, galactogogue, laxative, ophthalmic, vulnerary.

Digestion • Soothing aid to digestion and laxative. Relieves wind, constipation, inflammatory problems such as gastritis, colitis, acid indigestion, irritable bowel syndrome. Clears excess heat in the liver and gall bladder.
Respiratory system • Expectorant and soothing; helpful in sore throats, laryngitis, bronchitis, asthma, harsh dry coughs and pleurisy. • Reduces fevers and thirst.
Urinary system • Soothing diuretic; relieves fluid retention, cystitis and irritable bladder. • Aids the elimination of toxins via the kidneys, which helps skin problems and arthritis. • Traditional remedy for obesity.
Reproductive system • Traditionally a post-partum blood purifier. • Promotes milk flow in nursing mothers.
Skin • Excellent cooling remedy for inflammatory skin conditions such as eczema, heat rashes, urticaria, sunburn, boils and spots.
Externally • A specific for itchy skin conditions including eczema, roseola, fragile superficial veins, burns, scalds, ulcers, piles and abscesses. • Healing for wounds, and ulcers. • Expressed juice is used as an eyewash for inflammatory eye problems. • Poultice and strong infusions added to baths reduce inflammation and encourage tissue repair. • Helps bring poisons and pus to the surface.

CAUTION Excess doses can cause diarrhoea and vomiting. Avoid in pregnancy and breast-feeding.

Symphytum officinale
Comfrey

Comfrey is native to Europe and western Asia, growing wild in damp meadows and by streams. It is highly valued for its ability to promote the repair of wounds, ulcers and broken bones.

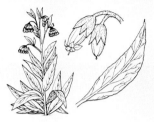

FAMILY Boraginaceae
PARTS USED Root (external use only), leaf
CONSTITUENTS Mucilage (mucopolysaccharides), gums, tannins, allantoin, inulin, resin, rosmarinic acid, pyrrolizidine alkaloids, essential oil, beta-sitosterol, triterpenes, silicic acid, calcium, iron, potassium, amino acids, vitamin B12, zinc.
ACTIONS Demulcent, emollient, haemostatic, nutritive, refrigerant, vulnerary, expectorant, astringent, pectoral tonic, alterative, anti-inflammatory.

Digestion • Mucilage soothes irritation and inflammation. • Astringent tannins stop bleeding and protect surfaces against inflammation and infection. • Cooling and soothing remedy for heartburn, gastritis, peptic ulcers, diarrhoea and ulcerative colitis. • Rich in nutrients, nourishing and restorative.
Respiratory system • Mucilage soothes irritation; relieves sore throats, laryngitis, tonsillitis, pleurisy, harsh, irritating coughs, bronchitis, whooping cough and asthma. • Rosmarinic acid decreases microvascular pulmonary injury.
Musculoskeletal system • Allantoin is a remarkable cell proliferant; stimulates the production of cells responsible for forming collagen and connective tissue, cartilage and bone and speeds repair in injury. Excellent for broken or fractured bones. • Rosmarinic acid decreases inflammation. Reduces pain and swelling in arthritis, gout, carpal tunnel syndrome, tendonitis, sprains and strains.
Urinary system • Soothes mucous membranes; relieves cystitis and irritable bladder.
Externally • Promotes wound healing and tissue regeneration. Prime first-aid remedy for healing cuts, wounds, bruises, burns, scalds, sunburn and ulcers, with minimal scar formation. Soothing and rejuvenating to dry, sore, scarred and wrinkled skin.

CAUTION Avoid root for internal use. Avoid use on broken skin and during pregnancy.

Tabebuia impetiginosa
Pau d'arco

An evergreen flowering tree native to Brazil and Argentina, famous as a strengthening tonic and immune enhancer, for fighting infection and preventing cancer.

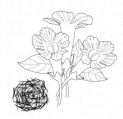

FAMILY Bignoniaceae
PARTS USED Inner bark
CONSTITUENTS Quinine compounds (naphthaquinones, lapachol, beta-lapachone, xyloidine and deoxylapachol), anthroquinone tabeuin, furonaphthoquinones.
ACTIONS Immune enhancing, antitumour, antioxidant, antimicrobial, antiparasitic, laxative, antimalarial, antischistosomal, anti-inflammatory, anticoagulant.

Digestion • Antimicrobial for infections associated with diarrhoea, dysentery and peptic ulcers. Combats intestinal parasites and candida[320]. • Beneficial action on the liver. • Reduces blood sugar; indicated in diabetes[321]. • Reduces inflammation; useful in gastritis, ulcers, acidity, colitis and enteritis. • Laxative.
Circulation • Increases oxygen supply to the body by enhancing blood and lymphatic circulation and red blood cell production[322]. Used for anaemia, lymphatic congestion and hypertension.
Respiratory system • Enhances immunity; wards off infections, fevers, colds, flu, coughs, bronchitis and chest infections. • Relaxes bronchi in asthma.
Musculoskeletal system • Anti-inflammatory and depurative for arthritis, osteomyelitis, rheumatism, lupus and rheumatism.
Immune system • Antibacterial, antifungal and antiviral; helpful in herpes, flu and colds[323]. • Lapachol, beta-lapachone and xyloidine all show activity against candida. • Lapachol has antioxidant, anticoagulant, antiviral, anti-inflammatory, antibacterial, antimalarial and anticancer properties[324]. • May inhibit the growth of tumours by preventing cancer cells from using oxygen[325]. • Useful for allergies and chronic fatigue. • Lapachol and beta-lapachone have antibacterial action[326].
Skin • Helpful in skin disease, including eczema, psoriasis, ulcers[327], infections, candida, athlete's foot, herpes, impetigo, boils and acne.
Externally • Applied to skin infections, eczema, psoriasis, cuts and sores and skin cancers.
CAUTION Avoid in pregnancy and blood-clotting disorders.
Drug interactions Avoid with anticoagulants.

Tanacetum parthenium
(also known as *Pyrethrum parthenium* and *Chrysanthemum parthenium*)
Feverfew

An attractive perennial with aromatic leaves and daisy flowers that are loved by bees. So named because of its ability to bring down fevers. It is an excellent remedy for headaches and migraine. As prevention the leaves can be eaten daily in a sandwich or with other food.

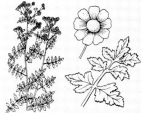

FAMILY Asteraceae
PARTS USED Aerial parts
CONSTITUENTS Sesquiterpene lactones, volatile oils, tannins, bitter resin, pyrethrin.
ACTIONS Diaphoretic, relaxant, uterine stimulant, anti-inflammatory, antihistamine, digestive bitter, nerve tonic, analgesic, depurative, decongestant, cholagogue.

Digestion • Enhances appetite and digestion and allays nausea and vomiting. • Clears heat and toxins. • Bitter liver tonic. • Reduces symptoms associated with sluggish liver, such as lethargy, irritability, headaches and migraines.
Mental and emotional • Nerve tonic; relaxes tension, lifts depression and promotes sleep. • Relieves nerve pain in shingles, trigeminal neuralgia and sciatica. • Used for oversensitivity to pain, irritability and anger. • Traditionally used for convulsions and fretful children.
Respiratory system • Hot infusion increases perspiration and reduces fevers. It is decongestant and clears catarrh and sinusitis. • Used for asthma, migraine and other allergies such as hay fever due to its sesquiterpene lactones, which inhibit the release of prostaglandins and histamine. • Indicated in dizziness and tinnitus.
Musculoskeletal system • Clears toxins and heat; useful anti-inflammatory for arthritis.
Externally • The fresh plant is used on insect stings and bites to relieve pain and swelling. • Dilute tincture can be used as a lotion to repel insects and for spots and boils.

CAUTION Avoid during pregnancy. The fresh leaves may cause mouth ulcers.

Taraxacum officinale
Dandelion

Dandelion is a native of many parts of Europe and Asia. The young leaves are traditionally eaten in the spring as a bitter detoxifying tonic to cleanse the body of wastes from the heavy, clogging food and more sedentary habits of winter.

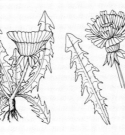

FAMILY Asteraceae
PARTS USED Leaf, root
CONSTITUENTS Terpenoids, acids (chlorogenic and caffeic), carbohydrates, vitamins A, C and B complex, minerals (potassium, zinc and manganese), phytosterols, flavonoid glycosides.
ACTIONS Digestive, bitter tonic, diuretic, mild laxative, cholagogue, depurative, anti-inflammatory, antilithic.

Digestion • Bitter digestive and liver tonic; enhances appetite and digestion, increases the flow of digestive juices and aids absorption. • Supports the liver as a major detoxifying organ; recommended in liver and gall bladder problems, hepatitis and problems associated with sluggish liver such as tiredness, irritability, headaches and skin problems. • The root is mildly laxative.
Immune system • The root is anti-inflammatory[328]; used for arthritis and rheumatism. • May increase insulin secretion from the pancreas; helpful in diabetes.
Urinary system • The leaves are diuretic; useful in water retention, cellulite and urinary tract infections. Their high potassium content replaces that lost through increased urination. • Dissolve stones and gravel. • Improves the elimination of uric acid; useful remedy for gout.
Skin • Detoxifying bitter tonic, increasing the elimination of toxins and wastes through the liver and kidneys, cleansing the blood and clearing the skin. For spots, acne, boils and abscesses.
Externally • White juice from the stems can be applied to warts. • Infusion of the leaves and flowers is used for skin complaints.

CAUTION Avoid in obstruction of bile ducts and gall bladder[329]. Milky latex in the leaves can cause dermatitis.

Thymus vulgaris
Thyme

An intensely aromatic small evergreen shrub native to the Mediterranean, found growing wild on warm, dry, rocky banks and heaths. It is widely cultivated for its powerful antiseptic properties.

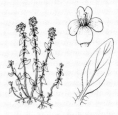

FAMILY Lamiaceae
PARTS USED Flowering aerial parts
CONSTITUENTS Tannins, bitters, essential oil, terpenes, flavonoids, saponins.
ACTIONS Antispasmodic, astringent, digestive, antiseptic, antibacterial, decongestant, circulatory stimulant, relaxant, immunostimulant, antioxidant.

Digestion • Enhances appetite and digestion and stimulates the liver. Used for indigestion, poor appetite, anaemia, liver and gall bladder complaints. • Flavonoids have relaxing effects and relieve wind, colic, IBS and spastic colon. • Astringent tannins protect the gut from irritation and reduce diarrhoea. • Antiseptic oils fight infections and help re-establish gut flora after antibiotics.
Circulation • Warming stimulant; prevents chilblains and combats the effects of cold in winter.
Mental and emotional • Strengthening tonic for physical and mental exhaustion. • Relieves tension, anxiety and depression. • Increases concentration and memory.
Respiratory system • For colds, sore throats, flu and chest infections, such as bronchitis, pneumonia and pleurisy. • Relieves asthma and whooping cough. • Expectorant action increases the production of mucous.
Immune system • Volatile oils have powerful antibacterial and antifungal effects. They support the body's fight against infections, particularly in the respiratory, digestive and genitourinary systems. • Anti-inflammatory, possibly by inhibition of prostaglandin synthesis[330]. • Antioxidant, protecting against degenerative problems. Increases longevity. • Increases perspiration and reduces fevers.
Urinary system • Diuretic; relieves water retention.
Reproductive system • Antispasmodic for dysmenorrhea. • Antimicrobial for infections such as candida and salpingitis.
Externally • Used in liniments for aching joints, muscular pain and to disinfect cuts and wounds. • Gargle used for sore throats; and douche for vaginal infections.

CAUTION Avoid large amounts in pregnancy.

Tilia europaea (also known as *T. americana* and *T. cordata*)
Lime flower

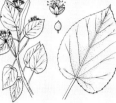

A deciduous tree native to Europe, western Asia and North America with a profusion of creamy flowers that smell like honey and are loved by bees. They make a delicious tea to reduce anxiety and fevers.

FAMILY Tiliaceae
PARTS USED Flower
CONSTITUENTS Essential oil (farnesol), tannins, flavonoids (hesperidin, quercitrin and kaempferol), mucilage, phenols (caffeic acid).
ACTIONS Antispasmodic, thymoleptic, cholagogue, emollient, expectorant, hypotensive, nervine, sedative, stomachic, vasodilator, demulcent, diaphoretic, diuretic, ophthalmic, vermifuge (root).

Digestion • Soothes and relaxes the gut; for digestive complaints associated with anxiety such as wind, colic, indigestion, diarrhoea, heartburn and acidity. • Roots act as a vermifuge for worms.
Circulation • Antispasmodic; opens the arteries, reduces hypertension. • Protects blood vessel walls by reducing cholesterol build-up and hardening of the arteries. • Useful for migraine. • Diaphoretic; increases blood flow to the periphery. Reduces fevers. • A decoction of the roots and the bark has been used in the treatment of internal haemorrhaging.
Mental and emotional • Antispasmodic and sedative; relieves tension, anxiety, insomnia, pain, nervous headaches, migraine, restlessness and agitation. Calms exam nerves.
Respiratory system • Decongestant and soothing expectorant for feverish colds, flu, catarrh, irritating coughs, bronchitis and asthma.
Urinary system • Soothing diuretic; clears toxins via the kidneys, relieves cystitis, urethritis and frequent urination due to nerves.
Externally • Infusion of leaves used as an eyewash; poultice for burns and scalds. • Infusion of the flowers is applied to spots, acne, boils, burns and rashes to clear heat and irritation. • Gargle used for mouth ulcers.
• Added to baths to calm restless children.

CAUTION Large doses may cause nausea. Excess use may damage the heart.

Tinospora cordifolia
Guduchi

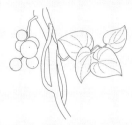

A vigorous creeper that grows in the forests of India. A renowned rejuvenative in Ayurvedic medicine, it is best when growing through neem trees, as their combined properties are strengthening and detoxifying.

FAMILY Menispermaceae
PARTS USED Stem, leaf
CONSTITUENTS Beta-sitosterol, alkaloids (including berberine and tinosporin), bitters, glycosides, diterpenes.
ACTIONS Adaptogen, digestive, astringent, anti-fungal, rejuvenative, alterative, diuretic, cholagogue, anti-inflammatory, antioxidant, probiotic, vermifuge.

Digestion • Enhances energy by improving appetite, digestion and absorption. • Reduces inflammation in acidity, gastritis, peptic ulcers, nausea and vomiting.
• Re-establishes gut flora. Dispels worms. Antifungal; helpful in candida. • Relieves constipation and clears toxins. • Used for chronic hepatitis and toxic damage. Aids liver tissue regeneration. • Stabilizes blood sugar.
Circulation • Reduces bleeding tendency such as in bleeding gums and haemorrhoids. Useful in anaemia.
• Lowers harmful cholesterol.
Mental and emotional • Adaptogenic; increases resistance to emotional and physical stress. • Increases energy yet relaxes tension.
Respiratory system • Helps resolve infections and catarrhal congestion. Indicated in coughs, colds, flu, sinusitis and allergies such as hay fever and asthma.
Musculoskeletal system • Anti-inflammatory for joint problems; used for gout and with Ginger for arthritis.
Immune system • Antioxidant and antitumour activity; reduces side effects of radiotherapy and chemotherapy.
• Stimulates antibody production and macrophage function. Improves resistance to infection.
• Lowers fevers. • Take prior to surgery to improve resistance to infection and post-operative complication.
• Helps autoimmune problems such as psoriasis and systemic lupus erythematosus.
Urinary system • Aids elimination of uric acid; helpful for arthritis and gout.
Skin • Clears skin problems such as eczema and psoriasis.

CAUTION Excessive doses can inhibit B vitamin assimilation and can cause nausea.

Trifolium pratense
Red clover

A perennial native to Europe,
North America and western
Asia, found growing wild in
meadows. It is known as
a cleansing and immune-
enhancing remedy, and for
women's health problems.

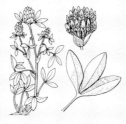

FAMILY Fabaceae
PARTS USED Flowering top
CONSTITUENTS Flavone glycosides, coumarins,
minerals (including calcium, iron, magnesium, sodium,
potassium, copper and zinc), saponins.
ACTIONS Alterative, antiscrophulous, antioxidant,
antispasmodic, aperient, antitumour, diuretic,
expectorant, sedative, oestrogenic.

Circulation • Helps prevent hypertension. Coumarins
may affect platelet activity and reduce lipids[331].
Respiratory system • Antispasmodic and expectorant
for catarrh, whooping cough, dry coughs, bronchitis
and asthma.
Immune system • Traditionally used as a detoxifying
herb for cancer of the breast, lung and lymphatic system.
Flavone glycosides have been shown to inhibit cancer by
inhibiting angiogenesis and cancer cell adhesion[332].
• Indicated in chronic degenerative diseases and
lymphatic congestion.
Musculoskeletal system • Beneficial to post-
menopausal women; may encourage calcium storage and
prevent osteoporosis. • Used for arthritis and gout.
Reproductive system • Flavone glycosides increase
follicle-stimulating hormones[333] and are oestrogenic;
useful for menopausal complaints such as hot flushes,
night sweats and insomnia. • Benefits lymphatic system;
helpful in mastitis. • Helps prevent prostate problems.
• Traditionally used for breast and ovarian cancer.
Skin • Clears toxins; helps resolve skin complaints,
especially eczema and psoriasis.
Externally • Poultices are applied to skin problems and
cancerous growths.

CAUTION Avoid in bleeding disorders, pregnancy and
breast-feeding. Diseased clover, even if no symptoms of
disease are visible, can contain toxic alkaloids.
Drug interactions Use with caution with anticoagulants
and contraceptives.

Trigonella foenum-graecum
Fenugreek

Fenugreek is a member of the
pea family and native to the
Mediterranean, Ukraine and India.
Highly nutritious, the seeds are
well known as a cooking spice
and are used in Africa as a
coffee substitute.

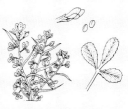

FAMILY Fabaceae
PARTS USED Seed
CONSTITUENTS Gallactomannans (including
mucilagin), pyridine alkaloids (including trigonelline,
gentianine and carpaine compounds), steroidal saponins
(including diosgenin, fenugreekine and tigogenin), fibre,
proteins, amino acids (including lysine and arginine),
flavonoids.
ACTIONS Digestive, laxative, demulcent, emollient,
nutritive, galactogogue, expectorant, cardiotonic,
diuretic, antiviral, antihypertensive, hypoglycaemic,
hypocholesterolaemic, oestrogenic.

Digestion • Enhances appetite, digestion and absorption.
• Mucilagin coats the gut lining, protecting it from irritation
and inflammation in gastritis, acid indigestion and peptic
ulcers. • Not absorbed, so adds fibre and acts as a bulk
laxative in constipation.• Possesses hypoglycaemic activity
by delaying gastric emptying, slowing carbohydrate
absorption and inhibiting glucose transport. It may also
increase insulin receptors in red blood cells and improve
glucose utilization in peripheral tissues.
Circulation • Lowers harmful cholesterol and
triglycerides. • Reduces blood pressure and inhibits
clotting; helps to prevent heart and arterial disease.
Respiratory system • Expectorant and immune-
enhancing for chronic coughs and bronchitis. • Antiviral.
Urinary system • Diuretic; aids elimination of toxins via
the kidneys.
Reproductive system • Diosgenin is used to create
semisynthetic forms of oestrogen. Can enlarge breast
size. • Reduces menopausal symptoms such as hot
flushes, night sweats, vaginal dryness and insomnia.
• Stimulates milk flow in nursing mothers.
Externally • Decoction used as a lotion for boils, ulcers
and eczema.

CAUTION Avoid in pregnancy.
Drug interactions Use with caution with antidiabetic and
anticoagulant drugs.

Trillium erectum
Beth root

A beautiful woodland plant native to North America, renowned among Native American tribes for lessening pain during childbirth and preventing post-partum bleeding.

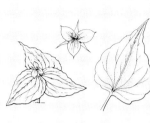

FAMILY Trilliaceae
PARTS USED Rhizome, root
CONSTITUENTS Steroidal saponins (diosgenin and trillarin), fixed oils, gum, volatile oils, tannins.
ACTIONS Astringent, partus praeparator, antiseptic, antifungal, uterine tonic, hormone regulator, antihaemorrhagic, alterative, expectorant.

Digestion • Astringent; tones and protects the gut lining, reducing inflammation and bleeding. Recommended in inflammatory bowel problems, diarrhoea, dysentery and bleeding.
Respiratory system • Astringent and expectorant; dries up excess secretions and reduces catarrh. Helpful in catarrhal coughs, asthma, chronic lung problems and haemoptysis.
Urinary system • Used for haematuria.
Reproductive system • Traditionally used to induce childbirth, stimulate contractions and reduce pain. • Regulates hormones and relieves menstrual problems. • Astringent; constricts blood vessels. Used for fibroids, heavy bleeding, dysfunctional uterine bleeding and post-partum haemorrhage. • Reduces perimenopausal flooding and menopausal symptoms. • Relieves sore nipples. • Aphrodisiac.
Externally • Lotion used to reduce bleeding speed, healing of ulcers, for inflammatory skin problems, haemorrhoids and varicose veins, tumours, insect bites and stings. • Antiseptic/antifungal douche used for vaginal infections such as candida and trichomonas; reduces discharges.

CAUTION Avoid during pregnancy and gastric reflux.
Drug interactions May decrease the effects of cardiac glycosides.

Turnera aphrodisiaca (also known as *T. diffusa*)
Damiana

A small shrub that grows throughout Mexico, Central America, the West Indies and South America. Recorded as an aphrodisiac as far back as the ancient Mayan civilization it has long been valued as a tonic for the hormonal and nervous systems.

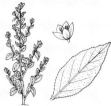

FAMILY Turneraceae
PARTS USED Aerial parts
CONSTITUENTS Volatile oils (including 1,8-cineole, p-cymene, alpha- and beta-pinene, thymol, alpha-copaene and calamene), tannins, flavonoids, beta-sitosterol, damianin, glycosides (gonzalitosin and arbutin).
ACTIONS Antispasmodic, thymoleptic, adaptogen, expectorant, astringent, digestive, laxative, bitter tonic, aphrodisiac, hypoglycaemic, sedative, tonic, diuretic.

Digestion • Reduces tension and spasm; for stress-related disorders, stomachache, colic, dyspepsia, peptic ulcers, diarrhoea and constipation. • Stimulates liver function and reduces blood sugar.
Mental and emotional • Nerve and brain tonic excellent for debility, headaches and convalescence. • Specific for anxiety and depression associated with sexual inadequacy. • Used for obsessive compulsive disorder, neurosis and paranoia. • Relieves excess mental activity and agitation.
Respiratory system • Astringent and expectorant; relieves colds, catarrh, coughs, asthma and bronchitis.
Urinary system • Antiseptic diuretic; soothes irritation; indicated in cystitis, fluid retention and infections. • Strengthens muscular control in incontinence and bed-wetting.
Reproductive system • Alkaloids have testosterone-like action. Used for impotence, erectile dysfunction, frigidity, anorgasmia, low libido, orchitis and spermatorrhea. • Used for dysmenorrhoea, menstrual headaches, acne, irregular periods, amenorrhoea and fertility problems. • Aids childbirth. • Useful during menopause for hot flushes, night sweats, insomnia and vaginal dryness.

CAUTION May interfere with iron absorption. Do not take with food. Avoid in pregnancy.
Drug interactions Use with caution with antidiabetic drugs.

Tussilago farfara
Coltsfoot

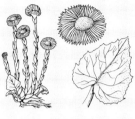

A perennial herb that grows throughout Europe, in North Africa and western and northern Asia in hedgerows, woodland and meadows. Its bright yellow flowers resembling dandelions appear before the leaves. It is famous as a remedy for respiratory problems, traditionally used in cough syrups or candied and sucked as a sweet.

FAMILY Asteraceae
PARTS USED Leaf, flower
CONSTITUENTS Flower: mucilage, triterpenes, carotene and other flavonoids, tannins, arnidiol, taraxanthin, pyrrolizidine alkaloids; leaf: zinc, magnesium, potassium, glycosidal, sitosterol, inulin.
ACTIONS Antispasmodic, anti-inflammatory, emollient, bronchodilator, demulcent, antitussive, diuretic, astringent, diaphoretic, expectorant, digestive.

Digestion • Improves digestion and appetite. Soothes irritation of the gut lining.
Respiratory system • Soothing, anti-inflammatory and expectorant for colds, catarrh, sore throats, tonsillitis, dry, persistent coughs, bronchitis and asthma. Particularly useful for relieving coughing in chronic emphysema and silicosis. • Rich in zinc it promotes tissue repair; indicated for susceptibility to coughs and chest infections due to damage to respiratory system following infection or from smoking. • Antispasmodic effects are helpful for relieving bronchospasm in asthma.
Immune system • Enhances immunity; helps resolve infection and prevents platelet aggregation[334].
Urinary system • Soothes irritation and inflammation; used for cystitis and urethritis.
Externally • Poultice of flowers soothes and promotes healing of skin disorders such as eczema, ulcers, sores, bites and other inflammation.

CAUTION Contains traces of liver-affecting pyrrolizidine alkaloids (largely destroyed when the plant is boiled to make a decoction). Potentially toxic in large doses. Take for a maximum of 28 days at a time. Avoid in liver disease, pregnancy and breast-feeding, and in children under 6.

Ulmus fulva (also known as *U. rubra*)
Slippery elm

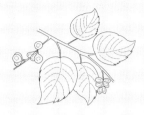

A handsome deciduous tree growing throughout Canada and the USA. The inner bark, collected from trees that are at least ten years old, was used by Native Americans to soothe an irritated digestive system and as a poultice for wounds and ulcers.

FAMILY Ulmaceae
PARTS USED Inner bark, generally as powder
CONSTITUENTS Mucilage (including polysaccharides, hexoses and pentosespolyuronide), tannins, calcium, chromium, iron, zinc, manganese, procyanidins, antioxidants.
ACTIONS Demulcent, emollient, nutritive, antitussive, antioxidant, anti-inflammatory, diuretic, expectorant, laxative, rejuvenative, vulnerary, probiotic.

Digestion • Polysaccharide molecules expand in water and create a gruel that coats the gut lining and soothes pain in inflammatory conditions, acid reflux, heartburn, nausea, gastritis, colitis, peptic ulcers, IBS, diverticulitis and leaky gut syndrome[335]. • Good bulk laxative for constipation. • Enhances growth of normal gut flora. • Nourishing food when weak, particularly good for infants and elderly, as it is easy to digest.
Respiratory system • Moistens and reduces heat irritation and inflammation in the throat and chest, relieves catarrh and dry coughs. • Traditionally used for bronchitis, pneumonia and pleurisy. • Relaxes throat and bronchi; used for sore throats, hoarseness, laryngitis, pharyngitis, asthma and whooping cough.
Musculoskeletal system • Rich in calcium for strengthening bones and promoting healing.
Immune system • Anti-inflammatory, enhances immunity. • Soothing and strengthening when recovering from illness or undergoing chemotherapy. Ingredient of the renowned anticancer formula Essiac.
Urinary system • Soothes the lining of the urinary tract; reduces pain and inflammation in cystitis and urethritis.
Externally • Used as a poultice for drawing out toxins in boils, abscesses and varicose ulcers. • Applied to wounds, burns and inflammation to reduce swelling and pain.

Drug interactions Separate from medicines taken by 2 hours; may inhibit absorption.

Uncaria tomentosa
Cat's claw

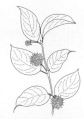

A climbing vine native to the Amazonian jungle, where it has been famous as a remedy for infections and inflammatory conditions as well as for contraception for centuries.

FAMILY Rubiaceae
PARTS USED Bark, root, leaf
CONSTITUENTS Pentacyclic and tetracyclic oxidole alkaloids, triterpenes, phytosterols, tannins, quercitrin, rutin, proanthocyanidins, catechin, polyphenols.
ACTIONS Immune enhancing, anti-inflammatory, hypotensive, antioxidant, antitumour, antimicrobial, depurative, diuretic, vermifuge.

Digestion • Strengthens the gut in Crohn's disease, inflammatory bowel disorders, diverticulitis and leaky gut syndrome[336]. • Used in gastritis, ulcers, diarrhoea, dysentery and candidiasis. • Enhances liver function.
Circulation • Inhibits blood platelet aggregation[337], strengthens blood vessels and helps prevent strokes.
Respiratory system • Gives immune support in asthma, bronchitis and hay fever.
Musculoskeletal system • Anti-inflammatory for osteo- and rheumatoid arthritis, lupus, bursitis and gout.
Immune system • Oxidole alkaloids stimulate immunity by enhancing the activity of phagocytes, macrophages, lymphocytes and leucocytes. Used for chronic immune deficiency and HIV[338], chronic fatigue, allergies and tendency to infections[339]. • Slows growth of leukaemia cells[340]. Used as a complement to cancer treatments[341]; protects against the effects of radiation and chemotherapy. • Combats bacterial and viral infections such as shingles; reduces fevers. • Traditionally used for deep wounds, abscesses and cysts.
Urinary system • Used for urinary tract infections.
Reproductive system • Regulates the menstrual cycle; relieves PMS. • Helpful in prostatitis.
Eyes • Reduces inflammatory problems such as conjunctivitis and iritis.
Externally • Lotions/creams used for acne, herpes, shingles, athlete's foot, haemorrhoids and cuts. • Eye lotion used for conjunctivitis.

CAUTION Avoid in pregnancy.
Drug interactions Use cautiously with immunosuppressive drugs.

Urtica dioica (also known as *U. urens*)
Nettle

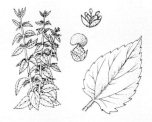

This much maligned perennial grows throughout Europe, Asia, North Africa and North America. It is highly nutritious, rich in vitamins A and C, and minerals.

FAMILY Urticaceae
PARTS USED Aerial parts of young plants, root, seed
CONSTITUENTS Amines (including histamine, 5-hydro xytryptamine and serotonin), minerals (including potassium, iron and calcium), rutin, quercetin, malic acid, formic acid, chlorophyll.
ACTIONS Alterative, astringent, haemostatic, diuretic, galactogogue, blood building, antihistamine.

Digestion • Astringent tannins protect the gut lining from irritation and infection. • Relieves diarrhoea and flatulence. • Stimulates liver and kidney function and clears toxins. • Reduces blood sugar. • Seeds improve thyroid function and reduce goitre.
Respiratory system • Clears catarrh in coughs, bronchitis, hay fever and asthma. • Seeds /fresh juice used for fevers and lung disorders.
Immune system • Detoxifying. • Antihistamine for allergies such as asthma and hay fever. • Flavonoids have immunostimulatory effects. • Antibacterial activity against *Staphylococcus aureus* and *S. albus*.
Reproductive system • Stimulates milk production in nursing mothers. • Regulates periods and reduces heavy bleeding. • Rich in iron.
Urinary system • Diuretic; relieves fluid retention, cystitis and urethritis. • Softens stones and gravel. • Helps prevent bed-wetting and incontinence. • Enhances excretion of uric acid; good for gout and arthritis. • Root used for benign prostatic hypertrophy.
Skin • Depurative and anti-inflammatory; clears skin in eczema, urticaria and other chronic skin problems.
Externally • Fresh juice/tea used for cuts, wounds, haemorrhoids, burns and scalds, bites/stings, including nettle sting. • Fresh nettles used to sting skin to stimulate the circulation and used for poor peripheral circulation and for pain and swelling in arthritis.

CAUTION Avoid in oedema from impaired cardiac or renal function.
Drug interactions Avoid with diuretics and antihypertensives.

Vaccinium myrtillus
Blueberry/Bilberry

A perennial shrub, native to Europe, bearing black shiny berries, which are a potent source of antioxidants. These reduce free radicals, helping to slow the ageing process and aiding the prevention of degenerative disease and cancer.

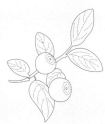

FAMILY Ericaceae
PARTS USED Fruit, leaf
CONSTITUENTS Flavonoids (more than 15 anthocyanosides), catechins, invertose.
ACTIONS Antioxidant, anti-inflammatory, astringent, vasoprotective, antispasmodic, diuretic, rejuvenative.

Digestion • Increases gastric mucous. Reduces inflammation of the stomach and intestinal lining, and protects the gut lining against excess acid. • Leaves are a traditional remedy for diabetes (rich in chromium), diarrhoea, vomiting, typhoid and stomach cramps[342]. • Berries reduce blood sugar and are mildly laxative and astringent; relieve both constipation and diarrhoea.
Circulation • Antioxidant; enhances circulation and protects arteries from free radical damage. Useful in Raynaud's disease, capillary fragility, bleeding gums, spider veins, haemorrhoids, varicose veins and venous insufficiency. • Anthocyanosides stabilize collagen and help rebuild capillaries. • Reduces platelet aggregation, prevents clots and protects against heart attacks and strokes without the risk of increased bleeding. • Useful to prevent and treat atherosclerosis.
Musculoskeletal system • Antioxidant and anti-inflammatory, stabilizes collagen; helpful in arthritis.
Urinary system • Anti-inflammatory; and diuretic used for bladder infections and stones.
Reproductive system • Antispasmodic; relieves dysmenorrhoea.
Eyes • Enhances circulation to the eyes, improves eyesight. • Antioxidant action prevents free radical damage that can cause cataracts and macular degeneration. • Used for diabetic or hypertensive retinopathy; strengthens collagen and protects eye tissue against glaucoma and eyestrain. • Regenerates rhodopsin, a pigment found in the retina that is vital to good night vision[343].
Externally • Promotes healing; useful after surgery. • Mouthwash used for inflammation of the mouth and gums; gargle for sore throats.

Valeriana officinalis
Valerian

A perennial wild plant with pretty pink flowers native to Europe, Asia and North America. The root is highly pungent with a smell that is disliked by many but loved by cats and apparently by rats, as it is said that the Pied Piper of Hamelin lured the rats away with Valerian.

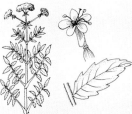

FAMILY Valerianaceae
PARTS USED Root, rhizome
CONSTITUENTS Volatile oils, valepotriates, valerianic acid, glycosides, alkaloids, choline, tannins, resins.
ACTIONS Anxiolytic, sedative, hypnotic, anodyne, anthelmintic, antibacterial, antispasmodic, astringent, bitter, carminative, diaphoretic, diuretic, hypotensive, nervine, restorative, stomachic, tonic.

Digestion • Antispasmodic and sedative. Relaxes tension and spasm in stress-related problems such as dyspepsia, intestinal colic and IBS.
Circulation • Lowers blood pressure. • Increases blood flow to the heart[344]. • Calms nervous palpitations.
Mental and emotional • Well-known sedative and nerve tonic; valepotriates are mainly responsible for its calming effects. Excellent for anxiety, nervous tension, agitation, panic attacks, irritability, insomnia, nervous headaches and exhaustion. • Strengthens and calms the heart. Relieves nervous palpitations. • Relaxing to smooth muscle; useful for stress-related disorders such as muscle tension, colic, IBS, period pain and headaches. • Useful in treatment of addiction (tobacco or tranquillizer), chronic aggression and ADD. • Historically an esteemed remedy for epilepsy, hysteria, convulsions, migraine, headaches and most nerve problems; used in World War I for shell shock and nerve strain caused by air raids.
Respiratory system • Antispasmodic for paroxysmal coughs and croup.
Reproductive system • Antispasmodic for period pain.

CAUTION Avoid prolonged use. Excessive doses may cause headaches, muscle spasm, insomnia or palpitations.

Verbascum thapsus
Mullein

This impressive biennial, with tall spikes of yellow flowers is native to Europe, Asia and North Africa. Its downy leaves and flowers make soothing medicine for irritating coughs and for relieving pain in ear infections.

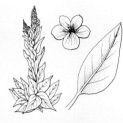

FAMILY Scrophulariaceae
PARTS USED Leaf, flower, root
CONSTITUENTS Mucilage, triterpenes, volatile oil, saponins, resins, flavonoids, iridoid glycosides.
ACTIONS Expectorant, astringent, vulnerary, sedative, demulcent, decongestant, anodyne, antispasmodic.

Digestion • Soothes the gut, eases peptic ulcers and curbs diarrhoea.
Mental and emotional • Painkiller for headaches, neuralgia, arthritis and rheumatism; encourages sleep.
• Specifically for earache; applied locally and taken internally for catarrhal deafness, tinnitus, ear infections, wax accumulation and head pain caused by ear congestion. • Relieves anxiety, nervous palpitations, heart irregularities, cramps and nervous colic. • Astringent properties curb nervous diarrhoea. • Root decoction was a traditional remedy for toothache and convulsions.
Respiratory system • Soothing expectorant for harsh, dry coughs, sore throats and inflammatory conditions such as pharyngitis, tracheitis, bronchitis and bronchiectasis. Traditional remedy for TB, whooping cough and pleurisy. • Relaxing and antiseptic; relieves colds, flu, asthma, croup and chest infections.
• Decongestant; clears phlegm, sinusitis and hay fever.
Immune system • Enhances immunity. • Anti-inflammatory; relieves the pain of swollen glands and mumps. • Antibacterial and antiviral activity against influenza strains and herpes simplex.
Urinary system • Soothing diuretic for burning and frequency of cystitis, and fluid retention. • Increases the elimination of toxins; useful for arthritis, rheumatism and gout.
Externally • Compress of leaves used for painful joints and muscles, asthma, headaches, swollen glands and mumps. • Speeds healing of wounds, burns, sores, ulcers and piles. • Flowers used for ringworm and other skin infections. • Mullein oil from the flowers used as eardrops for earache and eczema of the outer ear.

Verbena officinalis
Vervain

Native to Europe, this perennial has attractive spikes of mauve flowers in summer and is found growing wild from Denmark to North Africa and western Asia to the Himalayas. It was revered by the Romans as a cure-all.

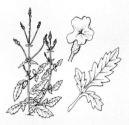

FAMILY Verbenaceae
PARTS USED Aerial parts
CONSTITUENTS Iridoid glycosides (verbenin, verbenalin and aucubin), flavonoids, triterpenes, sterols, volatile oil, tannins, alkaloids, mucilage, caffeic acid derivatives, adenosine, betacarotene.
ACTIONS Thymoleptic, nerve tonic, antioxidant, analgesic, antibacterial, anticoagulant, antispasmodic, antitumor, astringent, birthing aid, depurative, diaphoretic, tonic, hepatic, sedative, vulnerary, galactogogue.

Digestion • Enhances appetite and improves absorption. May be useful in anorexia, hypochloridia and indigestion.
• Bitters stimulate the liver and relieve headaches, lethargy, irritability and constipation. Used for liver disorders and gallstones. • Root is astringent; used for diarrhoea and dysentery.
Mental and emotional • Excellent tonic; calms irritability and anxiety, lifts depression and supports the body during stress. For stress-related symptoms such as headaches, indigestion, insomnia, high blood pressure, muscle pain and nervous exhaustion. • Helpful for convalescence after stress or illness and in chronic fatigue syndrome. • Verbenin is thought to block sympathetic innervation of the heart, blood vessels and intestines.
Immune system • Taken hot it reduces fevers.
Urinary system • Taken cool it has a diuretic and detoxifying action; useful for fluid retention and gout.
Reproductive system • Regulates periods and relieves PMS. • Enhances contractions during childbirth.
• Enhances milk supply in nursing mothers; for insufficient lactation associated with stress.
Externally • Astringent mouthwash used for bleeding gums and mouth ulcers. • Lotions used for cuts, insect bites, eczema, sores and neuralgia.

CAUTION Do not take simultaneously with mineral supplements. Avoid during pregnancy.

Viburnum opulus
Cramp bark

Native to Europe, North America and northern Asia, this striking tree, with its bright red berries, was prized among Native American and pioneer women to prevent miscarriage and relieve period pains.

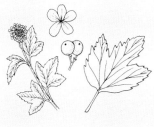

FAMILY Caprifoliaceae
PARTS USED Bark, stem bark[345]
CONSTITUENTS Coumarins (scopoletin and scopolin), catechin, epicatechin, bitters (viburnin), arbutin, valeric acid, salicylates, tannins, resin.
ACTIONS Antispasmodic, hypotensive, nervine, peripheral vasodilator, sedative, carminative, astringent, partus praeparator, anodyne.

Digestion • Relaxes tension and spasm. Relieves stress-related disorders such as colic, nausea, wind, abdominal cramps and IBS.
Circulation • Dilates the arteries, reduces blood pressure. • Used for palpitations and angina[346]. • Releases tension in arteries, relieves leg cramps, helpful in Raynaud's syndrome.
Musculoskeletal system • Used as a general muscle relaxant[347] for voluntary and involuntary muscular cramp[348] and tension. Famous as a remedy for leg cramps. • Used for tension headaches.
Reproductive system • Uterine sedative and tonic. Aesculetin and scopoletin have a powerful antispasmodic action, relieving cramps. Salicin is a good pain reliever. Used in spasmodic dysmenorrhoea for bearing-down pain, back and thigh pain, heavy bleeding, endometriosis, threatened/repeated miscarriage and to prepare for labour. • Helps prevent uterine irritability, over-strong contractions, false labour pains and afterpains. • Prevents excessive menstrual flow during the menopause[349]. • Used as an antispasmodic for benign prostatic hypertrophy. Astringent action is helpful in prolapse.
Respiratory system • Relaxes spasm in bronchi; useful for harsh irritating coughs and asthma as an adjuvant.

CAUTION The fresh berries are poisonous[350]. Avoid with anticoagulant drugs.

Viburnum prunifolium
Black haw

A small deciduous tree native to North America, where its medicinal benefits were taught by the Native American to the settlers. It was primarily used as a remedy for women, for preparing the uterus for childbirth, to relieve pain and reduce bleeding.

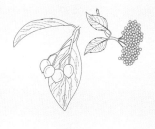

FAMILY Caprifoliaceae
PARTS USED Bark, root
CONSTITUENTS Flavonoids, coumarins (scopoletin), iridoid glycosides, triterpenes, tannins, fruit acids, bitter resins, arbutin.
ACTIONS Uterine antispasmodic, astringent, bronchodilator, hypotensive, diuretic, sedative, partus praeparator.

Digestion • Relieves the nausea of pregnancy. • Used for abdominal spasms, especially chronic hiccups, hiatus hernia and gastric or intestinal cramps[351] and diarrhoea[352].
Circulation • Lowers arterial blood pressure. • Useful for venospasm and as an adjunctive treatment for mild to moderate hypertension[353]. • Used for asthma.
Mental and emotional • Helps calm anxiety, particularly when related to miscarriage.
Reproductive system • Amphoteric effect on uterine muscles, toning over-relaxed muscles while relaxing tension in muscles causing spasm and pain. • Scopoletin and aesculetin have both been shown to have a sedative effect on the uterus[354]. Prepares the uterus for childbirth. • Improves circulation to the uterus and ovaries and promotes nutrition to the pelvic area. • Relieves dysmenorrhoea with scanty flow. • It can be used for threatened/repeated miscarriage and nocturnal leg cramps during pregnancy. • Eases childbirth, relieves false pains and labour pains and prevents post-partum haemorrhage. • Helps normal involution of the womb after childbirth. • Strengthening tonic after miscarriage.

CAUTION Use cautiously in cases of kidney stones[355].
Drug interactions Avoid with anticoagulants such as heparin and warfarin.

Vinca major and *V. minor*
Greater and Lesser periwinkle

Evergreen perennials with blue
windmill-shaped flowers that
grow wild throughout Europe.
The flowers and leaves were
traditionally chewed to stop
bleeding in the mouth, and to
relieve toothache.

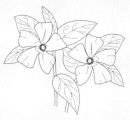

FAMILY Apocynaceae
PARTS USED Flower, leaf
CONSTITUENTS Tannins, alkaloids (including
pubescine, vinine and vincamine), flavonoids, pectin.
ACTIONS Astringent, sedative, hypotensive,
hypoglycaemic, thymoleptic, vulnerary.

Digestion • Astringent tannins curb diarrhoea and
dysentery, protect the gut wall from irritation and
infection and stop bleeding. • Healing remedy for
heartburn, gastritis, peptic ulcers and flatulence.
• May help regulate blood sugar and prevent diabetes.
Circulation • Improves blood flow to the brain;
recommended in cerebral arteriosclerosis and after
stroke. • Reduces high blood pressure and helps prevent
atherosclerosis.
Mental and emotional • Reduces tension, relieves
anxiety, lifts depression and SAD, clears the mind and
boosts energy levels.
Respiratory system • Astringent; clears chronic catarrh
and phlegm.
Immune system • *Vinca rosea* (now *Catharanthus
roseus*)/Madagascan periwinkle was discovered in the
1920s to reduce blood sugar in diabetics, and hailed as
a possible substitute for insulin. Lesser and Greater
periwinkles have also been used for diabetes. • Alkaloids
vinblastine and vincristine in *Vinca rosea* have been
extensively used to treat malignant tumours, leukaemia
and Hodgkin's disease.
Reproductive system • Reduces excessive menstrual
bleeding and vaginal discharge.
Externally • Leaves were traditionally inserted into the
nose to stop nosebleeds and bound to the skin to stop
bleeding from cuts and wounds. • Used to make vaginal
douches for discharges; lotions for haemorrhoids,
varicose veins and skin problems such as acne and
cradle cap; mouthwashes and gargles for mouth ulcers,
tonsillitis and sore throats. • Chewed to relieve toothache
and combat bleeding gums.

Viola odorata
Sweet violet

Native to Asia and Europe, the
sweet violet was traditionally
woven into garlands to cool
anger, cure headaches and
hangovers and induce sleep.
Hippocrates recommended it
for melancholia, bad eyesight
and inflammation of the chest.

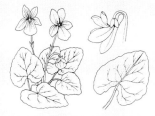

FAMILY Violaceae
PARTS USED Flower, leaf
CONSTITUENTS Saponins, salicylates, alkaloids, volatile
oils, flavonoids, mucilage, phenolic acids.
ACTIONS Expectorant, antitumour, demulcent,
diaphoretic, alterative, antifungal, anti-inflammatory,
antiseptic, antiscorbutic, astringent, emollient, febrifuge,
laxative, nutritive, restorative, vulnerary.

Digestion • Soothes irritation and inflamation in the gut.
• Gentle laxative.
Mental and emotional • Recommended for grief and
heartbreak[356] and to improve memory[357]. • Eases
headache from lack of sleep and helps moderate anger[358].
Respiratory system • Soothing expectorant for harsh,
irritating coughs and chest infections, pleurisy, chronic
bronchitis, tonsillitis, asthma and chronic catarrh; popular
in children's cough syrup. • Hot tea brings down fevers
and clears colds and congestion.
Musculoskeletal system • Cools heat and inflammation;
salicylates useful for arthritis.
Immune system • In Traditional Chinese Medicine used
for hot swellings, cysts and tumours. • Used in the
treatment of cancer (breast, lung, digestive tract, skin,
throat and tongue)[359]. • Deters infection[360].
Urinary system • Soothes inflamed and painful
conditions such as cystitis, trichomonas, urethritis[361] and
urinary tract infections[362].
Externally • Compress or poultice used to treat boils,
conjunctivitis, breast cysts, cancers and haemorrhoids[363].
• A cloth soaked in violet tea can be applied to the back of
the neck to treat headaches[364].

Viola tricolor
Wild pansy

Native to temperate parts of Europe, this charming plant was historically renowned for its ability to clear stubborn skin problems. It is often called heartsease because of its ancient reputation for curing affairs of the heart. Hippocrates used it as a cordial to lift the spirits and treat heart conditions.

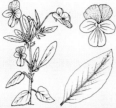

FAMILY Violaceae
PARTS USED Leaf, flower
CONSTITUENTS Flavonoids, mucilage, tannins, salicylates, saponins, alkaloids.
ACTIONS Anti-inflammatory, antirheumatic, expectorant, diuretic, alterative, laxative, antiallergenic, hypotensive, demulcent, decongestant.

Circulation • Enhances circulation, reduces blood pressure, strengthens blood vessels and helps prevent arteriosclerosis.
Respiratory system • Soothing and expectorant properties useful for inflammatory chest problems, bronchitis, harsh, irritating coughs, whooping cough, asthma and croup. • The saponins account for its expectorant action, while its mucilage content soothes the chest[365]. • Taken hot it relieves catarrhal congestion and brings down fevers.
Immune system • Used to reduce heat and inflammation and clear skin conditions. Helps clear chronic skin disorders with purulent sticky discharge, moist eczema, milk crust and ringworm[366]. • Traditionally used for skin cancer, seborrheic skin disease, acne, impetigo, pruritus vulvae and cradle cap[367]. • Salicylates are helpful for treating arthritis and gout.
Urinary system • Soothing diuretic; relieves cystitis and fluid retention, and clears toxins. • Relieves painful and frequent urination[368].
Externally • Lotion used for seborrheic skin disease, acne, impetigo, pruritus vulvae and cradle cap[369].

CAUTION Avoid if allergic to salicylates[370].
Drug interactions May increase actions of salicylates (aspirin)[371].

Viscum album
Mistletoe

An evergreen partial parasite native to Europe, North Africa and Asia, which draws nourishment and medicinal constituents from the host deciduous tree. When used medicinally, it is usually taken from apple trees.

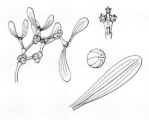

FAMILY Loranthaceae
PARTS USED Leaf, young twig
CONSTITUENTS Mucilage, lignans, phenylpropanoids, fixed oil, resin (viscin), saponins, tannins, alkaloids, flavanoids, polypeptides (lectins and viscotoxin), viscols A and B histamine (constituents vary according to the host tree), proteins, phytosterols, triterpenoids.
ACTIONS Vasodilator, hypotensive, diuretic, nervine, antispasmodic, immunostimulant, cardiotonic, antitumour, narcotic, sedative.

Circulation • Regulates heart and blood pressure, normalizes pulse and calms rapid heart and nervous palpitations. • Dilates arteries. • Useful for angina and helpful for arteriosclerotic narrowing of the arteries. • Strengthens capillary walls, improves circulation and relaxes muscles[372]. • Relieves headaches due to high blood pressure[373]. • Useful for varicose veins.
Mental and emotional • Sedative, muscle relaxant and nerve tonic; used for epilepsy, convulsions, panic attacks, nervous debility, tense, aching muscles, anxiety, insomnia, cramps, nervous headaches, migraines and vertigo. • Increases resilience to stress.
Immune system • Enhances immunity, specifically the function of the thymus gland and spleen, accelerating antibody production; used for lowered immunity, chronic candida, ME and HIV. • Cytotoxic alkaloids and lectins may have antitumour effects; the 'viscum therapy' of injecting fresh mistletoe extracts in cancer originated in Switzerland based on the findings of Rudolf Steiner. • Aids recovery of energy, health and appetite after orthodox cancer treatment. • May have anti-inflammatory effect in gout. • An injectable form of mistletoe lectins has been used to reduce the signs and symptoms of hepatitis[374].

CAUTION Raw mistletoe is toxic, as are the berries[375]. Only use under professional guidance and in small doses[376]. May cause temporary numbness, vomiting and reduced heart rate. Avoid during pregnancy[377].

Vitex agnus castus
Chaste tree

An attractive shrub, native to seashores of Europe, North Africa and Asia, with long spikes of mauve flowers and highly aromatic seeds. Its name derives from its reputation for calming sexual desires, particularly in men.

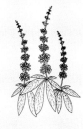

FAMILY Verbenaceae
PARTS USED Berry
CONSTITUENTS Essential oils (including monoterpenes and sesquiterpenes), flavonoids (casticin, isovitexin and orientin), alkaloids (vitticine), iridoglycosides (agnuside, aucubin and erostoside).
ACTIONS Carminative, diaphoretic, galactogogue, anaphrodisiac, antiandrogenic, aromatic, diuretic, emmenagogue, febrifuge, ophthalmic, phytoprogesteronic, sedative, stomachic, vulnerary.

Urinary system • Diuretic; relieves fluid retention, particularly accompanying PMS.
Reproductive system • Acts on the pituitary gland to regulate the production of follicle-stimulating hormone, luteinizing hormone and prolactin[378]. This leads to an increase in progesterone production during the second half of the cycle, balancing hormones that regulate menstruation and fertility[379]. • Relieves symptoms associated with high oestrogen and low progesterone, such as migraines, breast tenderness, bloating, mood swings, cramps, fluid retention, constipation, herpes (related to menses), premenstrual acne, PMS and threatened miscarriage[380]. • Taken over 3–6 months it regulates menstrual cycle and relieves painful periods, fibrocystic breast disease, PMS, acne and endometriosis. • Reduces prolactin secretion; useful for benign breast problems, fibroids, and prostatic hypertrophy[381]. • Enhances fertility and remedies amenorrhoea and menorrhagia caused by corpus luteum insufficiency[382]. • Useful in polycystic ovary syndrome, endometriosis, cysts (in breasts, ovaries and uterus) and threatened miscarriage. • Stimulates milk flow in nursing mothers. • Used for menopausal symptoms such as hot flushes, vaginal dryness and depression. • Regulates menstrual cycle in women coming off birth control pills[383]. • Beneficial after hysterectomy[384] and childbirth.

Drug interactions Avoid with HRT or the contraceptive pill.

Vitis vinifera
Red grape

The common grape vine is native to the Mediterranean, central Europe and south-western Asia. The seeds contain an oil that has antioxidant actions more powerful than vitamin C, helping to prevent damage to the body caused by free radicals.

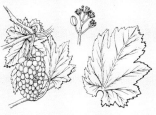

FAMILY Vitaceae
PARTS USED Seed and skin of fruit
CONSTITUENTS Polyphenols, catechin, epicatechin, oligomeric proanthocyanidins, flavonoids, resveratrol, essential fatty acids (linoleic, oleic and palmitic acid), tocopherols, tannins.
ACTIONS Antioxidant, astringent, collagen stabilizer, circulatory tonic, anti-inflammatory, probiotic.

Digestion • Astringent tannins protect the gastrointestinal tract from irritation and inflammation. • Used in gastritis, ulcers and pancreatitis. • Essential fatty acids and tocopherols protect the liver and prevent the oxidation of vitamin E. • Helps regulate gut flora in dysbiosis.
Circulation • Improves circulation and venous return; useful for peripheral vascular disease such as Raynaud's disease, venous insufficiency, varicose veins and haemorrhoids. • Strengthens blood vessel walls. Used for capillary fragility and diabetic and hypertensive retinopathy. • Protects collagen from degradation and reduces harmful cholesterol and blood pressure.
• Inhibits platelet activity without prolonging bleeding.
• Antioxidant; helps prevent cardiovascular disease.
Musculoskeletal system • Reduces pain and inflammation in joints and protects synovial fluid and collagen[385].
Immune system • Re-establishes normal bacterial population of the gut. • Antioxidants may protect against tumour formation[386] especially in the breast, stomach, colon, prostate and lung. • Good after radiation therapy for cancer. • May help protect liver damage from toxins and chemotherapy.
Reproductive system • Used for chloasma and congestive dysmenorrhoea.
Eyes • Inhibits macular degeneration and diabetic retinopathy; improves nearsightedness[387].
Externally • Strengthens connective tissue and promotes healing.

Withania somniferum
Ashwagandha/Winter cherry

Native to India, and one of the most important herbs in Ayurvedic medicine. As a restorative and rejuvenative it is esteemed as highly as Ginseng in Traditional Chinese Medicine. It boosts strength and vitality.

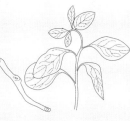

FAMILY Solanaceae
PARTS USED Root
CONSTITUENTS Steroidal lactones (withanolides), tropane alkaloids, phytosterols, saponins, iron.
ACTIONS Sedative, antispasmodic, anticonvulsant, nerve tonic, diuretic, astringent, nutritive, rejuvenative, anti-inflammatory, anticancer, cardioprotective, hypotensive, adaptogen, antioxidant, aphrodisiac, immunomodulatory, thyroid balancing.

Mental and emotional • Exceptional nerve tonic. Promotes energy and vitality. • Adaptogen; modifies the harmful effects of stress on mind and body. Engenders calmness and clarity of mind. Excellent for stress, anxiety, depression, overwork, panic attacks, nervous exhaustion and insomnia. • Used for behavioural problems, poor memory and concentration, ADHD and problems associated with drug abuse/addiction. • Used for problems associated with old age such as loss of energy and muscular strength, arthritis and insomnia.
Respiratory system • Immune enhancing and antimicrobial; increases resistance to infections.
• Relieves allergies such as, rhinitis and asthma.
Immune system • Anti-inflammatory for joint problems.
• Decreases free radical damage and slows the ageing process. • Enhances immunity; used for chronic immune deficiency, fibromyalgia, HIV, autoimmune problems such as MS, ankylosing spondylitis, lupus and rheumatoid arthritis. • May inhibit the growth of cancers. • Supports the system during chemotherapy and radiation therapy.
Genitourinary system • Used for urinary problems, dysmenorrhea, irregular and scanty periods and endometriosis. • Famous for infertility and as a male reproductive tonic.
Externally • Oil used for arthritic joints, frozen shoulder and nerve pain such as sciatica, muscle spasm and back pain. • Used for wounds, sores and dry, itchy skin conditions such as eczema and psoriasis.

CAUTION Avoid over 3 g daily in pregnancy.

Zanthoxylum americanum
Prickly ash

A tall shrub native to North America. It has warming and stimulating effects and was well known among Native Americans for relieving arthritic pain and toothache.

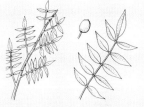

FAMILY Rutaceae
PARTS USED Bark
CONSTITUENTS Alkaloids, lignans, resins, essential oils, xanthoxyllin, alyklamides, tannin, coumarins, phenol.
ACTIONS Circulatory stimulant, diaphoretic, sialogogue, alterative, analgesic, anthelmintic, antibacterial, anti-inflammatory, antispasmodic, astringent, emmenagogue, immunostimulant, nervine, rubefacient, digestive.

Digestion • When chewed it stimulates the flow of saliva and other digestive juices. • Improves digestion and absorption, and increases pancreas and liver function.
• Used for constipation due to deficient secretions, colic, bloating and wind.
Circulation • Increases blood flow to the periphery; used for chilblains, intermittent claudication, Raynaud's disease, Buerger's disease, cerebrovascular disease, varicose veins, haemorrhoids and leg cramps. • Prevents blood platelet aggregation and regulates blood pressure.
• Stimulates lymphatic circulation. • Increases kidney output and cardiac function.
Mental and emotional • Strengthening stimulant; used for debility and nervous exhaustion. • Helpful in neuralgia and restless leg syndrome.
Respiratory system • Useful in chronic pharyngitis and post-nasal catarrh. • Diaphoretic when taken hot; helps resolve chills, colds, coughs, flu, fevers and sore throats.
Musculoskeletal system • Alterative properties are helpful for osteoarthritis, rheumatism, gout and lumbago.
Immune system • Enhances fight against infection and cancer. • Used as a capillary stimulant for resolving eruptive diseases such as measles and chickenpox.
Reproductive system • Stimulates blood flow to the uterus; relieves uterine cramps and dysmenorrhoea.
Externally • Rubefacient to improve circulation and relieve rheumatic pain, backache and toothache.

CAUTION Avoid in pregnancy and with gastrointestinal inflammation.
Drug interactions Avoid with anticoagulants and antihypertensives.

Zea mays
Corn silk

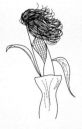

Corn silk is the yellow strands inside the husks of corn, harvested before pollination. Native to Central and South America, it is rich in nutrients and contains silicon, B vitamins, para-amino benzoic acid and small amounts of iron, zinc, potassium, vitamin K, calcium, magnesium and phosphorus. For best results use fresh.

FAMILY Poaceae
PARTS USED Style, stigma
CONSTITUENTS Mucilage, tannins, ascorbic acid, pantothenic acid, flavonoids (anthocyanins), malic acid, alkaloids, saponins, sterols (sitosterol and stigmasterol), allantoin, resin.
ACTIONS Urinary demulcent, antilithic, diuretic, liver tonic, hypoglycaemic, hypotensive, alterative, anti-inflammatory, antiseptic, galactogogue, tonic, vulnerary.

Digestion • Stimulates bile flow from the liver and aids the liver's detoxifying work. • Helps regulate blood sugar.
Circulation • Dilates arteries and reduces blood pressure and blood clotting time[388]. • Good source of vitamin K; helps control bleeding, for example during childbirth.
Urinary system • Demulcent diuretic for cystitis, dysuria, urethritis and bed-wetting. • Anti-inflammatory effects are useful in the treatment of acute and chronic prostatitis and inflammatory conditions of the bladder and kidneys. • Excellent for symptoms associated with benign enlargement of the prostate. • Reduces fluid retention and aids elimination of toxins and excess uric acid via the kidneys; helpful in gout and arthritis and chronic skin problems such as boils. • Helps to dissolve stones and gravel. • Useful in fluid retention associated with PMS.
Other • Anti-inflammatory for arthritis, skin problems and for carpal tunnel syndrome.
Externally • Applied powdered to soothe and speed healing of the skin.

CAUTION Avoid in corn allergies.

Zingiber officinale
Ginger

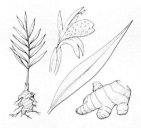

A wonderfully pungent spice native to South Asia. Its warming and energizing properties were mentioned in the writings of Confucius as early as 500 BCE and Chinese and Indian medical texts written 2,000 years ago.

FAMILY Zingiberaceae
PARTS USED Rhizome, leaf
CONSTITUENTS Volatile oils (including zingerone, gingerol, camphene, borneol, phellandrene and citral).
ACTIONS Circulatory stimulant, carminative, digestive, expectorant, diuretic, aphrodisiac, antiemetic, analgesic, anti-inflammatory, diaphoretic, antispasmodic, immune tonic, antimicrobial, antioxidant.

Digestion • Warming digestive stimulant; improves appetite and digestion. Useful in anorexia. • Removes accumulation of toxins, enhancing immunity. • Relieves pain and spasm, indigestion, distension and wind, nausea, IBS and food allergies. • Relieves griping from diarrhoea, travel and morning sickness and hangovers.
Circulation • Stimulates the heart and circulation, and reduces blood clotting; used for poor peripheral circulation, chilblains and Raynaud's disease.
Respiratory system • Antispasmodic and expectorant; relieves asthma, catarrhal coughs, chest infections, bronchitis and bronchietasis. • Hot tea taken at the onset of sore throat, cold or flu brings down fevers, clears catarrh and helps resolve infection.
Immune system • Volatile oils dispel acute bacterial and viral infections such as colds, flu, bronchitis, bacterial dysentery and malaria. Used in East for epidemics such as cholera. • Anti-inflammatory and antioxidant; inhibits prostaglandin synthesis and aids immunity and circulation; used for osteo- and rheumatoid arthritis.
Reproductive system • Promotes menstruation; used for delayed/scanty periods and clots. • Relieves spasm, pain at ovulation and menstruation and in endometriosis. • Ancient reputation as an aphrodisiac. Its invigorating properties are helpful for impotence.

CAUTION Avoid with peptic ulcers and gallstones.
Drug interactions Avoid with anticoagulants.

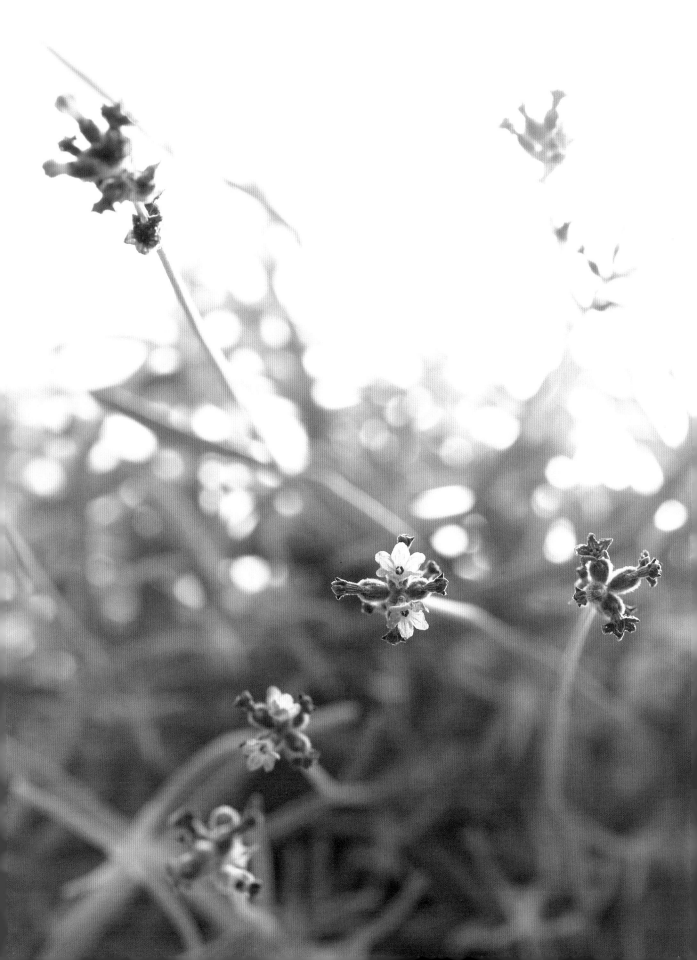

Treating common ailments

The most common health conditions that respond to herbal remedies are profiled in this chapter. The ailments are organized by body system, and each treatment protocol offers advice on herbs to be used and effective methods of their administration. Supportive action is suggested for each condition, including changes to diet and lifestyle and supplements that could augment herbal treatment. Brief case studies illustrate the effectiveness of these treatments.

The nervous system

Our nervous system is an amazing communication network by which the brain and nerve cells send messages via neurotransmitters across synapses from one nerve cell to another, or to a bunch of muscle fibres. It is a wonderful example of the intimate link between mind and body – in fact, they are one and the same thing.

Part of our physical body, the nervous system is made up of nerve cells (neurones) and fibres, which comprise the brain and spinal cord, the peripheral nerves and the autonomic nervous system. This body system is responsible for executing physical actions and registering sensations, while at the same time it is the tool we use both to experience and express all our thoughts and feelings. Physical discomfort and disease can affect the way we think and feel, and every thought and emotion we experience has a direct effect on our physical state. Negative thoughts and feelings, for example, sap our energy and vitality and reduce our natural resistance to disease, and they may be expressed in symptoms including migraine, peptic ulcer and heart disease. Happiness and positivity directly influence our physical bodies too, affecting the chemistry of our tissues and body secretions for the better, and helping to bring about health and vibrancy.

Nervous problems

Stress is part of our everyday lives, and there is very little chance of escaping it, and yet some of us are better at dealing with it than others. Our strength and resilience can be worn down by long-term mental or emotional difficulties, acute trauma, overwork, lack of sleep, chronic or regular illness, poor diet and digestive problems that inhibit the absorption of nutrients. When this occurs, we may have an exaggerated response to or an inability to deal with challenging situations, creating further stress. We have all experienced that tendency to be more irritable when we are tired or run-down. In the same situation, when our energy is optimal, we may not feel stressed in the least.

Stress-related physical problems can benefit from a psychological approach, such as counselling or psychotherapy, while stress and psychological problems can be helped by working through the body with, for example, massage, yoga, breathing exercises, relaxation and exercise, herbs and a good diet.

Good digestion and healthy eating can radically transform our mental and emotional state. Vitamins B, C and E, calcium, magnesium, zinc and essential fatty acids are all vital to the normal functioning of the nervous system and may need to be increased during times of stress, when the body's uptake of them can increase dramatically. Eating a diet high in foods devoid of nutrients – such as refined carbohydrates, sugar and junk foods – can result in deficiencies of essential nutrients, while caffeine can have a powerfully negative effect too, and is best avoided completely in order to optimize natural resilience.

Herbs and the nervous system

There are many wonderfully beneficial herbs that have a direct effect on the nervous system and the world of herbs offers a range of therapeutic strategies for dealing with specific nervous problems. There are herbs to lift the spirits, calm anxiety, relax muscles, increase memory and concentration and aid sleep. There are other herbs, known as adaptogens, that have an impressive ability to improve energy and vitality and enhance resilience to stress. There are even herbs that work on a more emotional level, for mending a broken heart and combating low self-esteem for example. Specific herbal recommendations are given for common complaints of the nervous system on pages 180–183.

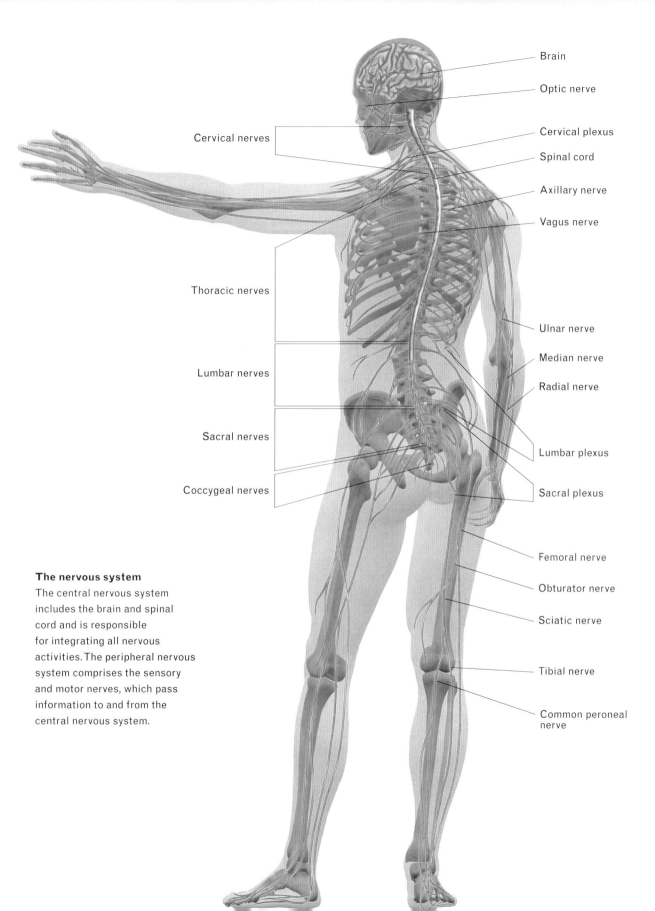

Cervical nerves

Thoracic nerves

Lumbar nerves

Sacral nerves

Coccygeal nerves

Brain

Optic nerve

Cervical plexus

Spinal cord

Axillary nerve

Vagus nerve

Ulnar nerve

Median nerve

Radial nerve

Lumbar plexus

Sacral plexus

Femoral nerve

Obturator nerve

Sciatic nerve

Tibial nerve

Common peroneal
nerve

The nervous system

The central nervous system
includes the brain and spinal
cord and is responsible
for integrating all nervous
activities. The peripheral nervous
system comprises the sensory
and motor nerves, which pass
information to and from the
central nervous system.

Tension and anxiety

Tension or anxiety is a normal response to a difficult situation, which should settle once the problem is resolved. It can become habitual when we are run-down either by long-term stress, nutritional deficiencies, excess alcohol and caffeine, or lack of exercise and sleep.

Treatment Effective calming herbs for acute anxiety are Passion flower, Wild lettuce, Skullcap and Wild oats taken every hour or 2 hours if necessary. Chamomile or Lemon balm tea is also soothing. For chronic problems, adaptogens like Ginseng, Ashwagandha, Bacopa, Polygonum, Schisandra, Shatavari, Bhringaraj, Liquorice and Holy basil will strengthen the nerves. Other good anxiolytic herbs include Vervain, St John's wort, California poppy, Rose, Motherwort, Lime flower, Hops, Lavender, Rosemary and Peony.

Hot herbal baths and massage using relaxing essentials oils of Holy basil, Nutmeg, Lavender, Rosemary, Rose or Chamomile in a base of sesame oil will ease muscle tension and soothe anxiety.

Other measures Regular aerobic exercise is advised to stimulate endorphins and increase resilience. Meditation cultivates calmness and a sense of control, Pranayama (breathing exercises) is calming, and inhalations of Frankincense oil deepen breathing. Avoid caffeine, sugar, alcohol and any unnecessary drugs, which can reduce resistance to stress.

Depression

Treatment Mood-elevating Wild oats, Vervain, Skullcap, St John's wort and Siberian ginseng taken 3 times daily can appreciably lift the spirits and replace essential nutrients necessary for the nervous system. Lemon balm, Damiana, Borage, St John's wort, Wild oats, Holy basil and Wood betony taken 3–6 times daily can help acute depression. Adding essential oils of Lavender, Rosemary, Chamomile or Rose to baths/massage oils can also help.

Rosemary, Rhodiola, Gotu kola, Siberian ginseng, Liquorice and Wild oats are great adaptogens, excellent for debility and depression following illness or long-term stress. Rose, Shatavari, Chaste tree, Evening primrose, Black cohosh and St John's wort are particularly appropriate for depression related to hormone imbalance (premenstrual or in menopause).

Other measures It is important to take regular exercise, which enhances the secretion of natural opiates (endorphins), creating a feeling of wellbeing.

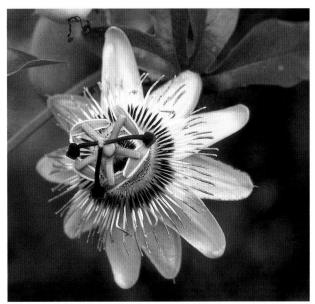

Passion flower is an effective herb for calming anxiety, relaxing tense muscles and promoting sleep.

CASE STUDY **ANXIETY**

CLIENT PROFILE
Kate, aged 42, had been feeling generally anxious since her husband had died two years ago and was having trouble sleeping. She would feel tired at night and fall asleep easily, but then wake in the early hours between 2 and 3 am and not get back to sleep until around 6 am.

THE HERBAL TREATMENT
I suggested that before going to bed at night Kate should drink hot rice or almond milk containing a teaspoonful of Ashwagandha powder and a little honey, and then massage herself with warm sesame oil. After 10–15 minutes, she should soak in a warm bath containing a few drops of lavender and rose essential oils. I made her a prescription to nourish her nervous system, including Wild oats, Skullcap, Passion flower, Holy basil, Liquorice and Ashwagandha, to take 3–6 times a day.

I recommended that she avoid all caffeine and try to set regular times for eating, exercising and sleeping to settle her nervous system and make sure she relaxed in the evening.

This treatment helped Kate to remain calm and increased her resilience to stress. She said that it helped her to sleep much better.

Insomnia

Treatment For problems getting off to sleep, use Hops, Passion flower, Chamomile, Lemon balm, Lime flower, Wild oats, Wild lettuce, Ashwagandha or Valerian as teas, or 1–3 teaspoons of tincture before bed. A teaspoonful of Ashwagandha or Nutmeg is good taken in hot milk at bedtime.

For problems staying asleep, try taking Ashwagandha, Bacopa, Wild oats, Skullcap, Hops, Passion flower, St John's wort or Valerian.

Nourishing nervines such as Wild oats, Skullcap, Vervain, Rosemary, Holy basil, Liquorice and Ashwagandha help when insomnia is related to being tired and run-down and these can be taken 3 times daily.

A warm sesame oil massage followed 10–15 minutes later by a bath before bed can work wonders. Add strong infusions/oils of Lavender, Chamomile, Neroli or Rose to the bath for added effect.

Other measures Allowing 45 minutes of quiet time before retiring is important. It is best to avoid all caffeine and have regular meals, exercise and sleep times and no sleep during the day, to settle the nervous system.

Headache and migraine

These may be warning signs of stress or fatigue, or related to eyestrain, sinusitis, hormonal imbalances, allergy, liver and digestive problems, dysbiosis, pollution, poor diet, high blood pressure, low blood sugar, alcohol or back problems. The best way to manage your headaches is to understand what causes them so that you can prevent them effectively.

Treatment Effective preventative herbs include Lemon balm, Rosemary, Feverfew, Wood betony, Gotu kola, Bacopa and Gingko.

At the first signs of pain, take relaxant and painkilling herbs such as Passion flower, California poppy, Hops, Pasque flower, St John's wort, Wild lettuce, Rosemary, Skullcap, Chamomile or Vervain and repeat as necessary. You can also use anti-inflammatory herbs: Meadowsweet, Black willow, Ginger, Cayenne pepper or Lavender. Inhale Lavender, Peppermint or Rosemary oils, or massage them into the temples.

Liver herbs Dandelion, Burdock, Vervain, Holy thistle and Milk thistle are important to detoxify the system. Chaste tree, Shatavari or Wild yam and Evening primrose oil will help address hormone imbalances. Massage, particularly of the head and neck, and feet with Gotu kola oil can bring relief.

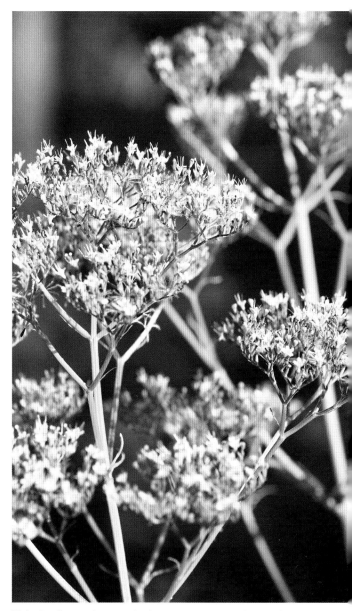

Valerian has sedative and relaxant properties and is used to promote sleep.

Other measures Avoid all caffeine and sugar as well as known migraine triggers – chocolate, cheese, alcohol and citrus fruits.

Poor memory and concentration

The brain can be affected by long-term stress, drugs, smoking, dietary and environmental toxicity and free radical damage, which over time can affect blood flow to the brain and impair brain function. Poor memory and concentration can also result from the mind being overloaded when stressed, tired or run-down from illness, nutritional deficiencies, hormonal changes including low thyroid function, PMS or the menopause.

Treatment Some herbs, including Bacopa, Gotu kola, Rhodiola, Peppermint, Rosemary, Periwinkle and Gingko, have the ability to increase brain function by increasing the flow of blood and nutrients to the brain, enhancing the production of neurotransmitters.

Antioxidant herbs such as Gingko, Ginseng, Hawthorn, Ashwagandha, Thyme, St John's wort, Rhodiola, Amalaki, Polygonum and Schisandra protect the brain cells and artery walls by preventing damage from free radicals. Other good brain tonics include Wild oats, Damiana, Lemon balm, Wood betony, Skullcap and Vervain.

Other measures Supplements of B vitamins, antioxidant vitamins A, C and E, zinc, selenium, choline, lecithin, coenzyme Q10 and omega-3 essential fatty acids can be helpful.

ADD and ADHD

Attention deficit disorder (ADD) and attention deficit hyperactivity disorder (ADHD) have been linked to toxic metals, dysbiosis, food sensitivities, nutritional deficiencies (B vitamins, magnesium, essential fatty acids, iron and zinc) and excess sugar. Impaired glucose metabolism may also be a major contributory factor, caused by excessive intake of simple carbohydrates and nutrient-poor junk foods. Lack of fresh air and exercise, hypoglycaemia and over-exposure to smoky atmospheres, noise, computers and television can all affect the brain adversely.

Treatment Red clover, Pau d'arco, Coriander leaf, Bladderwrack and Nettle aid the elimination of heavy metals. These can be combined with cleansing herbs Milk thistle, Turmeric, Common grape vine, Barberry, Dandelion or Burdock to detoxify the system and protect against toxic damage.

Nervines to promote normal brain function and neurotransmitter production are important, such as Gotu kola, Bacopa, Ginkgo, St John's wort, Wild oats, Skullcap and Vervain.

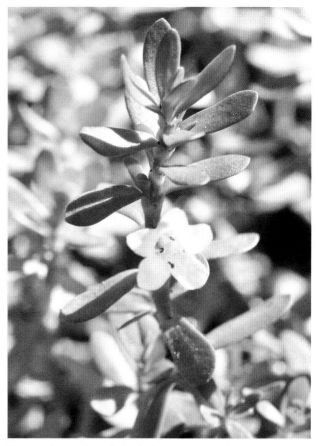

Bacopa is popular in India for boosting mental acuity, including concentration and memory recall.

To aid sleep, use Ashwagandha, California poppy, Chamomile, Passion flower, Hops or Lime flower. Liquorice is helpful as an adaptogen and adrenal tonic.

Other measures Avoiding allergenic foods including food colourings and additives, dairy produce, salicylates, wheat or gluten, corn, chocolate, caffeine, eggs and citrus fruits can be helpful. Supplements of B vitamins, magnesium and omega-3 essential fatty acids are recommended.

Neuralgia and sciatica

Inflammation or injury of a nerve can cause excruciating pain, as experienced by anyone who has suffered from sciatica, lumbago or trigeminal neuralgia. Nerves can be traumatized by injury, burns, cuts, slipped discs, vertebrae out of alignment, a tumour or muscle spasm. Heavy metals such as lead or mercury can damage nerves, as can alcoholism and diabetes. To ensure recovery, the cause of the pain needs to be identified and treated. Where there is pressure on a nerve from a spinal problem, consult a chiropractor or osteopath.

Treatment To relieve nerve pain, try California poppy, Hops, St John's wort, Wood betony, Pasque flower, Feverfew, Meadowsweet or Black cohosh, in acute doses if necessary. Cramp bark, Valerian, Passion flower, Skullcap, Lavender, Rosemary, Chamomile or Wild yam will help relax tense and painful muscles. Wild oats are wonderful 'nerve food' and help repair nerve tissue. Where circulation to the area is poor, Hawthorn, Cinnamon and Ginger will bring blood and nutrition to the area.

Externally, St John's wort oil, gently massaged into the area, is specific for damaged nerves and neuralgia, and is an excellent pain reliever. A few drops of Cayenne pepper tincture added to the oil will increase its pain-relieving properties. Start with 1–2 drops and gradually build up the ratio of Cayenne pepper, as it may have a tendency to cause a burning sensation in some people with hypersensitive nerves.

Other pain-relieving essential oils that can be used for massage in a base of sesame oil include Ginger, Rosemary, Lavender, Peppermint, Chamomile and Coriander.

Shingles

Shingles is a painful inflammatory nerve problem, caused by a reactivation of the latent varicella zoster virus that causes chickenpox. This herpes virus produces a rash along a nerve pathway often on the abdomen or the face, which results in tingling and pain, often severe, followed by the appearance of fluid-filled blisters (vesicles) on the skin. Tiredness, stress, poor nutrition and depleted immunity increase the risk of developing shingles after contact with chickenpox.

Treatment Antiviral herbs such as St John's wort, Lemon balm, Barberry, Lavender, Pau d'arco, Andrographis, Neem, Echinacea or Olive leaf will help combat the herpes infection. To reduce nerve pain and inflammation, use California poppy, St John's wort, Passion flower, Skullcap, Pasque flower, Meadowsweet or Gotu kola, in acute doses if necessary.

Adaptogenic herbs Liquorice, Ashwagandha, Shatavari, Aloe vera, Wild oats and Shiitake and Reishi mushrooms strengthen immunity, help speed recovery and prevent post-herpetic neuralgia.

Externally, St John's wort oil with a few drops of essential Lavender oil (5 drops per 5 ml/1 teaspoon) can be applied gently to the rash. Aloe vera gel can also be soothing.

Other measures When infection occurs, avoid foods that inhibit immunity and stimulate inflammation, such as saturated fats, refined foods and sugars, caffeine and alcohol. A diet low in the amino acid arginine, which can activate the virus, and high in lysine, which can suppress it, is recommended.

Supplements of betacarotene, zinc and vitamin C and E enhance immunity and speed healing of the skin.

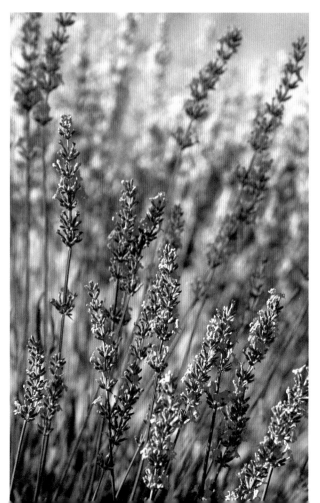

Lavender helps to reduce pain and has a soothing effect on the nervous system; it is also antiviral and antibacterial.

The immune system

The immune system consists of the lymphatic system, white blood cells, and specialized cells and chemicals including antibodies. When infection threatens to overcome our homeostatic mechanisms – which maintain the stable state of the body and are vital for health – and invade the body, the immune system rallies its defences to deal with it.

In response to infection, the lymphatic system produces an increased amount of lymphocytes and macrophages, which work with cytokine chemicals to destroy the invaders. The thymus gland aids the production of and stores white blood cells known as T-cells, which attack cells infected by bacteria, fungi and viruses. The spleen, liver, tonsils, adenoids and wall of the intestine also contain lymphatic tissue. The lymphatic tissue lining the gut is responsible for maintaining lymphocytes capable of responding to all the infecting organisms (antigens) that are introduced to the body through food entering the digestive tract.

Should these protective mechanisms fail, specific immune responses occur. Molecules on the surface of antigens stimulate lymphocytes and produce antibodies to destroy the antigens. These have a memory, so that antigens are recognized should infection reoccur, ensuring that the body is able to respond effectively to the pathogenic organisms before an infection develops.

Everyday maintenance

A healthy lifestyle is the key to an efficient immune system. It is essential to eat plenty of nutritious, natural, preferably organic food and to have a balance of work and play, exercise and relaxation, sufficient sleep, and a minimum of pollution in the environment. It is also important to engender a positive attitude to dealing with stress, as well as to cultivate practices that promote peace of mind. A positive outlook, fun, laughter, serenity, being in beautiful, peaceful surroundings and clean air can all boost immunity. Our natural immunity is lowered by physical or emotional stress, overworking or -playing, poor diet, toxins, smoking and drinking excess alcohol.

The importance of good digestion is often overlooked when considering immunity. If our 'digestive fire' is good, the food eaten will be efficiently digested and assimilated, and the residue of wastes remaining to be eliminated

from the body will be minimal. If, however, the digestive fire is low, much of what is eaten will remain in the gut as partially digested or undigested food, which ferments and produces toxins that can undermine the local immune mechanisms in the gut. These toxins can permeate the body and in turn lower resistance to a range of immune problems.

To maintain good digestion, it is best to avoid eating heavy, rich foods such as fatty meats, cream and cheese, bread, pastries and sugar, and drinking alcohol and excess cold water. Better to eat plenty of steamed vegetables, grains and pulses, and drink warming herbal teas to enhance digestion. Spices such as Ginger, Cinnamon, Cardamom, Coriander, Clove, Black pepper and Asafoetida are some of the best remedies for the digestion and for raising immunity.

The world of herbs is replete with immune stimulants that perform their work in a variety of ways. Some herbs increase the production and activity of macrophages – cells that the immune system sends to digest invaders – while others also stimulate the production of defence substances, such as interferon, which protect non-infected cells from viruses. Herbs can also enhance the production and function of T-cells – vital immune cells that kill viruses, fungi and certain bacteria. Immune-enhancing herbs include Ginseng, Guduchi, Cat's claw, Aswagandha, Liquorice, Astragalus, Echinacea, Olive leaf, Garlic, Shiitake and Reishi mushrooms and Turmeric.

A network of vessels produce and carry lymphocytes around the body. These white blood cells contain antibodies that give protection against bacteria and viruses.

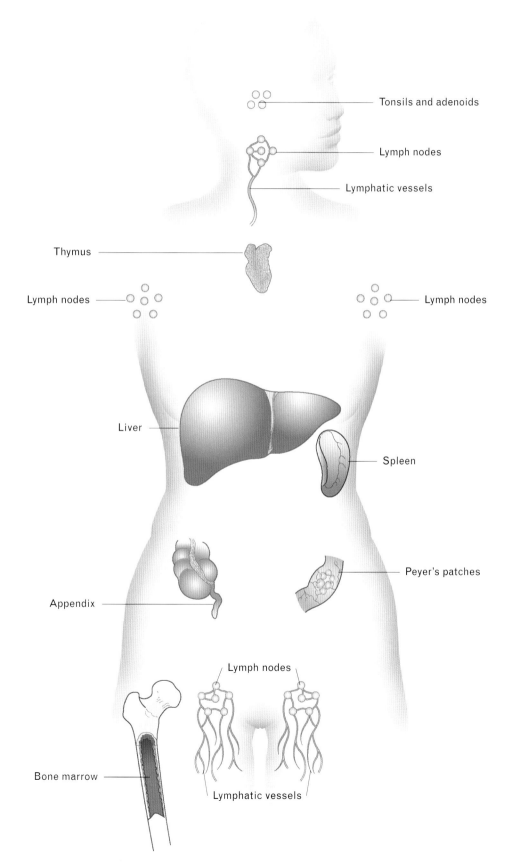

Tonsils and adenoids

Lymph nodes

Lymphatic vessels

Thymus

Lymph nodes

Lymph nodes

Liver

Spleen

Peyer's patches

Appendix

Lymph nodes

Bone marrow

Lymphatic vessels

Fevers

A fever is the body's vital reaction to an infection and a symptom that the body is fighting invaders, whether they are bacterial, viral or fungal. Raising the internal thermostat enables the body to fight off the infection quickly, as it has a natural antibiotic and antiviral effect.

Treatment At the first sign of fever it is best to fast in order to boost the immune system and drink plenty of fluids to aid elimination of toxins. If uncomfortable, take hot teas of diaphoretics like Chamomile, Lime flower or Meadowsweet every couple of hours to bring heat to the surface, cause sweating and hasten the elimination of heat and toxins.

Other good fever-reducing herbs include Willow bark, Vervain, Cleavers, Rose, Holy basil, Boneset, Elderflower, Yarrow, Peppermint, Lavender and Lemon balm. Take singly, or in combinations every 2 hours and sponge the body with tepid infusions. Also take ½ teaspoon of either Echinacea, Andrographis, Pau d'arco, Neem, Myrrh or Cat's claw tincture every 2 hours to fight off infection.

Caution Do not give herbs containing salicylates to children under 12.

Infections

Treatment There are many immune-enhancing herbs that strengthen and support our innate defence mechanisms and help prevent infection. Many have powerful antiviral and antibacterial effects should we succumb. As prevention, add immune-enhancing spices, such as Ginger, Nutmeg, Coriander, Turmeric, Long pepper or Cinnamon to cooking daily, and drink Ginger tea before breakfast. Adaptogenic herbs such as Shiitake and Reishi mushrooms, Cat's claw, Astragalus, Guduchi, Bhringaraj, Ashwagandha, Shatavari and Ginseng are great preventatives.

At first signs of infection, fast to boost immunity, drink plenty of fluids to aid the elimination of toxins and take ½ teaspoon of Echinacea, Wild indigo, Golden seal, Myrrh, Barberry, Andrographis, Pau d'arco or Boneset tincture every 2 hours. Add a little Liquorice, which has antiviral and immune-enhancing properties.

Drink antimicrobial teas through the day: Dill, Marigold, Wild celery, Lemon balm, Chamomile, Lavender, Sage, Thyme, Elecampane, Rosemary or Rose.

Other measures A healthy diet, good digestion (much of our immunity lies in the gut) and adequate exercise and rest and relaxation will support the immune system.

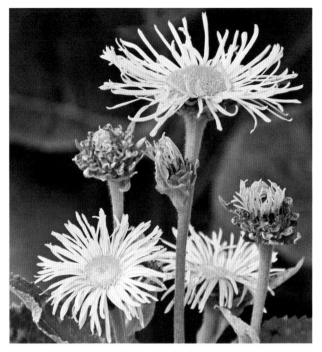

Elecampane is an excellent tonic for the respiratory system, combating infection and clearing congestion.

MRSA

Methicillin-resistant *Staphylococcus aureus* (MRSA) is a 'superbug' that is resistant to antibiotics, including methicillin. The implicated bacteria is *Staphylococcus aureus*, which is found on the skin in about one in three people and generally causes no problems unless immunity is lowered and the bacteria penetrate a break in the skin. Then it can cause boils and abscesses or more serious infections in the bloodstream, bones or joints. Outbreaks in hospitals are common.

Treatment Despite the fact that MRSA is resistant to drugs, it is not resistant to antimicrobial herbs, including Pau d'arco, Garlic, Milk thistle, Golden seal, Turmeric and Myrrh. These can be taken internally 3–6 times daily and used in washes for the skin.

Immunostimulating herbs like Ginseng, Echinacea, Astragalus, Guduchi, Ashwagandha, Liquorice and Shatavari will enhance resistance and help prevent infection. Recent research has demonstrated that beta-glucans from medicinal mushrooms such as Shiitake and Reishi can significantly enhance immunity by activating white blood cells.

Green tea, Tea tree oil, Manuka honey, Grapefruit seed extract and sea salt are all excellent used externally.

Allergies

If a person's immune system reacts against substances that are not infectious or harmful, they have an allergy. Allergic symptoms include sneezing, runny nose, nasal congestion, itchy nose and eyes, digestive disturbances, eczema and asthma. Stress, poor diet, nutritional deficiencies, environmental pollution, drugs, injury, surgery, digestive problems, dysbiosis and genetic tendencies can all predispose to allergies. Treatment involves improving nutrition, temporarily avoiding the allergen and balancing digestive and immune systems.

Treatment Adaptogenic herbs Ashwagandha, Guduchi, Amalaki, Liquorice, Shiitake and Reishi mushrooms, Shatavari, Aloe vera and Ginseng increase immunity and help prevent allergic reactions.

Cat's claw, Walnut, Burdock, Turmeric, Ginger, Myrrh, Cinnamon and Andrographis will combat dysbiosis, which predisposes to leaky gut syndrome and allergies.

Chamomile, Nettle, Lemon balm and Yarrow soothe the allergic response and inhibit histamine, which is responsible for inflammatory symptoms.

Evening primrose oil or Borage seed oil will provide gamma-linolenic acid (GLA), deficiency of which is implicated in several allergic conditions.

Other measures Minimize allergenic foods such as dairy produce, citrus fruits, chocolate, peanuts, wheat or gluten, shellfish, food colourings and preservatives. Avoid caffeine, alcohol, tobacco, sugar and junk foods, which increase susceptibility to allergies.

The severity of the inflammatory response can be diminished by vitamin C (500 mg twice daily) plus bioflavonoids and magnesium (500 mg daily), which are natural antihistamines. Quercetin, a bioflavonoid found in citrus fruits, helps to inhibit the secretion of histamine, leukotrienes and prostaglandins. Other flavonoid-containing foods and herbs could also prove helpful, as they have anti-inflammatory, antioxidant and immunoregulating properties. Capillary-strengthening magnesium with vitamins B and C has an antihistamine action[1] and can be taken at the onset of symptoms.

Chronic fatigue syndrome (CFS)

Also known as post-viral fatigue syndrome or ME (myalgic encephalomyelitis), CFS is common between the ages of 25 and 45, and is characterized by prolonged fatigue and other symptoms including poor memory and concentration, swollen glands, muscle/joint pain, headaches, poor sleep and malaise after exertion. It tends to follow an acute viral infection when immunity has been compromised by toxicity, drugs or alcohol, poor diet, depression, dysbiosis or stress caused by a major life event like bereavement or job loss.

Treatment Adaptogenic herbs Ashwagandha, Shatavari, Astragalus, Liquorice, Guduchi, Amalaki, Rehmannia, Shiitake and Reishi mushrooms, Rhodiola or Siberian ginseng are excellent for increasing resistance to stress and strengthening immunity.

Ginkgo and Gotu kola enhance memory and concentration and relieve depression. St John's wort, Lemon balm and Vervain are good antidepressants.

Black cohosh, Turmeric, Frankincense, Devil's claw, Skullcap and Ginger help alleviate joint and muscle pain.

Take Ginger tea before breakfast to improve digestion and Andrographis, Cat's claw, Burdock, Neem, Myrrh and Olive leaf to combat dysbiosis.

Other measures Eliminate inflammatory foods including refined carbohydrates, saturated fats, alcohol and caffeine, and take vitamin supplements, coenzyme Q10, magnesium, B vitamins and zinc to support the immune system and increase energy. A supplement of bromelain from pineapple is recommended for easing joint and muscle pain.

Shiitake mushrooms are adaptogens, enhancing immunity and increasing the body's ability to cope with stress.

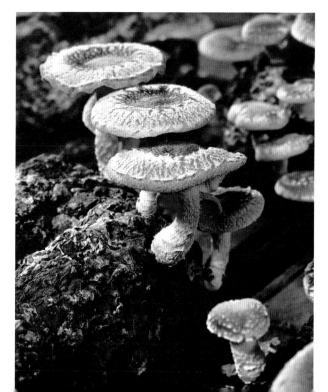

The respiratory system

The respiratory system is responsible for supplying the blood with oxygen. The blood then conveys oxygen to the cells of the body that need it in order to carry out their vital functions. As they use oxygen they give off carbon dioxide as a waste product, which is subsequently carried to the lungs, where it is exhaled.

Oxygen is breathed in through the mouth and the nose and then passes through the larynx and trachea into the chest cavity. The trachea divides into two bronchi that branch into numerous bronchial tubes leading to the lungs, where they divide into many smaller tubes that connect to tiny air sacs called alveoli. Our lungs contain about 600 million alveoli, and these allow oxygen to diffuse through them into the surrounding capillaries and carbon dioxide from the veins to enter the respiratory system to be exhaled by the same pathway. Breathing is brought about by movements of the diaphragm, a sheet of muscle lying at the base of the chest. When it contracts, oxygen is pulled into the lungs; when it relaxes, carbon dioxide is pumped out.

The breath of life

We may be able to go for days without food and water, but can survive only a few minutes without air. To ensure sufficient intake of oxygen we need to maintain a healthy respiratory system, to have plenty of fresh air and exercise and also to breathe properly. Congestion of the airways from excess catarrh reduces the amount of oxygen we take in. The quality of the air is also of vital importance. Environmental pollutants, cigarette smoke, carbon monoxide, lead from car fumes and so on bring pollution into the lungs, which is then transported in the blood around the body and into the cells.

In India air is called 'prana', or 'breath of life', which includes gases vital for normal functioning of our cells and tissues, as well as the energy of the atmosphere around us that radiates from the trees and other green plants and ultimately from the sun. Correct breathing is important for our nerves and muscles to enable relaxation and rest, and also to engender a clear, alert mind. In many cultures and religions the use of the breath is central to spiritual practices such as yoga and meditation, and to traditional movements like T'ai chi and Qi Gong.

Protective measures

The respiratory system is open to the atmosphere via the nose and mouth, and is therefore vulnerable to airborne irritation and infection. It also functions as a pathway for the elimination of toxins, along with the skin, the bowels and the urinary tract. If the body is overloaded with toxins, it can overburden the respiratory system and lead to problems. For this reason our overall health needs to be considered when treating respiratory disorders.

A healthy diet with plenty of fresh fruit and vegetables rich in antioxidants including vitamins A, C and E is essential for a healthy respiratory tract and to protect it from infection and the effects of pollution. Nutritional deficiencies, low hydrochloric acid levels in the stomach and a lack of zinc and magnesium are often found in people who suffer from respiratory diseases. If you have a tendency to respiratory problems, it is best to avoid mucus-forming foods, particularly wheat, milk and sugar and junk foods. The herbal approach to the treatment of respiratory problems is firstly prevention through diet, lifestyle and herbs to maximize immunity and resistance to infections. Herbs such as Echinacea, Garlic, Thyme, Ginger and Turmeric all have effective immunostimulatory as well as antimicrobial actions.

The respiratory system
Oxygen is inhaled as air through the nose and mouth and taken to the lungs, where it is diffused through the alveoli walls into the blood cells. At the same time, carbon dioxide is absorbed from the blood into the alveoli, to be expelled through exhalation.

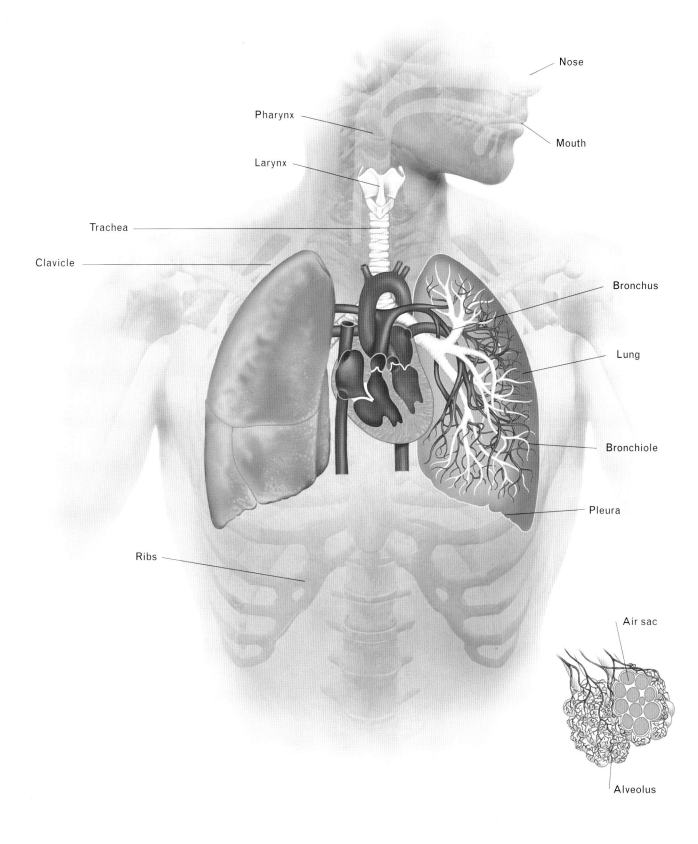

Nose

Pharynx

Mouth

Larynx

Trachea

Clavicle

Bronchus

Lung

Bronchiole

Pleura

Ribs

Air sac

Alveolus

Colds and flu

The common cold virus can thrive only where the conditions in the body are right, and this is more likely when we are run-down, stressed, take insufficient exercise, have sluggish bowels, a poor diet, dysbiosis, or we are overloaded with toxins. The resulting symptoms, particularly fevers and catarrh, are the body's way of clearing toxins.

Treatment At the first signs of infection, take a hot infusion of Boneset, Elderflower, Peppermint and Yarrow every 1–2 hours to relieve aches and pains, reduce fever and clear catarrh. Ginger tea or hot Lemon with honey is also excellent. At the same time take ½ teaspoon of Echinacea tincture and 500 mg of vitamin C every 2 hours. Other immune-enhancing, antimicrobial and decongestant spices, like Cinnamon, Cardamom, Fenugreek, Turmeric and Coriander, improve digestion and balance the gut flora and can be taken similarly. Andrographis, Elderberry and Elderflower, Garlic, Golden seal, Lemon balm, Pau d'arco, Cat's claw, Amalaki and Wormwood are other effective remedies to combat infection and reduce fevers.

Aromatic inhalations or hot foot baths of Rosemary, Lavender, Thyme, Cinnamon or Chamomile will reduce swelling of mucous membranes and loosen and clear catarrh. A Ginger or Mustard foot bath can be effective, too.

Other measures Supplements of vitamin C and zinc will help to prevent and decrease the duration of a cold.

Catarrh and sinusitis

Irritation and inflammation of the nasal passages and sinuses from infection or inhaled pollutants causes extra secretion of mucus as a protective mechanism, which accumulates as catarrh. This can lead to sinusitis, which can be very painful and result in headaches and post-nasal drip, causing recurrent throat and chest problems. Chronic catarrh and sinusitis can be due to infection, pollution, poor diet or food allergy, or a sign of intestinal dysbiosis and toxicity.

Treatment Take antimicrobial herbs Golden seal, Wild indigo, Elderberry, Andrographis, Echinacea, Neem, Amalaki, Turmeric, Garlic or Myrrh to enhance immunity, combat infections in the respiratory system and clear toxicity from the gut. These are best combined with decongestants and astringents taken in hot teas, such as Ginger, Cinnamon, Coriander, Thyme, Ground ivy, Yarrow, Elderflower, Chamomile, Eyebright, Agrimony, Meadowsweet and Peppermint.

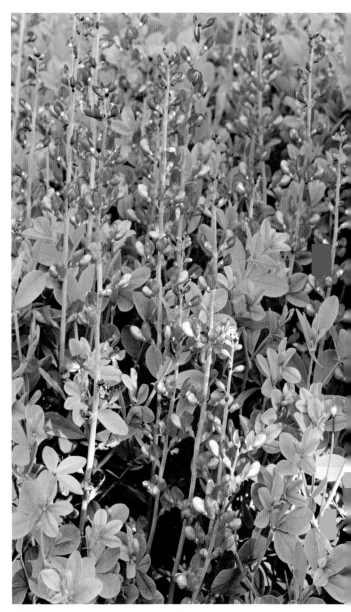

Wild indigo is an antimicrobial herb with antiseptic properties used to boost the body's immune responses.

Demulcents like Slippery elm, Marshmallow, Mullein and Plantain soothe irritation and pain in the sinuses.

Oils of Lavender, Peppermint, Rosemary, Thyme or Chamomile are good in inhalations and baths, or for massage around the nose and sinuses.

Other measures Washing the sinuses by sniffing salt water can work wonders. Omitting wheat or gluten, dairy produce and sugar from the diet and taking a supplement of vitamin C is recommended.

Earache

This can arise from pain and inflammation in the throat, tonsils, gums, teeth or parotid glands, or inflammation of the outer ear. Acute middle ear infection (otitis media) causes acute pain and is common in children. Children treated with antibiotics are prone to recurrent antibiotic-resistant strains of ear infection and glue ear. Other underlying causes include dysbiosis, passive smoking, chronic catarrh and throat, tonsil and sinus infection.

Treatment For ear infections, use a combination of internal and local herbs. Chamomile is an excellent antimicrobial, anti-inflammatory and pain reliever for children. Echinacea enhances the immune system's fight against infection. Elderberry, Garlic, Golden seal, Andrographis, Wild indigo and Cat's claw are also good antimicrobials and will combat infection and reduce fevers. Elderflower, Plantain, Thyme, Ground ivy and Meadowsweet help clear catarrh and alleviate pain. Pasque flower is specific for pain. Cleavers, Dandelion, Blue flag and Poke root help reduce swollen glands that can cause congestion in the middle ear.

Provided there is no pus from a perforated eardrum, drop warm Mullein, St John's wort or Olive oil with a few drops of either Lavender, Garlic or Chamomile oil into the ear and plug it with cotton wool to relieve inflammation or infection. Avoid mucus-producing foods, such as sugar, junk foods and dairy produce.

Tonsillitis and laryngitis

Acute throat infections can be caused by viral or bacterial infection. Tonsillitis causes swollen and pus-filled tonsils, quite severe throat pain, difficulty swallowing, fever and malaise. Laryngitis is inflammation or infection of the larynx, which causes a sore throat aggravated by talking, dry cough, hoarseness and fever. The tonsils are bundles of lymphatic tissue whose role it is to clear the blood of toxins. Chronic tonsillitis develops when other eliminative pathways (bowels, kidneys and lungs) are overburdened, putting the lymphatic system under extra pressure, and is often related to allergies.

Treatment Potent antimicrobials such as Garlic, Andrographis, Neem, Golden seal, Wild indigo, Echinacea, Poke root, Cat's claw, Pau d'arco, Turmeric, Wormwood or Myrrh taken every 2 hours at the first signs will help combat acute infections.

Marshmallow, Slippery elm, Mullein, Aloe vera, Liquorice, Coltsfoot or Comfrey soothe soreness and pain, and can be combined with painkilling herbs like Pasque flower, Black cohosh or Chamomile. In acute infections use gargles, sprays or steam inhalations of Myrrh, Sage, Thyme, Raspberry leaf, Marshmallow, Plantain or Turmeric, or essential oils of Lavender, Thyme or Chamomile every 2 hours.

For chronic tonsillitis, immune-enhancing Shatavari, Ashwagandha, Guduchi, Shiitake and Reishi mushrooms, Schisandra or Amalaki will help reduce allergies and chronic inflammation, while lymphatic stimulants Cleavers, Poke root, Marigold, Blue flag, Burdock and Red clover enhance detoxification and immunity.

Other measures Avoiding dairy produce, sugar and junk food is recommended.

Caution Seek medical attention for acute tonsillitis to rule out streptococcal infection, which can cause serious secondary infections.

Echinacea, well-known as a herbal immune stimulant, is prescribed to prevent and treat all acute respiratory infections.

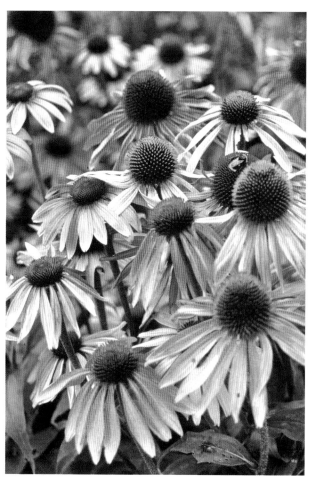

Sore throat and swollen glands

Generally a prelude to a bacterial or viral infection, sore throats can also be caused by irritation of the throat lining by tobacco smoke, post-nasal drip, allergies, acid reflux, dry heat and shouting. Swelling of lymph glands in the neck indicate that the body is attempting to fight off infection, or is overloaded with toxins and increasing the work of the lymphatic system in carrying away waste products.

Treatment Antimicrobial herbs Echinacea, Wild indigo, Turmeric, Garlic, Wormwood, Cat's claw, Pau d'arco, Myrrh or Andrographis can be taken at the first signs to ward off infection.

Immune-enhancing Ashwagandha, Shatavari, Guduchi, Baikal Skullcap, Astragalus, Rehmannia, Shiitake and Reishi mushrooms, Schisandra and Amalaki help reduce allergies and inflammation caused by environmental irritants.

Demulcents Marshmallow, Slippery elm, Mullein, Aloe vera, Liquorice, Coltsfoot and Comfrey moisten and soothe irritation of the mucous membranes of the throat.

Cleavers, Poke root, Marigold, Blue flag, Burdock and Red clover enhance the lymphatic system in its cleansing and immune work.

Gargling or spraying the throat with Sage, Thyme, Sweet marjoram, Turmeric, Myrrh or salt water will also help.

Other measures Supplements of vitamins A, B and C also enhance immunity.

Caution If a child runs a fever with an acute sore throat and swollen tonsils, seek professional help. It could indicate a streptococcal infection with risk of further complications such as nephritis and rheumatic fever.

Asthma

This is caused by the release of inflammatory chemicals that inflame and narrow the bronchial tubes, making it difficult to breathe. Increased mucus production blocks the airways still further. Asthma can be triggered by food allergies, environmental pollutants, respiratory infections, immune problems (caused by suppression of eczema and chest infections for example), emotional problems, digestive disturbances or dysbiosis. Prevention is the best line of treatment. Herbs can be taken in conjunction with other medication or inhalants, and may need to be taken over several months. Treat the first signs of respiratory infection vigorously to prevent asthma from getting progressively worse.

Treatment Expectorant herbs such as Elecampane, Thyme, Hyssop, Garlic, Coltsfoot, Ginger, Garlic, Liquorice and Mullein liquefy and clear mucus from the bronchial tubes, and strengthen and relax bronchial muscles, opening the airways. Thyme, Elecampane, Pleurisy root, Angelica, Pau d'arco and Sweet marjoram are excellent for combating chest infections.

Adaptogens Schisandra, Ashwagandha, Shatavari, Liquorice, Turmeric or Shiitake and Reishi mushrooms enhance immunity, reduce inflammation and increase resilience to stress.

Ginkgo, Chamomile, Yarrow, Feverfew, Baikal Skullcap or Nettle help decrease allergic responses that may trigger asthma.

Relaxing herbs like Skullcap, Holy basil, Rose, Lavender, Honeysuckle, Wild oats or Chamomile help reduce tension.

Caution Seek medical attention in cases of acute asthma.

CASE STUDY **ASTHMA**

CLIENT PROFILE
David, aged 8, suffered from wheezing and a dry cough every time he exerted himself, such as running during school sports or playing football. He also tended to wake in the early hours of the morning with mild asthma. His symptoms worsened during cold winter weather and when he was anxious.

THE HERBAL TREATMENT
I made David a prescription of antispasmodic and demulcent herbs to relax and soothe the bronchi and open the airways. It included Marshmallow, Elecampane, Thyme, Hyssop, Coltsfoot, Liquorice and Mullein. I added Ashwagandha and Shatavari to enhance immunity and increase resilience to stress, a little Ginger to aid digestion and elimination of toxins from the gut, and suggested he drink Chamomile and Nettle tea to decrease any allergic response that may trigger his asthma.

I recommended that David's parents remove dairy products and wheat from his diet, as he frequently ate pizza and pasta. I also suggested that they ensured David had plenty of calcium in his diet from other sources, such as green vegetables, bony fish, nuts and seeds.

With this treatment, David's asthma was better within a few weeks.

Hay fever

Hay fever, which is also known as allergic rhinitis, is a common atopic condition that mostly occurs when high concentrations of pollens are released during late spring and summer, especially during hot weather. The familiar symptoms are caused by the release of histamine and other inflammatory chemicals, and are generally worse in the morning and evening, which coincides with the changes in air temperature. House dust and animal hair can also produce similar reactions. Hay fever as well as other atopic conditions like eczema and asthma tend to be genetic and occur when immunity is lowered, for example by long-term stress and dysbiosis.

Treatment As a preventative, take immunostimulants Ashwagandha, Astragalus, Guduchi, Amalaki, Siberian ginseng or Echinacea and 1–2 dessertspoons of local honey in honeycombs with each meal for 2–4 months before the hay fever season.

Antihistamine and anti-inflammatory herbs Turmeric, Echinacea, Golden seal, Chamomile, Nettle, Lemon balm, Feverfew, Baikal skullcap or Yarrow with a little Liquorice help to reduce symptoms once they start and can be taken every 2 hours if necessary. They can also be used as teas for inhalations to ease symptoms.

Agrimony, Elderflower, Plantain and Eyebright tone mucous membranes and desensitize them to allergens. Marshmallow and Slippery elm soothe irritation of the mucosa.

Ginger, Garlic, Thyme, Burdock or Marigold combat dysbiosis, while Burdock, Dandelion, Agrimony and Milk thistle support the liver.

Other measures Supplements of vitamin C and magnesium are recommended. Cutting out wheat or gluten and dairy foods is also helpful. Sunglasses may help to reduce eye irritation.

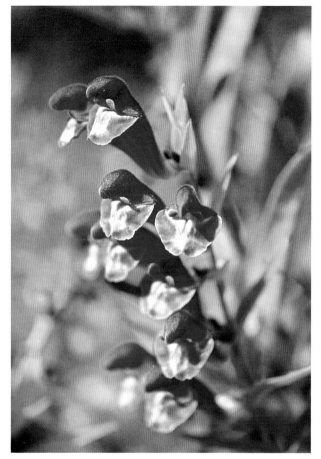

Baikal skullcap has antihistamine effects useful in the treatment of hay fever.

Coughs and bronchitis

A cough is a reflex response designed to remove irritants such as dust, toxins, micro-organisms or mucus blocking the throat or bronchial tubes, but it can become chronic and debilitating, disturbing sleep. Coughs can be aggravated by stress and cold weather.

Treatment Demulcent herbs like Marshmallow, Mullein, Plantain, Liquorice, Coltsfoot or Slippery elm soothe irritation and inflammation in dry, tickly coughs.

Expectorants and decongestants including Thyme, Elecampane, Ground ivy, White horehound, Hyssop, Ginger, Angelica and Sweet marjoram liquefy and clear phlegm. Vitamin C in Elderberries and Blueberries/Bilberries, as well as infusions of Rose petals, stimulate the mucociliary escalator, clear phlegm and protect the lungs from infection.

Nervous coughs can be eased with relaxing herbs such as Chamomile, Lemon balm and Holy basil. Antimicrobials including Thyme, Elecampane, Hyssop, Cat's claw, Pau d'arco, Garlic, Cinnamon and Pleurisy root combat infection and support the immune system. A cough formula will need to consist of mixtures of these, depending on the nature of the cough.

Essential oils of Rosemary, Rose, Thyme, Ginger or Cinnamon can be used in baths and inhalation.

Caution Fever and malaise with cough, green phlegm or breathlessness may indicate acute bronchitis or pneumonia. Seek medical attention.

The digestive system

Efficient digestion is absolutely essential to good health. The digestive system enables our bodies to convert the food we eat into the energy needed for all the minute biochemical reactions that keep us alive. It also provides the major pathway for the elimination of toxins from the body.

Health and vitality largely depend not only on an excellent diet but also on how efficiently our digestion makes the nutrients from food available to us and, in turn, passes out undigested food residues and the waste products of metabolism.

The digestive tract is lined with a protective mucous membrane, which also serves to secrete digestive juices that contain enzymes designed to break down food into a form our bodies can absorb. Other digestive enzymes are supplied to the digestive tract by the liver, gall bladder and pancreas. The conversion of food in the digestive tract provides energy, but it also requires energy to carry out all the essential biochemical reactions involved in the process. If our digestive energy is low or upset, it can lead to digestive symptoms such as bloating, stomachaches, IBS (irritable bowel syndrome), diarrhoea and constipation, and can also fundamentally affect our general health and energy, predisposing to lethargy, lowered immunity, nervous problems, poor concentration and sleep disturbances.

Influencing factors

Good digestion and elimination depend on several factors. We need to eat sufficient fibre from whole foods, fruit and vegetables and to drink plenty of fluids to ensure regular peristaltic movements that propel food along the alimentary canal. The right diet is vital to the health and normal function of the digestive tract. Over-refined foods, excess sugar, fizzy drinks, ice creams and fermented and fried foods can all irritate and create disturbances. Indigestible foods, such as bread, cheese, red meat and excess hard, raw foods, can leave partially digested or undigested food residues in the gut that are prone to fermentation and predispose to a toxic state in the gut. We need to eliminate food residues as well as the waste products of cellular metabolism every day to help prevent fermentation and toxicity and the absorption of these toxins into the body. Dysbiosis, or a toxic state of the bowel involving a disturbance of the bacterial population of the gut, is increasingly being recognized as the underlying cause of many health problems including IBS, allergies, autoimmune disease and obesity.

There is constant interaction between the brain and the digestive system, making digestion susceptible to the effects of the mind and emotions, and therefore to stress of various kinds. The nervous system regulates the circulation to and from the digestive tract, as well as the secretion of digestive juices. Tension and anxiety can reduce the flow of digestive enzymes and inhibit good digestion. Alternatively, stress may trigger excess secretion of hydrochloric acid in the stomach, which can irritate, inflame and, in some cases, ulcerate the lining of the stomach or intestine.

The herbal materia medica offers a huge range of remedies for almost every kind of digestive disorder. For example, warming spices such as Ginger, Cinnamon and Long pepper will stimulate the secretion of digestive enzymes; mucilage-rich herbs including Slippery elm and Marshmallow soothe irritation; Fennel, Peppermint and Chamomile ease pain and spasm, and bitter herbs such as Dandelion, Agrimony and Burdock support the liver.

The digestive system
Ingested food is broken down in the alimentary canal to a form that can be assimilated by the body. Digestion begins in the mouth with the action of saliva on food, but most of the process takes place within the stomach and small intestine.

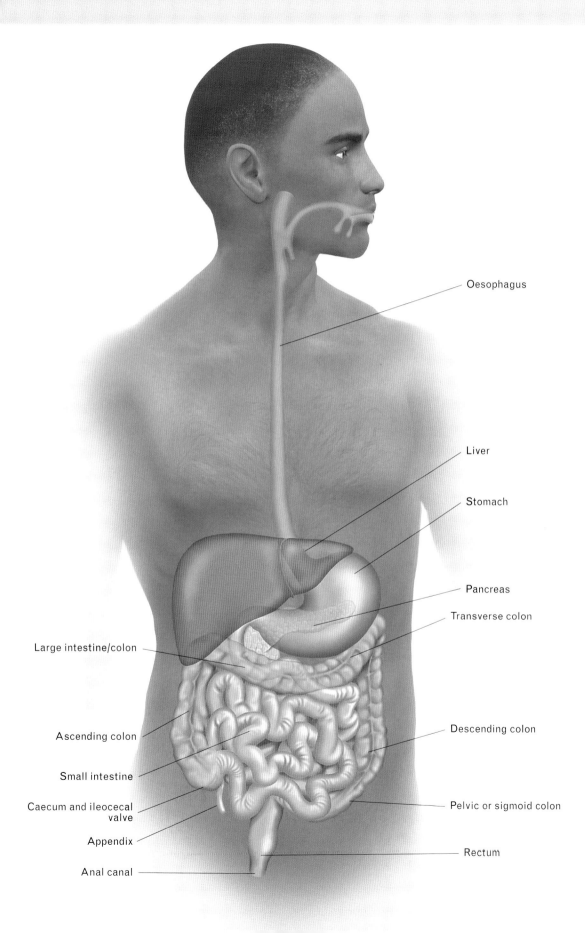

Oesophagus

Liver

Stomach

Pancreas

Transverse colon

Large intestine/colon

Ascending colon

Small intestine

Caecum and ileocecal valve

Appendix

Anal canal

Descending colon

Pelvic or sigmoid colon

Rectum

Dysbiosis

Intestinal bacteria in a healthy gut synthesize vitamins, break down dietary toxins, making them less harmful, and stimulate local immunity (inhibiting infections like salmonella, decreasing the risk of food poisoning) and enhance general immunity. Four-fifths of the body's immune system is found in the gut lining. Use of antibiotics and steroids, as well as poor digestion and stress, leads to the proliferation of pathogenic yeasts and bacteria, which create toxins, destroy vitamins, inactivate digestive enzymes and lead to the formation of carcinogenic chemicals. They provoke inflammatory diseases such as ulcerative colitis, Crohn's disease and arthritis by causing autoimmune reactions and leaky gut syndrome as well as liver problems. Symptoms of yeast overgrowth include vaginal thrush, chronic diarrhoea, allergic reactions, asthma, hives, psoriasis, eczema, migraine, recurrent infection, abdominal pain, cystitis, catarrh, depression and lethargy.

Treatment Cat's claw, Garlic, Myrrh, Andrographis, Golden seal, Olive leaf and Reishi mushroom are excellent for combating pathogenic micro-organisms. Oregon grape, Elecampane, Dill, Burdock, Bearberry, Marigold, Echinacea, Fennel, Amalaki and Bladderwrack act similarly.

Aloe vera juice (25 ml/1 fl oz twice daily) is soothing, immune enhancing and combats dysbiosis.

Antimicrobial spices Turmeric, Cinnamon, Ginger and

Reishi mushrooms can help overcome intestinal dysbiosis by fighting growth of pathogenic micro-organisms.

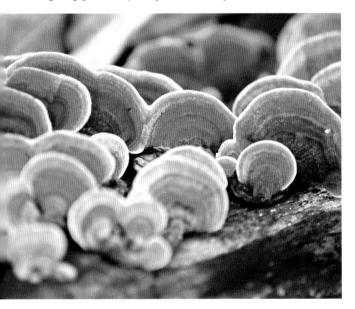

Long pepper enhance secretion of digestive enzymes and can be added daily to food. Evening primrose and Linseed oil are also helpful.

Other measures Supplements of *Lactobacillus acidophilus* help restore normal bacterial population of the gut. Taking vitamin C (500 mg daily) and caprylic acid (1 g with meals) is also beneficial.

Constipation

It is important to ascertain and treat the causes of constipation and not become reliant on laxative medicines, which can be taken short term but may aggravate the problem in the long run. Causes include lack of exercise, ignoring the urge, old age, piles, IBS, diverticulitis, food allergy, dysbiosis, nutritional deficiency, excess refined foods, insufficient fibre from fruit, vegetables and whole grains, and tension in the bowel due to stress. It is important to remedy constipation otherwise toxins from reabsorption in the bowel may cause chronic disease.

Treatment Use Linseed, Fenugreek or Psyllium seeds to bulk out bowel contents and push them along. Soak 1–2 teaspoons of seeds in a cup of hot water for 2 hours, add lemon and honey if you like and drink at bedtime. It is important to drink plenty of water. Liquorice, Dandelion root and Burdock root taken as decoctions 3 times a day are also effective for mild constipation. If necessary, add more stimulating laxative herbs such as Yellow dock or Senna pods with a little Ginger for a week or two.

For stress-related constipation, add Chamomile, Lemon balm, Dill, Hops or Cramp bark. Garlic, Thyme, Burdock or Marigold work well for dysbiosis.

Other measures Live yogurt, lacto-acidophilus or Grapefruit seed extract can also help candida, which can predispose to constipation. Taking 30 minutes of exercise daily is recommended.

Caution If constipation is persistent, develops suddenly or with pain, seek medical attention.

Diarrhoea

Diarrhoea represents the body's attempt to rid itself of poisons or irritants (including drugs, chemicals and allergens), inflammation or infection in the gut, so it is important not to stop it but to address the underlying causes. It is vital to drink plenty of fluids to replace lost water and electrolytes.

Treatment Use astringent herbs Agrimony, Bayberry, Cinnamon, Raspberry leaf or Yarrow to dry up secretions and tone the gut. Demulcent herbs Slippery elm and Marshmallow soothe irritation and act as prebiotics to support beneficial flora in the gut. Chamomile, Hops, Wild yam, Dill and Lemon balm reduce anxiety in stress-related diarrhoea. Digestives Ginger, Cinnamon, Turmeric and Coriander, taken regularly as teas or in food, enhance the secretion of digestive enzymes.

For infection causing gastroenteritis and dysbiosis, use antimicrobials including Golden seal, Thyme, Chamomile, Cinnamon, Pau d'arco, Garlic and Ginger.

Antispasmodics such as Peppermint, Ginger, Dill and Chamomile relieve cramping pain and Chamomile, Hops, Golden seal, Meadowsweet and Yarrow relieve inflammation.

Other measures Wheat or gluten and dairy foods can cause food intolerances, while red meat and too much hard, raw food can be indigestible and aggravate the condition, so these are best avoided until fully recovered. Acidophilus supplements are also useful.

Caution If diarrhoea persists or is accompanied by fever, or if there is mucus or blood in stools, seek medical attention.

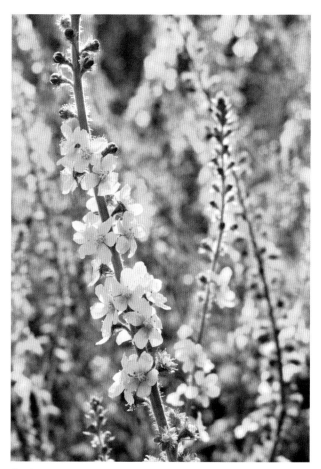

Agrimony is a good astringent and digestive tonic and can be helpful in relieving diarrhoea.

Irritable bowel syndrome (IBS)

The bowel can become irritated by poorly digested and putrefying foods caused by weak digestion, stress, poor diet and disturbance of gut flora by, for example, antibiotics. Accumulated toxins, loss of beneficial flora and increase of pathogenic organisms cause dysbiosis, which leads to leaky gut syndrome, food intolerances and lowered immunity. Resulting symptoms include alternating diarrhoea and constipation, flatulence and abdominal discomfort.

Treatment Anti-inflammatory and antispasmodic herbs such as Chamomile, Wild yam, Cramp bark, Meadowsweet, Peppermint, Hops or Myrrh can be helpful. Demulcents like Slippery elm, Aloe vera and Marshmallow are soothing and healing, while astringent Yarrow, Thyme, Agrimony and Bayberry protect the gut wall from irritation. Relaxants such as Lemon balm, Vervain, Dill, Hops or Valerian can help reduce stress. Blueberries/Bilberries are helpful for diarrhoea and Burdock or Liquorice can be taken for constipation.

To address dysbiosis and enhance immunity, Cat's claw, Chamomile, Cinnamon, Golden seal, Echinacea, Myrrh, Amalaki, Aloe vera, Olive leaf, Common grape vine, Garlic or Turmeric are recommended.

Drinking Ginger tea before meals and adding mild spices to cooking will stimulate the secretion of digestive enzymes and help maintain healthy gut flora.

Other measures Food intolerance is implicated in many cases, so temporarily omitting tea, coffee, dairy products, eggs and wheat or gluten from your diet is advisable.

Caution If there is mucus or blood in stools or severe abdominal pain, consult your doctor.

Poor absorption

A healthy digestive system removes nutrients from food so that they can be absorbed into the bloodstream. Poor secretion of digestive enzymes and damage to the villi in the small intestine where nutrients are absorbed can lead to poor absorption, fermentation and gas, increased acidity and weight gain, and reduces antioxidants in the body. Stress, illness, tiredness, old age, dysbiosis and chronic diarrhoea can inhibit digestive enzymes, and damage to villi can be caused by inflammation, infection, sudden changes in diet, excess wheat or gluten intolerance as in coeliac disease.

Treatment To improve digestion and absorption, start the day with tea made from fresh Ginger or hot water with a squeeze of lime juice. Chewing or adding seeds such as Dill, Cardamom, Fennel and Coriander to cooking stimulates the flow of digestive enzymes and promotes absorption. Long pepper is one of the best herbs for improving absorption.

CASE STUDY **POOR ABSORPTION**

CLIENT PROFILE
Peter, aged 35, consulted me about his bowel problems. He was suffering from intermittent abdominal pain, irregular bowel movements with hard, pellet-like stools, wind and bloating. He felt it had been worse since he had gastroenteritis while in Egypt. His tongue was pale with a white coating at the back, indicating poor digestion and bowel toxicity, and tooth marks around the edge of the tongue revealed poor absorption of nutrients.

THE HERBAL TREATMENT
I made Peter a prescription of antispasmodic, digestive and probiotic herbs to regulate his digestion and re-establish his gut flora. It included Ginger, Dill, Marshmallow, Chamomile, Liquorice, Amalaki and Turmeric.

I suggested that Peter should temporarily remove wheat and dairy produce from his diet and stop drinking coffee. I recommended drinking Chamomile, Mint and Fennel tea instead and taking Aloe vera juice in Ginger tea in the morning before he ate breakfast. I mentioned adding mild spices to his cooking to enhance the digestion and absorption of nutrients.

This treatment helped Peter's bowels to return to normal within a month.

Hot teas of Peppermint, Chamomile, Holy basil, Fennel, Rosemary, Thyme, Ginger or Cinnamon before and after meals will aid digestion. Relaxants such as Chamomile, Lavender, Lemon balm, Hops, Vervain, Fennel and Rose are recommended for stress.

For dysbiosis, Cat's claw, Cinnamon, Echinacea, Myrrh, Amalaki, Aloe vera, Olive leaf, Common grape vine, Garlic or Turmeric will help to re-establish beneficial gut flora.

Other measures Avoid indigestible foods such as salads, raw seeds and nuts as well as cheese and bread until digestion improves.

Obesity

Obesity can predispose to high blood pressure, raised cholesterol, heart disease, strokes, cancer and diabetes, especially if these run in the family. It is related to a complex interaction between hormones, digestion, metabolism, liver function and toxicity, as well as dietary factors and lack of exercise. A marginally underactive thyroid and insulin resistance (syndrome X) are often implicated in the condition.

Treatment Bladderwrack, Guggulu and chromium supplements help to regularize thyroid hormones and raise metabolism. Hawthorn, Gotu kola, Neem, Fennel, Amalaki, Cinnamon and Turmeric taken regularly and spices like Cayenne pepper, Garlic, Coriander, Ginger, Cinnamon and Turmeric in food will stimulate digestion and metabolism.

Teas of Cleavers, Dandelion leaf and Chickweed have a reputation for aiding weight loss and excess fluid through diuretic action.

Metabolism often changes after the menopause, causing weight gain. Wild yam, Chaste tree, Motherwort, Fennel and Black cohosh help to regulate hormone levels.

Gymnema is helpful in syndrome X and blocks sweet receptors on the tongue, helping to curb sweet cravings. Forskohlii is becoming well known for its effect on thyroid metabolism and syndrome X.

Other measures Essential fatty acids in oily fish, nuts, seeds, whole grains, Evening primrose and Flax seed oil help to raise metabolic rate. It is important to lose weight gradually, no more than 1 kg (2 lb) a week.

Inflammatory bowel disease (IBD)

Chronic inflammation of the gut is a serious problem that can involve ulceration and bleeding that sometimes necessitates surgery. It is indicated by severe abdominal pain, nausea, diarrhoea or constipation, blood in the stools, poor appetite, weight loss, fever as well as lethargy. The most common forms of IBD are autoimmune problems such as ulcerative colitis and Crohn's disease, which can be sparked off by a bacterial or viral infection and may cause poor absorption and nutritional deficiencies that in turn lead to anaemia and osteoporosis.

Treatment Turmeric and Frankincense are wonderful anti-inflammatory herbs and can be very effective for reducing pain and inflammation. Chamomile tea taken frequently through the day is excellent. Liquorice, Cat's claw, Golden seal, Myrrh, Hops, Peppermint, Yarrow, Meadowsweet and Sarsaparilla are also helpful. Ground Flax seed in water or Flax oil, Aloe vera juice, Marshmallow and Slippery elm soothe the gut lining and help regulate the bowels.

Lemon balm, Hops, Chamomile, Skullcap, Wild oats, Ashwagandha and Passion flower reduce tension and anxiety.

Other measures Avoid possible food allergens, particularly wheat or gluten and dairy products, as well as acidic and spicy foods, citrus fruits, tomatoes, alcohol and coffee. Bromelain from pineapple and papain from papaya help resolve inflammation and speed healing. Also, try to avoid getting tired and stressed, as this can aggravate symptoms.

Caution Seek medical attention if there is blood in the stool, a change in bowel habits lasting longer than 10 days or any of the above symptoms that do not improve with treatment.

Nausea and vomiting

These may be due to adverse reactions to foods or drugs, nervous tension, migraine or infections causing irritation and inflammation in the stomach. Other causes include early pregnancy, travel sickness, peptic ulcers, gastritis, shock, intestinal obstruction, pressure on the brain by fluid in altitude sickness or a tumour, or loss of balance caused by inner ear infection. It is important to drink plenty of fluid to prevent dehydration.

Treatment The best and most delicious remedy is fresh Ginger, sipped in tea or simply chewed. This is

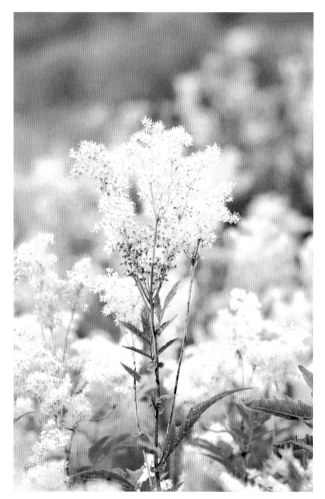

Meadowsweet reduces acidity in the stomach and has an anti-inflammatory action on the intestines.

particularly useful in pregnancy when other herbs might be contraindicated. Teas of Chamomile, Fennel or Peppermint can also settle the stomach.

If caused by emotional stress, teas or tinctures of Lemon balm, Chamomile, Lavender, Hops, Dill or Passion flower can help.

For an infection or food poisoning, take Garlic, Turmeric, Chamomile, Echinacea, Cinnamon, Pau d'arco or Golden seal every 2 hours.

Feverfew, Wood betony or Rosemary are best when there are headaches or migraine, while Marshmallow and Slippery elm will soothe irritation, and Meadowsweet, Gentian and Burdock can reduce heat and inflammation in the stomach.

Caution If symptoms persist or there is severe vomiting with high fever, seek medical attention.

Mouth ulcers

Ulcers can be caused by minor injuries from a sharp edge on a tooth or bad dentures for example, or they can be aphthous ulcers, indicating that immunity is lowered from physical or psychological stress, or there is a deficiency in vitamin B12, folic acid or iron. Aphthous ulcers can also be caused by viruses such as herpes and hand, foot and mouth disease, food allergies, dysbiosis, adverse drug reactions to medications or mercury fillings, cigarettes, alcohol, ulcerative colitis or Crohn's disease.

Treatment Soothing mouthwashes of Lavender, Marigold, Marshmallow or Chamomile used 3 times daily will help relieve pain and inflammation. Antiseptic mouthwashes of Sage, Echinacea, Pau d'arco, Thyme, Lemon balm, Myrrh and Blueberry/Bilberry combat infection and can be taken internally as teas to boost immunity.

Skullcap, Siberian Ginseng, Wild oats, Vervain and Ashwagandha are nourishing nerve tonics when run-down. Shiitake and Reishi mushrooms and Rhodiola also boost immunity.

Aloe vera gel is soothing and healing, as it forms a protective layer over the ulcer. A local spray of Golden seal, Liquorice or Myrrh will act as an anaesthetic and speed healing. Nettle is a good source of iron if deficiency is a contributing factor.

Other measures Supplements of vitamins B and C and folic acid are recommended.

Caution Ulcers that do not heal should always be checked by a doctor, since they may indicate mouth cancer.

Heartburn and acidity

These indicate a disordered stomach, hyperacidity and gastro-oesophageal reflux, which can be caused by chronic constipation, obesity or stress. They can also be triggered by alcohol, chocolate, sugar, refined carbohydrates, tea, coffee, cigarettes, rich, fatty, spicy and acidic foods such as tomatoes and citrus fruits, emotional upset and eating too fast. Heartburn and acidity can be aggravated by bending over, sitting hunched up and lying in bed.

Treatment Try sipping Chamomile tea frequently. Meadowsweet is also cooling and soothing. Surprisingly, some people find that chewing fresh Ginger can ease their feelings of discomfort.

Demulcent herbs such as Marshmallow or Liquorice

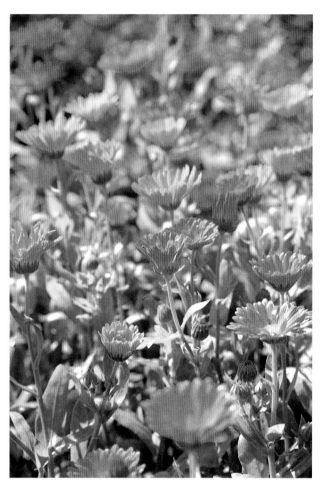

Marigold improves digestion and can help fight infection caused by diverticulitis.

can soothe pain and reduce acidity. A gruel made with 1–2 teaspoons of Slippery elm powder mixed with warm water can bring almost instant relief. Taking 25 ml (1 fl oz) Aloe vera juice twice daily can also be effective, cooling heat and inflammation and combating symptoms caused by dysbiosis.

Peppermint, Lemon balm, Holy basil and Dill are excellent digestives and reduce tension in the gut, while bitter herbs like Dandelion root and Burdock are gently laxative, enhance digestion and reduce heat and burning. Chamomile, Hops, Vervain or Lemon balm are good when heartburn is related to stress.

Diverticulitis

This is inflammation and infection that develops in small pockets in weakened areas of the bowel wall. It tends to occur more in people over 50, often as a result of lack of exercise, an over-refined diet and long-term constipation. It can cause quite severe cramping pains, irregular bowels, sometimes bloody stools, flatulence and fever.

Treatment Flax or Psyllium seeds soaked in water and allowed to swell into a gel, or Slippery elm powder mixed with water, can be taken at night to regulate and soothe the bowels. Marshmallow and Aloe vera are also antibacterial and demulcent.

Chamomile is anti-inflammatory and antiseptic, and is excellent sipped throughout the day. Wild yam and Hops are antispasmodic and anti-inflammatory, and can be combined with Liquorice and Peppermint.

Cat's claw, Turmeric, Marigold, Echinacea or Pau d'arco help combat infection and are particularly useful in acute attacks taken every 2 hours.

Other measures Eat plenty of high-fibre foods, but avoid wheat, dairy and irritating foods such as bran, nuts and seeds, hard raw vegetables and fruits with seeds like raspberries, tomatoes and blackberries. Drink plenty of fluids to ensure regular bowel movements. Avoid caffeinated drinks and take plenty of exercise.

Wind and bloating

Most wind is produced in the intestines by fermentation of undigested carbohydrates. The gut does not produce sufficient enzymes to digest certain carbohydrates, particularly those from beans and brassicas. It can also be indicative of dysbiosis, food intolerances to wheat and dairy foods for example, bad eating habits, low digestive enzymes, stress, gastritis and peptic ulcers, gall bladder disease, constipation and IBS.

Treatment Carminative herbs are specific for relieving wind and bloating, and act by improving digestion and absorption and reducing inflammation and dysbiosis. Recommended carminatives are Fennel, Dill, Rosemary, Peppermint, Ginger, Cinnamon, Lemon balm and Chamomile. Coriander, Cardamom, Fennel and Dill seeds are excellent when chewed or added to food. Ginger tea is recommended before meals.

Antimicrobial herbs such as Pau d'arco, Amalaki, Garlic, Burdock, Echinacea, Olive leaf, Golden seal, Turmeric, Rosemary, Chamomile, Thyme or Sweet marjoram will help clear toxins and putrefactive bacteria.

Gentle massage of the abdomen clockwise using dilute

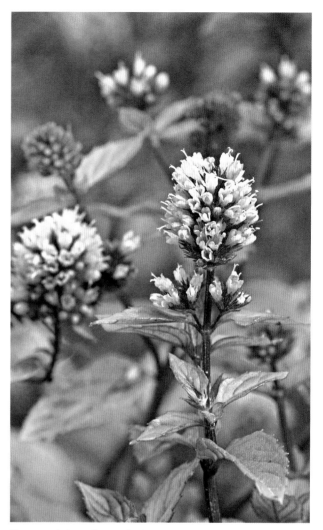

Peppermint soothes and relaxes the digestive system, and reduces bloating and wind.

oils of Cinnamon, Ginger, Cloves or Peppermint can be very effective for relieving wind and discomfort.

Other measures It is important to eat slowly and when relaxed, not to eat late at night and to take plenty of exercise to enhance digestion. Eliminating wheat or gluten and dairy foods from the diet can be helpful.

Gastritis and peptic ulcers

The stomach may become irritated and inflamed through weak digestion, poor diet, drugs (such as ibuprofen and aspirin) or stress, which causes over-secretion of hydrochloric acid in the stomach, and this leads to gastritis. As the condition worsens, ulceration of the lining of the stomach or small intestine can develop. Stomach ulcers can also result from infection by *Helicobacter pylori*. Gastritis and peptic ulcers tend to be aggravated by smoking, drinking alcohol, tea and coffee, and eating refined foods, pickles and acidic fruit like oranges and tomatoes.

Treatment The herbal approach to gastritis and ulceration aims to resolve the inflammation and heal the damaged stomach lining, while relieving tension and stress. Chamomile is an excellent antiulcer herb, either taken as a strong tea or ½ teaspoon of tincture in a glass of warm water on an empty stomach 4 times a day. Liquorice, Plantain, Marshmallow and Comfrey are wonderfully soothing.

Astringent herbs like Meadowsweet, Elderflower, Yarrow and Thyme protect the gut lining from irritation and inflammation, while Golden seal, Myrrh, Turmeric, Pau d'arco and Marigold, with their antimicrobial actions, resolve infection.

Slippery elm gruel made from 1–2 teaspoons of powder in warm water provides quick relief from pain and, by coating the gut lining, protects it from irritation and acidity. Take 25 ml (1 fl oz) Aloe vera juice twice daily to reduce heat and inflammation.

To reduce anxiety and tension, Chamomile, Lemon balm, Hops, Ashwagandha or Vervain are all recommended.

Caution Acute abdominal pain, with a known history of ulcers, may indicate perforation and requires immediate medical attention.

Gallstones and gall bladder problems

The gall bladder stores bile supplied by the liver until it is required for breaking down dietary fats. It can become infected or inflamed, causing indigestion and stomach and gall bladder pain, especially after eating fatty food. Gallstones form from excessive concentration of bile and calcium salts or cholesterol and if one becomes lodged in the bile duct, which takes bile to the small intestine, it causes great pain.

Treatment For acute biliary colic, anti-inflammatory and pain-relieving herbs are needed. Chamomile and Wild

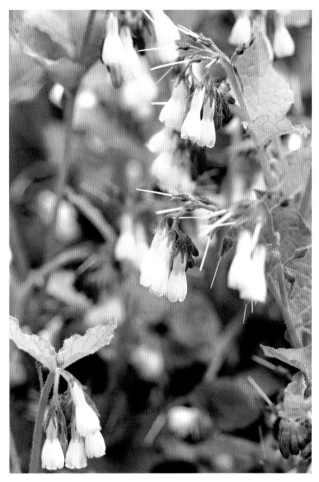

Comfrey with its anti-inflammatory effect and ability to repair damaged tissue is used to treat peptic ulcers.

yam are excellent when taken every 2 hours. Herbs with an affinity for the gall bladder and an ability to dissolve stones and resolve inflammation like Dandelion root, Peppermint, Rosemary, Agrimony, Oregon grape root or Marigold can also be taken singly or in combinations. For intense pain, add Pasque flower, Valerian or Wild yam.

For chronic, intermittent pain provoked by eating fatty foods, take the above herbs 3 times a day until all symptoms subside. Globe artichoke, Milk thistle, Turmeric, Goldenrod and Vervain stimulate the flow of bile from the liver and prevent stagnation in the gall bladder, and are especially helpful in preventing a reoccurrence of symptoms.

Caution Development of jaundice may indicate obstruction by gallstones and requires medical intervention.

Liver problems

The liver is the largest and perhaps most overworked organ in the body and performs many vital functions, including filtering and breaking down toxins from the blood, making amino acids for protein production, metabolizing carbohydrates, protein and fats, storing nutrients absorbed from the gut, producing cholesterol and bile, and manufacturing urea. Liver disease is mainly caused by alcohol, hepatitis, autoimmune diseases, poisons or drugs, and inherited disorders. Less serious but widespread is poor liver function, causing a wide range of metabolic and hormonal problems, poor immune function, skin problems and allergies.

Treatment Cholagogues are bitters such as Barberry, Yellow dock, Oregon grape, Rosemary, Vervain, Wormwood, Burdock, Dandelion and Guduchi, and can be taken to stimulate the flow of bile and support the liver in its work.

Barberry, Golden seal, Turmeric, Milk thistle, Marigold, Liquorice, Bhringaraj, Neem, Amalaki and St John's wort are antivirals that can be used for acute liver infections.

Some amazing adaptogenic herbs, including Guduchi, Andrographis, Neem, Milk thistle, Schisandra, Astragalus, Globe artichoke, Shiitake and Reishi mushrooms, Sarsaparilla and Rehmannia, protect the liver from damage from drugs and toxic chemicals.

Other measures It is important to avoid alcohol, unnecessary drugs, caffeine and junk foods.

Parasites

Most people have some kind of intestinal parasite, such as threadworms, roundworms or tapeworms, or protozoa such as amoeba and giardia. Their presence increases allergic tendencies, bleeding, loss of nutrients, bowel disturbances, aches and pains, and even migraine. Parasites spread easily, often via pets. Their eggs may be ingested with vegetables or fruit, or by putting contaminated fingers in the mouth. If someone has worms, treat the whole family and pets too.

Treatment Anthelmintic herbs eliminate parasites and need to be taken for 1–2 weeks. Take 1–2 Garlic cloves, finely chopped, in 1 teaspoon of honey or warm milk 30 minutes before breakfast. Olive leaf, Pau d'arco, Bhringaraj, Andrographis, Neem, Myrrh, Wormwood, Barberry, Marigold, Gotu kola, Ginger, Wild carrot, Holy basil, Elecampane or Walnut are also effective taken on an empty stomach. Add laxatives Liquorice, Yellow dock or Dandelion root to speed the expulsion of worms.

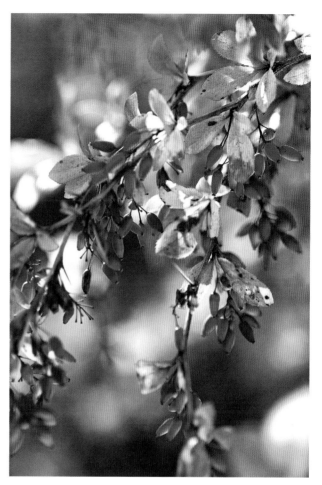

Barberry stimulates the liver to secrete bile and the gall bladder to regulate its flow, helpful in treating problems in these organs.

Apply oil of Lavender, Neem, Rosemary or Thyme in ointment to the anus at night to prevent worms from laying eggs and relieve itching.

Horseradish, Long pepper and Cayenne pepper are all toxic to worms and can be added to food, along with pumpkin seeds, raw onion, grated carrot and carrot juice.

Check the stools daily for worms and repeat treatment after 2 weeks.

Other measures Avoid sugary foods and refined carbohydrates, and eat live yogurt daily.

The urinary system

The urinary system consists of the kidneys, bladder and ureters. During circulation, blood passes through the kidneys, which act as an elaborate filtering system. They remove used and unwanted water, minerals, urea and wastes from the blood, which then becomes urine, and they reabsorb what is still required by the body back into the bloodstream.

As well as controlling the amount of water and salts that are absorbed back into the blood and what is excreted as waste, the kidneys also help maintain the correct acid/alkali balance in the body. They funnel the urine into the bladder along two tubes – the ureters. The bladder stores the urine until muscular contractions push it out through the urethra. Each day, your kidneys produce about 1.5 litres (2¾ pints) of urine. The Chinese value the kidneys as the seat of vital energy known as kidney 'jing', which promotes longevity and immunity.

Urinary problems

The urinary tract is prone to damage from the effects of an unhealthy lifestyle, poor diet and pollution. Solvents, paint, synthetic fragrances and colours, preservatives and nitrogenous waste from a high-protein diet have to be eliminated from the body via the urine and all impose a strain on the kidneys and can contribute to urinary problems. Urinary tract infections can affect the urethra and can subsequently pass into the bladder, causing cystitis. From the bladder, infection can pass along the ureters to the kidneys and cause pyelonephritis.

Other kidney infections can develop as secondaries from infection such as streptococcal throat infection, causing tonsillitis. Infections in babies and children may be related to structural abnormalities. Infections are most frequently caused by *E. coli* bacteria from the bowel that creep round from the anus, their journey aided by wiping from back to front rather than vice versa after urination or a bowel movement. Urinary tract infections tend to affect girls more than boys due to their anatomical differences, in that the passage from the urethra to the bladder is much shorter in girls. Vaginal infections such as thrush can also be related to urinary tract infections.

It is important to drink plenty of fluids to assist the kidneys in their cleansing work, to flush through toxins and the waste products of metabolism and to prevent them from causing irritation of the urinary tract along the way. Many herbs that exert their action on the urinary system can be used preventatively and therapeutically. Mucilaginous herbs such as Marshmallow, Corn silk, Comfrey leaf and Wild oats soothe irritation and inflammation. Aromatic herbs rich in antimicrobial volatile oils with a diuretic action, including Chamomile, Fennel, Lemon balm, Thyme and Coriander, taken regularly as teas or in food are excellent for helping to prevent infection. Cranberry and Blueberry/Bilberry are also valuable, helping to prevent infection by preventing pathogenic bacteria from sticking to the walls of the urinary tract. During any kind of infection or inflammatory process, diuretic herbs to increase the flow of urine such as Wild celery seed, Cleavers, Dandelion leaf, Corn silk, Couch grass and Bearberry can help the body to throw off accumulated toxins and debris produced as a result of the immune system's fight against infection and inflammation.

The kidneys These organs are responsible for the excretion of nitrogenous wastes, principally urea, from the blood. Nephrons within the cortex and medulla filter the blood under pressure and then reabsorb water and other useful substances back into the blood.

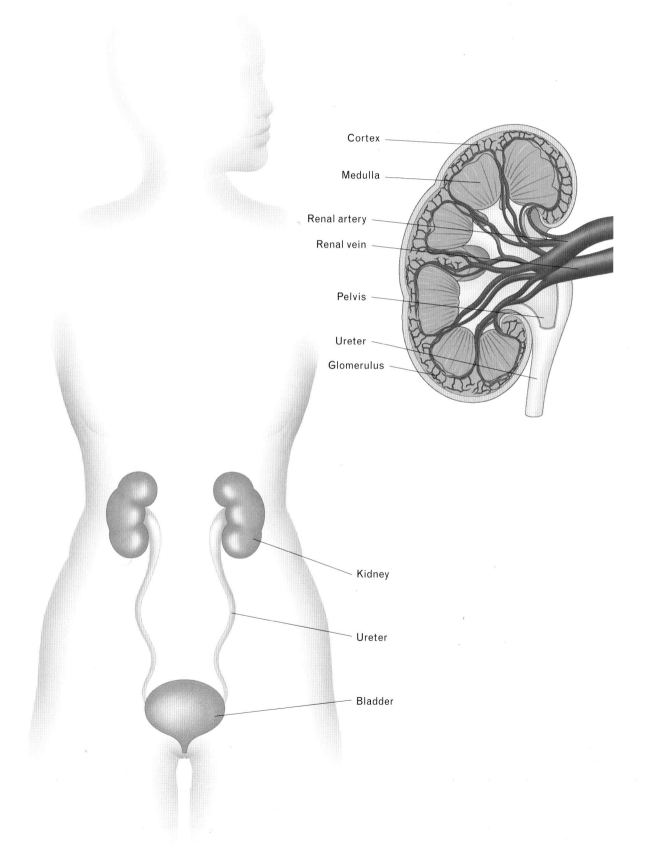

Cortex

Medulla

Renal artery

Renal vein

Pelvis

Ureter

Glomerulus

Kidney

Ureter

Bladder

Urinary tract infections

Infections tend to affect women more than men due to anatomical differences, but in men they can be caused by prostate problems. Cystitis refers to unpleasant urinary symptoms caused by irritation as well as infection, which are mostly from *E. coli* bacteria. Underlying causes include lowered immunity, dysbiosis, nutritional deficiencies, insufficient fluids, stress, excess alcohol and caffeine, blood sugar problems and sex.

Treatment Antiseptic diuretics Buchu, Bearberry, Golden seal, Goldenrod, Chamomile, Fennel, Coriander, Sarsaparilla or Yarrow help combat infection and flush out bacteria, debris and irritants. Soothing Marshmallow, Plantain, Slippery elm, Comfrey leaf, Corn silk and Couch grass relieve irritation, pain and inflammation. Horsetail is soothing and healing, particularly useful for repairing damage after repeated infection. For irritation causing incontinence or bed-wetting, use Marshmallow, Bayberry, Horsetail, Gravel root or Yarrow.

Drink lukewarm-to-cool teas of any of these every 1–2 hours in acute infections and 3 times daily in chronic problems. To relieve the burning/passing-broken-glass sensation, sit in a bath of strong Chamomile tea for 10–15 minutes.

Blueberries/Bilberries prevent bacteria from sticking to the walls of the urinary tract and are excellent as a preventative. Soups and juices made from Carrots, Parsley, Asparagus, Celery, Leeks and Garlic are also helpful.

Other measures To prevent infection and irritation, drink 3–4 litres (5¼–7 pints) fluid daily to flush toxins and bacteria out of the body. During infection, drink plenty of water, herb teas or soothing barley water throughout the day.

Fluid retention

Excess water in the tissues causes oedema, cellulite, swelling and discomfort, particularly in the feet and legs, where fluid accumulates first (due to gravity). It can occur temporarily in women premenstrually and during pregnancy, hot weather and long flights. More chronic fluid retention can be caused by thyroid problems, obesity, poor circulation, varicose veins and poor diet, especially insufficient protein. Oedema can indicate kidney and heart problems, which require professional treatment.

Treatment Diuretics including Dandelion leaf, Wild celery seed, Nettle, Cleavers, Fennel, Coriander, Buchu, Meadowsweet, Corn silk, Chamomile and Bearberry aid the elimination of water through the kidneys and help reduce fluid retention. Add Chaste tree and Lady's mantle for premenstrual problems, including tender, swollen breasts.

Yarrow, Gingko, Gotu kola, Golden seal, Garlic, Lime flower and Hawthorn improve venous circulation and relieve swelling and discomfort in the legs and ankles. Antioxidants such as Blueberry/Bilberry, Elderberry and Horse chestnut strengthen and heal blood vessels. Bladderwrack and Guggulu are helpful for treating low thyroid function and aiding weight reduction.

Other measures Excess sodium in salty foods increases fluid retention, so should be avoided, while potassium in foods like bananas, tomatoes and green vegetables encourages the elimination of sodium. It is important to take plenty of exercise, to raise the feet when sitting and avoid tea, coffee and alcohol. For premenstrual problems, take supplements of B-complex vitamins.

Bearberry acts as a disinfectant for the urinary tract thanks to its antibacterial properties.

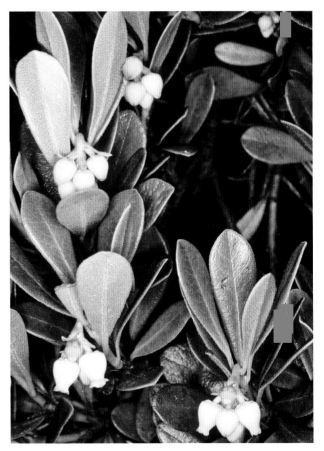

Kidney stones

Infection and irritation in the kidney and insufficient fluids can lead to the formation of crystals, which develop into stones and gravel. They are mostly formed from calcium oxalate, calcium phosphate and uric acid. When they move they cause sudden, excruciating pain, which passes once the stones have passed out of the bladder.

Treatment Use antilithic and diuretic herbs including Wild carrot, Gravel root, Blueberry/Bilberry, Buchu, Dandelion leaves, Goldenrod or Bearberry to dissolve and facilitate the passing of stones and gravel. These also combat urinary tract infection.

Demulcent diuretics Marshmallow, Comfrey leaf, Corn silk and Couch grass reduce inflammation, soothe and heal irritated urinary tubules, dissolve stones and gravel and ease their passing.

Antispasmodics Chamomile, Cramp bark, Wild yam, Passion flower and Valerian can help reduce pain and muscle spasm in the urinary tract caused by passing stones.

Other measures Plenty of fluids and foods rich in magnesium and B vitamins help reduce the formation of stones.

Prostate problems

The prostate is a walnut-sized gland surrounding the urethra, which carries urine from the bladder to the penis. An enlarged or swollen prostate obstructs the flow of urine and causes sensations of pressure, hesitancy or urgency to empty the bladder. Incomplete bladder emptying predisposes to urinary infections and disturbs sleep through frequent trips to the toilet. Benign prostatic hypertrophy (BPH) commonly affects men from their late 40s and is related to dwindling testosterone levels and conversion of testosterone into dihydrotestosterone (DHT), which is linked to deficiencies of zinc, vitamin B6 and essential fatty acids. Infection (prostatitis) and cancer can also cause enlargement of the prostate.

Treatment The best herb for shrinking the prostate is Saw palmetto when taken long term. Liquorice prevents conversion of testosterone to DHT and so prevents enlargement. Other useful herbs include Golden seal, Nettle root, Red clover, Horsetail, Dandelion, Gravel root, Siberian ginseng, Red grape seed extract, Evening primrose oil or Borage seed oil, Chinese angelica, Echinacea or Goldenrod.

For prostatitis, use Nettle root, Echinacea, Golden seal, Garlic, Buchu, Bearberry, Chamomile or Couch grass, in

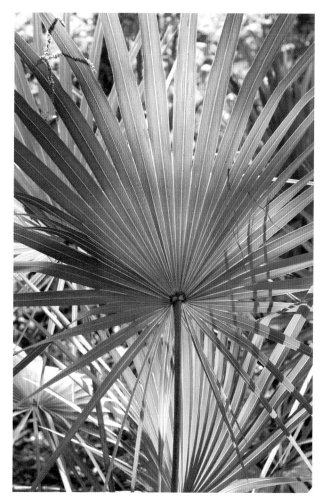

Saw palmetto is traditionally thought of as a man's herb and is prescribed to reduce enlarged prostate glands.

acute doses if necessary, and drink Cranberry or Blueberry/Bilberry juice and plenty of water.

For cramping pain caused by infection or inflammation, use Cramp bark, Chamomile or Chinese angelica.

Other measures A high-protein diet helps to maintain good testosterone levels. Increase zinc and essential fatty acid intake by eating pumpkin seeds daily and cooked tomatoes, which are rich in lycopene, as well as taking supplements of vitamins A, C and E, selenium and zinc.

Caution If you suspect prostate problems, you should seek medical attention.

The circulatory system

Each of us contains about 5 litres (8¾ pints) of blood, consisting of plasma, red blood cells, white blood cells and platelets, which is continually transported around the body via the circulatory system. Its purpose is to carry oxygen, hormones, gases and nutrients to every cell of the body and to take away the waste products of metabolism.

The blood is also responsible for maintaining correct body temperature and pH of the body. The circulatory system additionally includes the transportation of lymph around the body. The lymphatic system distributes immune cells called lymphocytes, which protect the body against infection, absorbs lipids from the gut and carries them to the blood. With the circulatory system it returns fluids and plasma proteins from cells and tissues to the blood and thus maintains fluid balance.

The heart pumps oxygen and nutrient-rich blood into the aorta, the main artery, from where it flows about 60,000 miles (96,000 km) through arteries and capillaries, a vast network of vessels of different sizes, to reach and nourish all the tissues of the body. Once the waste products, including carbon dioxide, are collected from the cells, the deoxygenated blood flows into the veins and is circulated back to the heart and the lungs, where carbon dioxide and oxygen are exchanged. On its journey around the body, the blood passes through the kidneys, which filter much of the waste from the blood. It also passes through the small intestine and into the portal vein, which passes through the liver, where sugars from the blood are filtered and stored.

Causes of circulatory problems

Most circulatory problems occur as a result of blocked arteries, caused by atherosclerosis or hardening of the arteries. For the heart muscle to work efficiently, it requires its own supply of oxygenated blood, which is carried through four small coronary arteries. Should these become blocked and prevent blood flow to the heart muscle, serious damage to the heart may occur.

There are several factors that contribute to circulatory problems, including high blood pressure, high blood cholesterol, smoking, obesity, heredity, lack of exercise and emotional stress. Damage or stress to the inner lining of the blood vessels can cause inflammation and lead over time to a build-up of debris and narrowing of the arteries, predisposing to blockage. High homocysteine levels increase the build-up of plaque in the arteries, and emotional stress can cause the release of biochemicals that contribute to the damage to arterial tissues. LDL (low-density lipoprotein) cholesterol from excess dietary animal fats or errors in the liver's metabolism of cholesterol can also line and narrow the arteries, making them susceptible to plaque deposits. It is therefore sensible to reduce the intake of animal fats and increase consumption of polyunsaturated and monosaturated fats. Folic acid and other B vitamins help lower cholesterol and homocysteine levels.

Fruit, vegetables and herbs, including Blueberry/ Bilberry and Ginkgo, that are rich in antioxidants protect arteries from oxidation and reduce plaque deposits, while several other herbs, such as Lime flower, Gotu kola and Hawthorn, have the ability to regulate blood pressure, nourish the heart and strengthen the arteries. Fibres in complex carbohydrates such as Wild oats carry cholesterol out of cells, tissues and arteries to the liver, where it is excreted. Limiting salt and sugar intake, taking regular aerobic exercise and maintaining ideal body weight are also good preventative measures against circulatory disorders.

The circulatory system A complex network of veins, arteries and capillaries allows blood to circulate all around the body. This enables the transportation of nutrients and oxygen to every part of the body, as well as the removal of waste products.

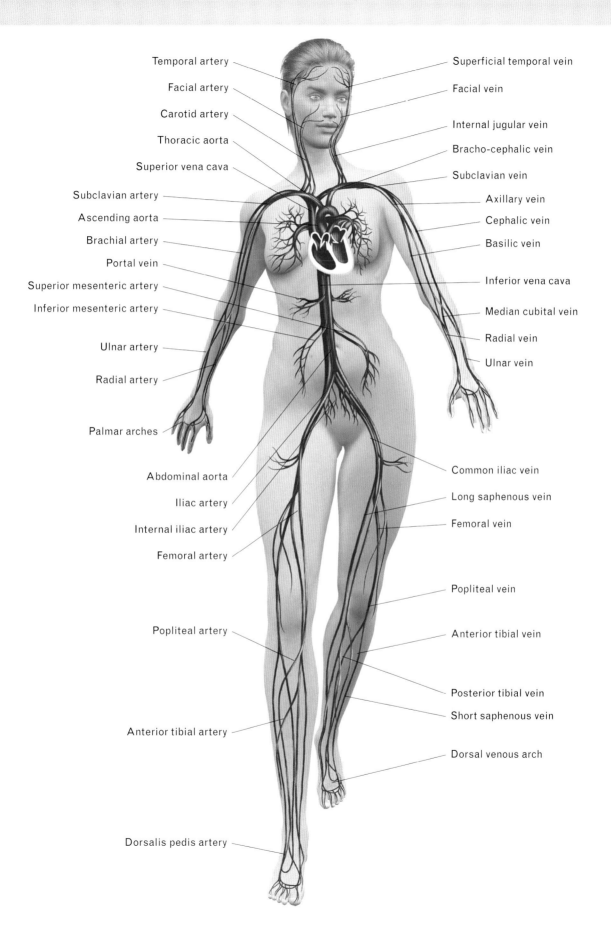

Temporal artery

Facial artery

Carotid artery

Thoracic aorta

Superior vena cava

Subclavian artery

Ascending aorta

Brachial artery

Portal vein

Superior mesenteric artery

Inferior mesenteric artery

Ulnar artery

Radial artery

Palmar arches

Abdominal aorta

Iliac artery

Internal iliac artery

Femoral artery

Popliteal artery

Anterior tibial artery

Dorsalis pedis artery

Superficial temporal vein

Facial vein

Internal jugular vein

Bracho-cephalic vein

Subclavian vein

Axillary vein

Cephalic vein

Basilic vein

Inferior vena cava

Median cubital vein

Radial vein

Ulnar vein

Common iliac vein

Long saphenous vein

Femoral vein

Popliteal vein

Anterior tibial vein

Posterior tibial vein

Short saphenous vein

Dorsal venous arch

Anaemia

Lack of dietary iron, excess loss of blood (from heavy periods, haemorrhoids, bleeding gums or peptic ulcers) and digestive problems resulting in iron deficiency are the most common causes of anaemia. Vitamin B12 or folic acid deficiency can also cause anaemia, while other more serious problems, such as leukaemia or radiation therapy, can result in disturbance to red blood cells.

Treatment Ashwagandha, Dandelion leaves, Blueberry/Bilberry, Raspberry leaves, Nettle, Yellow dock root, Codonopsis, Amalaki, Guggulu and Coriander leaves are all rich in iron and folic acid. Chinese angelica is rich in vitamin B12 and folic acid, and increases red blood cell production.

To improve iron absorption, take iron-rich digestive herbs like Burdock, Vervain, Hawthorn, Skullcap, Gentian or Hops. Drinking a hot cup of tea made from fresh Ginger before meals will also aid iron absorption. Siberian ginseng increases resilience and strength in anaemia.

Other measures Eat plenty of vitamin C-rich foods such as red, yellow and green vegetables and dark red fruit such as Blueberries/Bilberries, blackberries and blackcurrants, to enhance iron absorption. Avoid tea, coffee and alcohol, as they can inhibit iron absorption. Make sure that your diet is rich in iron, folic acid, protein and vitamins E and B12.

Heart conditions

There is much that can be done to prevent and heal heart problems, including dietary changes, exercise, nutritional supplements and herbs. Antioxidant herbs Turmeric, Blueberry/Bilberry, Hawthorn, Shiitake and Reishi mushrooms and Ginkgo can reduce oxidative damage to the heart and blood vessels caused by free radicals and strengthen the heart muscle by improving blood flow through the coronary arteries.

Treatment Many herbs, such as Guggulu, Olive leaf, Hawthorn, Cayenne pepper, Red grape seed extract, Ginger, Turmeric, Evening primrose, Chinese angelica and Garlic can significantly lower blood pressure and low-density lipoprotein (LDL) cholesterol and prevent, and even reverse, atherosclerotic plaque from forming, thereby reducing the tendency to heart attacks.

Forskohlii relaxes the arteries, lowers blood pressure and improves blood flow through the heart, and is indicated in congestive heart failure, arteriosclerosis and angina. Angelica is a calcium-channel blocker in the heart, useful for high blood pressure, angina and heart arrhythmias. Astragalus is a good antioxidant and diuretic, and lowers blood pressure. It improves blood flow through the heart and heart function, and reduces ischaemic heart disease and angina.

Hawthorn, Motherwort, Lime flower, Lemon balm, Passion flower and Rosemary steady heart contractions and reduce palpitations. When these are related to menopausal flushes, add Sage or Black cohosh.

Other measures Reduce or stop caffeine intake such as coffee, cola and tea.

Caution If you are on medication for a heart condition, check with your practitioner before taking herbs.

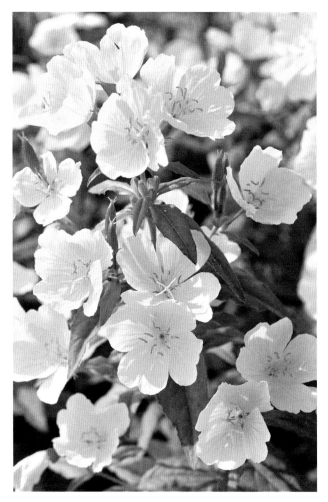

Evening primrose is prescribed to help lower blood pressure and keep platelets from clumping in the blood vessels.

Poor circulation

Poor circulation to the extremities causes cold hands and feet and increases the tendency to chilblains and cramp. Chilblains are itchy, sore red lumps on fingers or toes that develop due to insufficient oxygen and nutrients being carried to the area by the blood. Poor circulation is caused by constriction of the arteries and can be inherited. It is aggravated by lack of exercise, smoking, caffeine, poor diet, tiredness and stress. Raynaud's syndrome and circulatory problems associated with heart or arterial disease can also cause circulatory problems.

Treatment Circulatory stimulants include Ginger, Garlic, Cayenne pepper, Gotu kola, Coriander, Cinnamon, Prickly ash and Hawthorn. Hot teas of Yarrow, Peppermint, Elderflower, Rosemary and Lime flower increase blood flow, dilate arteries and reduce cramp. Blueberry/Bilberry and Horse chestnut improve circulation and strengthen blood vessels. Evening primrose and Borage seed oil also improve circulation.

Warm baths, foot baths or massage with oils of Ginger, Cinnamon, Coriander, Sweet marjoram, Thyme or Rosemary relax tense muscles and stimulate blood flow. Marigold cream and Gotu kola and Lavender oil soothe chilblains.

Other measures Supplements of vitamin C and bioflavonoids, omega-3 fatty acids and regular exercise are recommended.

Cramp

This is caused by muscular spasm and can be very painful. Pregnant women and the elderly are more likely to suffer from cramp, and it may be a sign of low calcium levels, deficiencies of vitamins B or D, low digestive enzymes, poor absorption or circulatory problems. Varicose veins, tiredness, lack of exercise, insufficient fluids and nervous tension may also be contributory factors to getting cramp.

Treatment Circulatory stimulants include Ginger, Garlic, Gotu kola, Turmeric, Gingko, Hawthorn, Prickly ash, Cinnamon and Cayenne pepper. Amalaki, Guggulu and Coriander are also helpful. Hot teas of Ginger, Cinnamon, Cardamom, Yarrow, Peppermint and Elderflower also promote circulation and prevent cramp. Gotu kola, Blueberry/Bilberry and Gingko will aid venous return if there are varicose veins.

For cramps related to stress, tension and tiredness, use Cramp bark, Passion flower, Rosemary, Skullcap, Gotu kola, Holy basil, Lime flower or Ashwagandha.

Nettle, Dill, Wild oats, Wild celery seed, Borage, Meadowsweet, Dandelion leaves and Buchu are all rich in calcium and can be taken regularly as teas.

Massage with essential oils of Ginger, Cinnamon, Rosemary, Thyme or Sweet marjoram in a base of sesame oil to swiftly relieve pain.

Other measures Moving the affected limb briskly, and walking and stretching are advisable. Take supplements of vitamin B and C, calcium and magnesium to support the nervous system and aid circulation.

CASE STUDY **POOR CIRCULATION**

CLIENT PROFILE
Donald is a writer who consulted me about the poor circulation in his hands. The minute he sat down to write at his computer in the morning, his fingers would turn blue and then white, and then feel numb and prevent him from working. He said that he felt the cold generally and tended to get anxious, especially when he couldn't get on with his work.

THE HERBAL TREATMENT
I recommended a warm Ginger footbath every morning for 10–15 minutes and asked Donald to massage his legs at night with warm sesame oil and a few drops of Ginger and Rosemary essential oils. I made him a prescription of circulatory stimulants combined with antispasmodics to relax tense muscles, including those in the arteries. It was also intended to enhance concentration and reduce mental tension. It contained Cramp bark, Gotu kola, Ginkgo, Coriander, Thyme, Prickly ash, Ashwagandha and Hawthorn.

I suggested that Donald should take supplements of vitamin C and bioflavonoids, and omega-3 fatty acids. I also recommended regular exercise and time to relax, and mentioned avoiding caffeine and junk foods and drinking plenty of Ginger and Cinnamon tea.

This prescription worked wonders for Donald!

Altitude sickness

High-altitude areas in mountainous regions contain less oxygen than lower areas, and when travelling or climbing in such situations it is advised to make the ascent gradually to allow the body time to acclimatize. A rapid ascent causes fluids to move from the blood to the tissues, which results in dehydration, and this is aggravated by vigorous exercise and alcohol. As the blood thickens from fluid loss, it inhibits the elimination of toxins and causes headaches, fatigue, malaise and extreme thirst. One of the best preventative measures is to drink plenty of liquid.

Treatment Cloves, Wild carrot seed, Cinnamon and Sweet marjoram contain eugenol, which helps thin the blood. Garlic, Ginger, Dill, Fennel, Cayenne pepper and Wild celery seed act similarly. Garlic, Ginger, Cayenne pepper, Gotu kola and Gingko increase blood flow and oxygen supply throughout the body, including the brain.

Adaptogens Rhodiola, Reishi mushroom, Siberian and Korean ginseng, Ashwagandha and other herbs rich in antioxidants like Hawthorn, Milk thistle and Schisandra increase the body's ability to adapt to changes in oxygen levels, as many of the symptoms of altitude sickness appear to be related to free radical activity.

Other measures Supplements of vitamin C and E, alpha-lipoic acid, coenzyme Q10, glutathione, l-glutamine and flavonoids can aid endurance of higher altitudes.

High blood pressure

An increase in pressure inside narrowed arteries weakens the heart and arteries, impedes blood flow to vital organs such as the kidneys, brain and eyes, and predisposes to heart attacks and strokes. The most common causes of high blood pressure are hereditary tendency, stress, obesity, kidney problems, excess alcohol and smoking and hardening of the arteries.

Treatment The best antihypertensive herbs that relax and dilate arteries include Hawthorn, Lime flower, Garlic, Gingko, Motherwort, Cramp bark, Valerian and Gotu kola. Antioxidant herbs Amalaki, Holy basil, Selfheal, Turmeric, Cayenne pepper, Shiitake mushroom, Blueberry/ Bilberry, Elderberry, Ginger, Red grape seed extract and Guggulu prevent damage to arteries from free radicals and reduce the risk of heart attacks and strokes.

For problems related to anxiety and tension, add to your prescription Cramp bark, Rosemary, Wild oats, Chamomile, Passion flower or Skullcap. Lime flower tea is relaxing and dilates the arteries, reducing blood pressure.

For excess fluid, take diuretic herbs such as Dandelion leaves, Corn silk, Bearberry, Cleavers or Goldenrod.

Other measures A largely vegetarian diet and cold-pressed vegetable oils are recommended. Avoid tea, coffee, alcohol and smoking, and take regular aerobic exercise. Meditation and yoga can be very helpful.

Caution Seek medical attention if you suffer from high blood pressure.

Arterial disease

Hardening of the arteries (arteriosclerosis) and deposits of cholesterol (atherosclerosis) in the artery walls cause the arteries to narrow, limiting blood flow to the tissues and resulting in poor circulation to the limbs, as in Buerger's disease. When the arteries in the heart are narrowed, lack of blood to the heart muscle causes anginal pain, and increases the risk of heart attack. Arterial disease is related to high blood pressure, blood sugar disorders, high homocysteine levels, over-consumption of animal fats, refined carbohydrates, sugar and alcohol, excess smoking, lack of exercise and obesity.

Treatment Antioxidant herbs prevent damage to artery walls that can lead to plaque development and oxidation of low-density lipoprotein (LDL) cholesterol, which forms deposits. Hawthorn improves blood flow through the heart and arteries, reducing inflammation in the arteries, regulating blood pressure, lowering cholesterol and preventing the build-up of deposits and formation of clots. Other beneficial herbs include Cayenne pepper, Turmeric, Shiitake mushroom, Blueberry/Bilberry, Elderberry, Garlic, Ginger and Red grape seed extract. Guggulu lowers cholesterol and scrapes existing plaque from the arteries. Ginger, Ginkgo, Turmeric, Blueberry/Bilberry and Elderberry are antioxidants that strengthen and stabilize artery walls and prevent clots.

Other measures Supplements of B vitamins, coenzyme Q10, selenium, omega-3 oils and antioxidants are recommended. Avoid tea, coffee, alcohol and cigarettes, and take regular exercise.

Raised cholesterol

There are two types of cholesterol: low-density lipoproteins (LDL), which increase the risk of heart attacks, and high-density lipoproteins (HDL), which actually reduce it. Cholesterol is a fatty, waxy substance, 25 per cent of which comes from food and the rest is manufactured in the liver. Excess sugar, refined carbohydrates and fats and errors of liver metabolism are largely to blame for high LDL.

Treatment Antioxidant herbs including Hawthorn, Cayenne pepper, Red grape seed extract, Guggulu, Blueberry/Bilberry, Elderberry, Ginger, Evening primrose, Chinese angelica and Liquorice protect arteries, inhibit formation of atherosclerotic plaque, lower cholesterol and help prevent cardiovascular disease.

Shiitake and Reishi mushrooms and Wild oats contain beta-glucans, which help lower cholesterol. A garlic clove a day can substantially lower cholesterol levels, and Red clover reduces its absorption.

Other measures Niacin (vitamin B3) lowers total cholesterol as well as LDL cholesterol, triglycerides and fibrinogen, a blood protein responsible for forming clots. It also raises HDL. Take in a B-complex supplement. Reduce high-fat foods, red meats and fried foods. Replace saturated oils with monosaturated ones like Olive and Avocado oils and polyunsaturated fats as in nuts, seeds, Flax seed and fish oils. Plant fibres can lower cholesterol, so a diet high in fruit and vegetables and whole grains with minimal fats helps maintain normal cholesterol levels. Take regular aerobic exercise.

Varicose veins, ulcers and haemorrhoids

Dilation and enlargement of veins in the legs cause varicose veins, and when they occur in the anal area they cause haemorrhoids. They tend to be hereditary, and can also be caused by stagnation of blood in the veins and aggravated by too much standing, not enough exercise, pregnancy, constipation, obesity, shallow breathing and stress. Where there is poor circulation in the legs, often associated with varicose veins, the tissues and skin begin to break down. If the leg is knocked, the skin will break easily and can become ulcerated, and can take a long time to heal.

Treatment For prevention and treatment use Yarrow, Ginkgo, Gotu kola, Golden seal, Garlic, Lime flower or Hawthorn to improve venous circulation and relieve pain and discomfort. Antioxidants such as Blueberry/Bilberry,

Elderberry and Horse chestnut strengthen and heal blood vessels. In addition, Horse chestnut improves the tone of veins and circulation through them, and can improve chronic venous insufficiency dramatically.

Use astringent herbs such as Marigold, Witch hazel, Rose, Agrimony, Horsetail and Comfrey externally in creams and lotions to tone and soothe varicose veins and haemorrhoids. Aloe vera gel can also be helpful.

Comfrey and Marigold poultices alternated night and morning speed healing of varicose ulcers and relieve pain and inflammation. The area can be bathed with Chamomile or Marigold tea between dressings. If an ulcer is infected or inflamed, add Garlic, Pau d'arco, Neem, Echinacea and Marigold to the internal formula.

Other measures Supplements of vitamin E and C, bioflavonoids and zinc will help strengthen the veins. Manuka honey is also recommended. Regular exercise, fibre-rich foods and avoiding sitting or standing for long periods are all important.

Elderberries are rich in flavonoids and oxidants and tone the walls of the small blood vessels.

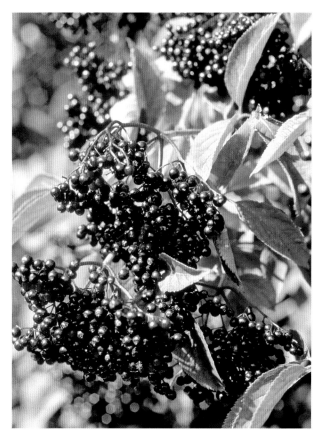

The musculoskeletal system

Our musculoskeletal system consists of bones, muscles, tendons, ligaments, joints, cartilage and other connective tissue that together provide the form and stability of the body and enable movement. Bones provide the structure of the body and protect the delicate internal structures such as the brain, spinal column, lungs and heart. They contain bone marrow, where specialized cells including stem cells manufacture red blood cells.

Although bone seems hard and rigid, bone cells are constantly being made and replaced, and bone is completely re-formed every ten years. The hard outer part is mainly made of protein, such as collagen, and hydroxyapatite, which largely consists of calcium and other minerals. Bones depend on minerals such as calcium and vitamin D for their density and strength, and also on activity and weight-bearing exercise, as well as the action of hormones including growth and parathyroid hormone, oestrogen, testosterone and calcitonin. They need a good blood supply, which is brought to them by vessels that enter via their outer membrane, the periosteum, where most of their nerve supply is located.

The junctions between bones are joints, some of which move and allow a wide range of movement, such as the shoulder and knee joints, and others, like those in the skull, that are immobile. Joints are designed to provide stability and protect against damage from use. They are lined with synovial fluid, which provides nourishment to cartilage on the end of bones and prevents friction as they move. Cartilage is a tough and resilient tissue composed of collagen and proteoglycans, which also prevents friction as the joints move. Ligaments are strong, elastic fibrous cords composed largely of connective collagen surrounding the joints, acting to strengthen and stabilize them. Their elasticity allows movement and protects the joints by ensuring that these movements take place in only certain directions.

There are three types of muscle: skeletal, smooth and cardiac. Skeletal muscles are bundles of elastic fibres attached to bones and joints that contract and relax, enabling smooth, controlled movements and maintaining posture. The action of skeletal muscle is voluntary, controlled by the conscious brain, unlike smooth muscle in the blood vessels, chest and abdominal organs and cardiac muscle in the heart, which is involuntary. The growth, strength and elasticity of the muscles all depend on growth hormone and testosterone, and are maintained and increased by regular exercise.

Alleviating problems

The health of our musculoskeletal system depends on good diet and efficient digestion, absorption and elimination. Overusing or neglecting certain groups of muscles, posture and the amount of fresh air and exercise we take all have their effect. Stress and the inability to relax put a strain on the system and can contribute to joint and muscle problems, but the biggest factor is age. From around the age of 30 our bone density diminishes and accelerates in women after the menopause, meaning that our bones become more fragile and prone to fractures and breaks. Changes in cartilage and connective tissue affect the strength and stability of the joints. Thinning of the cartilage makes the joint more susceptible to damage and to wear and tear, predisposing to osteoarthritis. The connective tissue in the ligaments and tendons becomes less elastic, which can cause stiffness and limited movement. Muscle tissue is also affected and the size and strength of muscles gradually diminishes, which means less support and stability generally, particularly of the joints, making them more prone to damage. Regular moderate- or low-impact exercise, however, can go a long way to slowing down this process. Massage, stretching, manipulation, rest and certain herbs can also be helpful.

Horsetail and Comfrey nourish the bones, Aloe vera, Wild celery seed, Burdock, Devil's claw and Liquorice help prevent and remedy joint problems, while Cramp bark, Rosemary, Skullcap, Hops and St John's wort help to relax tense muscles and prevent them from damage.

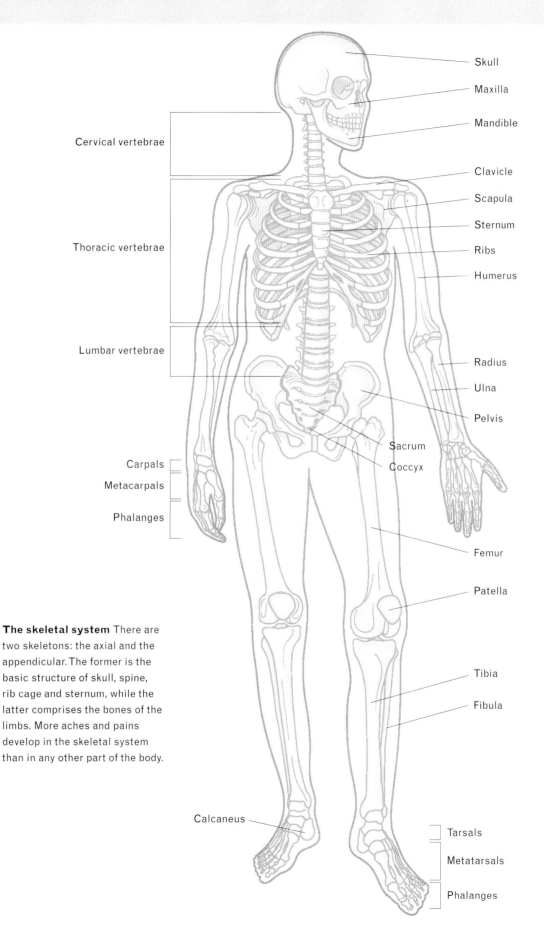

Cervical vertebrae

Thoracic vertebrae

Lumbar vertebrae

Carpals

Metacarpals

Phalanges

Skull

Maxilla

Mandible

Clavicle

Scapula

Sternum

Ribs

Humerus

Radius

Ulna

Pelvis

Sacrum

Coccyx

Femur

Patella

Tibia

Fibula

Calcaneus

Tarsals

Metatarsals

Phalanges

The skeletal system There are two skeletons: the axial and the appendicular. The former is the basic structure of skull, spine, rib cage and sternum, while the latter comprises the bones of the limbs. More aches and pains develop in the skeletal system than in any other part of the body.

Arthritis

Arthritis causes joint stiffness and inflammation, and can lead to degeneration of the joints, disfigurement and pain. Osteoarthritis involving wear and tear is most common; rheumatoid arthritis is a more serious and progressive autoimmune disease. Underlying causes include poor diet, digestive problems, dysbiosis, toxicity, free radical damage, age, stress and chronic infection. Poor digestion and constipation cause nutritional deficiency and accumulation of toxins in the gut, which are absorbed into the circulation and contribute to joint problems.

Treatment Turmeric and Frankincense can be used for osteoarthritis and rheumatoid arthritis, as they are potent antioxidants, enhance immunity, reduce pain and inflammation and have an affinity with muscles and bones. Devil's claw and Myrrh are excellent anti-inflammatories that reduce pain and stiffness. Black cohosh is anti-inflammatory and analgesic, excellent for post-menopausal arthritis. Liquorice has cortisone-like anti-inflammatory actions and increases tolerance to physical and emotional stress. Ashwagandha, with its painkilling and anti-inflammatory action and immunostimulating properties, is ideal for autoimmune problems like rheumatoid arthritis. Long pepper, Turmeric and Cinnamon improve digestion, while Burdock, Nettle, Yellow dock, Marigold and Cleavers

Nettles have been shown in studies to relieve the pain of arthritis; they also have diuretic and cleansing properties.

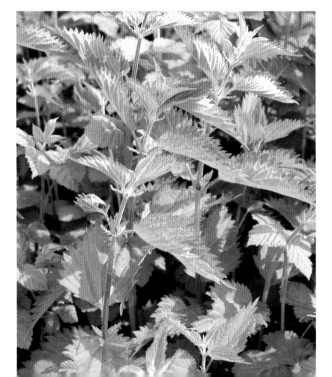

clear toxins. Other beneficial herbs include Meadowsweet, Bladderwrack, Gotu kola, Shiitake mushroom, Echinacea, Wild yam, Feverfew, Willow and Angelica.

Take Ginger tea daily as an anti-inflammatory and antioxidant to reduce pain and swelling and the associated bursitis.

Massage with liniments containing essential oils of Rosemary, Peppermint, Lavender or Sweet marjoram with a few drops of Cayenne pepper tincture to increase circulation to the joints and decrease pain.

Other measures Supplements of Evening primrose oil, glucosamine sulphate, methylsulfonylmethane (MSM), Rose hip, omega-3 oils and selenium protect and promote repair of cartilage.

Gout

Gout is caused by a build-up of uric acid in the blood. Uric acid is a by-product of protein metabolism in the liver, and when this reaches a certain level, uric acid crystals form and collect in joints, causing intense pain, swelling and inflammation. It usually starts in the big toe first. It tends to run in families, is more common in men who are overweight and associated with high blood pressure and triglycerides.

Treatment Diuretics, especially Wild celery seed and Nettle, but also Gravel root, Fennel, Wild oat straw, Cleavers or Goldenrod help the kidneys eliminate excess uric acid and other toxins. You can combine these with anti-inflammatory Devil's claw, Turmeric, Liquorice, Cat's claw, Rose hip, Olive leaf, Willow, Meadowsweet, Frankincense, Ginger, Sarsaparilla or Wild yam to reduce joint pain and swelling, along with herbs to support the liver such as Burdock, Gentian, Milk thistle or Rosemary.

Externally painful joints can be massaged with essential oils of Peppermint, Rosemary or Lavender oil in sesame oil.

Other measures Gout is related to excess fatty foods, purines (from red meat, organ meats and shellfish), nightshades (potatoes, peppers, aubergines and tomatoes), cheese, citrus fruits and alcohol (particularly beer), so adjust your diet accordingly. It can also be triggered by certain drugs, crash diets and exercise, therefore take pre-emptive action. Bromelain from pineapple is excellent for acute attacks and can be taken as a supplement along with quercitrin and vitamin C from cherries to prevent future attacks.

Osteoporosis

Loss of bone tissue actually begins in our 30s, but is hastened through lower oestrogen levels after the menopause. Other contributing factors are poor digestion and absorption, lack of calcium and other important bone nutrients including essential fatty acids, vitamin D, magnesium and boron in the diet, smoking, lack of exercise and a history of total hysterectomy. Women who are underweight, who have dieted frequently or suffered from coeliac disease are more at risk, as oestrogen is stored in fat tissue. It is indicated by a tendency to fractures, back pain, loss of height due to compression of the spine and muscle spasm.

Treatment Use oestrogenic herbs like Shatavari, Chinese angelica, Red clover, Marigold, Wild yam, Liquorice, Sage, Hops or Siberian ginseng, combined with herbs to improve digestion and absorption, including Long pepper, Ginger, Fennel or Coriander.

Evening primrose oil or Borage seed oil will help hormone balance.

Calcium-rich herbs are also important such as Nettle, Dandelion leaf, Horsetail, Bladderwrack, Dill, Wild celery seed, Wild oats, Borage, Codonopsis, Hawthorn and Amalaki.

Other measures Plenty of exercise and supplements of vitamins E and D, magnesium and boron are recommended.

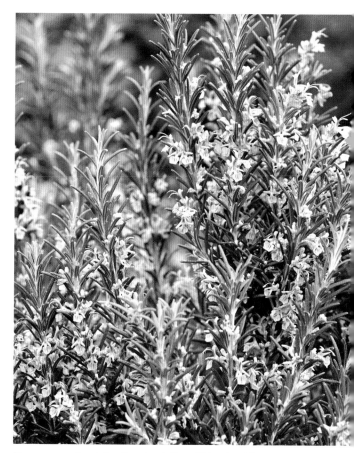

Rosemary stimulates the circulation of blood and has a restorative effect on body and mind.

Muscle pain and fibromyalgia

Tender, stiff and aching muscles can occur after unaccustomed exercise, while more extreme muscle pain is caused by cramp, muscle strain or other injuries such as a compressed nerve; the muscles affected or those nearby can go into spasm, which further increases the pain. If muscle tension or spasm is prolonged, tender lumps, which are fibrositic nodules, may develop. Generalized muscle pain combined with fatigue and malaise can be a symptom of chronic stress, overwork, tiredness, flu and fibromyalgia (which is associated with post-viral fatigue syndrome).

Treatment Massage tense and aching muscles with essential oils of Rosemary, Thyme, Holy basil, Lavender, Chamomile or Ginger diluted in sesame oil. This will increase circulation to the affected area, ease tension and spasm and reduce pain. Sesame oil is rich in calcium and magnesium, which help release muscle tension. Muscle-relaxing herbs Rosemary, Thyme, Chamomile, Ginger, Lavender, Holy basil, Skullcap, Black cohosh, Wild yam and Ashwagandha can be taken internally; the latter has a special affinity with muscle tissue.

For inflammation after an injury or muscle strain, use anti-inflammatory Frankincense, Devil's claw, Liquorice, Meadowsweet, Ginger, Black willow, Turmeric, Black cohosh or Cat's claw.

Adaptogenic, immune-enhancing and tonic herbs such as Ashwagandha, Siberian ginseng, Shiitake mushroom and Astragalus are helpful for states of depletion and fibromyalgia.

Other measures Rest aching muscles if they develop from overuse, but only for 2–3 days, after which gently start to stretch them. Supplements of calcium and magnesium can help to reduce muscle pain and spasm.

The skin

Our skin is a mirror of our health and plays many important roles in the body. It protects us against dirt, infection, extremes of temperature and climate, sunlight, pollution and physical injury. It secretes antiseptic substances to ward off infection, backed up by beneficial flora that live on the skin and the acid mantle formed by sweat that also helps to inhibit infection.

Below the outer layer of skin, the epidermis, is the dermis – a thick, strong and elastic layer of tissue richly supplied with blood vessels, sweat and oil glands and nerve endings. In cold weather the blood vessels contract to keep heat inside the body, and when it is hot, they dilate to bring blood to the surface to help the body lose heat and maintain its correct temperature.

The several million sweat glands enable the skin to be a major organ of excretion. Sweat contains water, mineral salts and nitrogenous wastes and other toxins, and is similar in content to urine. Most adults excrete about 600 ml (1 pint) of fluid through the skin daily and up to ten times more when taking vigorous exercise or in hot weather. It is important to take sufficient exercise to produce sweat on a regular basis in order to clear toxins and prevent overburdening the other pathways of elimination, the kidneys and bowels. Sweat production also helps maintain a stable inner environment by regulating the water and electrolyte balance in the body, and in this way it works hand in hand with the kidneys.

The skin is also a sense organ, richly endowed with nerve endings, which relay messages to the brain about sensations from the environment, heat or cold, pleasure or pain. It can be a useful diagnostic tool, reflecting the effects of our outer environment as well as the condition of our inner state, physical and emotional. When we are healthy, our skin glows; when unwell, it may look more sallow. Rashes and eczema may be related to contact with outside allergens, micro-organisms, chemicals, sunlight, pollutants or poor diet, or may be associated with emotional problems such as anxiety or grief.

Maintaining healthy skin

The skin's resilience to external and internal disturbance relies on nutrients brought to it by underlying blood vessels, which also remove waste products. Healthy skin will not let infection proliferate because its local immune mechanisms work well, but impaired skin function allows infection to spread, unable to rally its defences to resolve the infection without outside help. To maintain good blood flow, take regular exercise and avoid smoking, which constricts blood vessels and prevents the flow of blood, oxygen and nutrients to the skin.

To keep your skin healthy, eat a well-balanced diet that includes plenty of protein, essential fatty acids, particularly omega-3s from oily fish and flax seeds, and antioxidants from fresh organic fruit and vegetables.

Deficiencies of minerals, vitamins and trace elements and excess junk foods that create toxicity can impair the skin's resilience and predispose it to a number of disorders. Herbs can increase blood flow to the skin, providing vital nutrients and helping clear toxins.

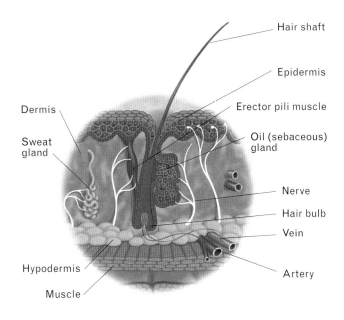

Labels:
Hair shaft
Epidermis
Erector pili muscle
Oil (sebaceous) gland
Nerve
Hair bulb
Vein
Artery
Dermis
Sweat gland
Hypodermis
Muscle

Skin has three layers, the epidermis, dermis and sub-cutaneous tissue. The hypodermis connects the skin to muscle and bone.

Eczema

Eczema is a systemic problem, not simply an external irritation. An allergic reaction to foods such as wheat, gluten or dairy foods or other external irritants such as animal dander and house dust mites is often involved. The local immune mechanisms in the skin may be put under pressure by underuse of the other eliminative pathways, the bowels and kidneys, or immunity may be lowered by dietary deficiencies, chronic toxicity, poor digestion, dysbiosis and stress. Adverse drug reactions and irritants such as washing powder can be implicated.

Treatment To soothe the allergic response, use antihistamines Chamomile, Yarrow, Feverfew, Nettle, Baikal skullcap or Lemon balm. Adaptogenic herbs Ashwagandha, Guduchi, Amalaki, Schisandra, Liquorice,

CASE STUDY **ECZEMA**

CLIENT PROFILE
Daisy, aged 3, had red inflamed eczema over her face, limbs and abdomen. It began when she was weaned on to solids at four months old and worsened in heat. Several times her skin had become infected from scratching, for which she was prescribed antibiotics orally and in creams. As quite a determined and fiery child, she found her itchy skin very irritating, and it often made it difficult for her to fall asleep, especially after a hot bath.

THE HERBAL TREATMENT
In Daisy's prescription I combined Nettle, Burdock, Guduchi, Chamomile, Liquorice, Gotu kola and Cleavers with a glycerite of Rose to sweeten the taste of the herbs, making them more palatable. I also gave Daisy a cream containing Neem, Turmeric and Rose to soothe the inflammation and prevent infection, plus a supplement of Evening primrose oil.

I recommended to Daisy's parents that they temporarily omit dairy products, sugar and bread from her diet, as she was likely to have a dairy allergy and some degree of dysbiosis from the antibiotics. I also suggested that they avoid sour fruit such as citrus, blackcurrants and tomatoes as well as salty foods like crisps and Marmite, which can have a heating effect. I asked them to give Daisy Chamomile tea at least 3 times a day to help soothe the allergic response and cool the heat.

With this prescription Daisy's skin was much better within three weeks.

Shiitake and Reishi mushrooms, Aloe vera and Ginseng increase general immunity and improve resilience to stress. Gentle relaxants Chamomile, Passion flower, Skullcap, Vervain, Lavender and Rosemary reduce tension and anxiety.

Cleansing herbs support the liver's detoxifying work, taking the strain off the skin. Burdock, Red clover, Cleavers, Nettle, Neem, Dandelion, Globe artichoke, Milk thistle and Aloe vera clear heat and inflammation.

Creams or oils containing Chamomile, Evening primrose oil, Marigold, Chickweed, Comfrey, Lavender, or Aloe vera gel, can soothe inflammation. Evening primrose oil or Borage seed oil will provide gamma-linolenic acid (GLA), often deficient in eczema.

Other measures Vitamins A, B, C and E, zinc magnesium, calcium and iron are also essential.

Acne

Overactive sebaceous glands due in part to hormonal changes especially during adolescence make the skin oily. The sebum blocks hair follicles, causing them to become inflamed and infected, producing the characteristic blackheads and spots. Acne is also indicative of nutritional deficiencies, toxicity, dysbiosis, stressed adrenals, PCOS and food allergies.

Treatment It is important to support the liver and bowels in their detoxifying work to take the load off the skin as an eliminative organ and prevent a build-up of hormones in the body. Use Burdock, Milk thistle, Dandelion root, Red clover, Guduchi, Cleavers, Liquorice or Yellow dock. For constipation, take 1–2 teaspoons of Linseeds or Psyllium seeds soaked in a little warm water before bed.

To clear the skin, use antimicrobial and anti-inflammatory herbs like Echinacea, Neem, Myrrh, Turmeric, Amalaki, Oregon grape and Wild indigo. Other cleansing herbs include Nettle, Bhringaraj, Borage, Aloe vera, Pau d'arco, Cat's claw, Wild pansy and Andrographis Hormone. Balancing herbs include Chaste tree, Wild yam, Evening primrose oil and Saw palmetto.

Leave the skin alone; clean it daily with Rose water, apply infusions of Marigold, Elderflower or Lavender afterwards and never squeeze pimples. Once the skin has cleared, use a few drops of either Neroli or Lavender oil in aqueous cream, Comfrey or vitamin E cream, to heal the scars.

Other measures Avoid fatty foods, dairy produce, chocolate, alcohol, sweets, red meats, iodine-rich foods, tea and coffee.

Infections of the skin

A variety of micro-organisms can invade the skin. Boils and abscesses arise from infections of the hair roots and sweat glands caused by staphylococcus bacteria and dead white corpuscles. Impetigo is a highly contagious bacterial infection that starts as a rash of small blisters and then forms yellow scabs around the lips, nose and ears. It can develop as a secondary infection on the skin where it is already disturbed, as in eczema, scabies and cold sores. Ringworm or athlete's foot is a contagious fungal infection that spreads in warm, moist conditions such as around swimming pools and in bathrooms, and can be resilient to treatment. Caused by tiny mites burrowing into the skin, scabies is an intensely itchy condition and highly contagious. When the eggs hatch, they can be passed on easily by direct contact or from bed linen, clothing (where they can survive for about two weeks) or from pets.

Treatment Echinacea, Marigold, Thyme, Sage, Pau d'arco, Cat's claw, Wild indigo or Turmeric are useful antimicrobial herbs for enhancing immunity and combating infection. Garlic is excreted via the pores, disinfecting the skin as it goes.

Cleavers, Nettle, Chickweed, Dandelion, Burdock, Milk thistle or Red clover help clear heat and toxins from the system that predispose to infection and boost immunity.

Externally, applying hot poultices of Marshmallow or Burdock with antiseptic oils of Lavender or Thyme will bring boils to a head. In addition, infected skin can be bathed with warm teas of Marigold, Myrrh, Golden seal, Echinacea, Cat's claw or Neem, or dilute oils of Lavender, Rosemary or Peppermint.

Caution Repeated attacks of boils indicate a run-down condition that requires further investigation and could be a sign of diabetes.

Warts and veruccae

Warts are small growths composed of dead cells and caused by a virus (HPV, or human papilloma virus). They are spread easily by direct contact or in wet places, such as in bathrooms and around swimming pools, and are most common on the hands and feet when they are called plantar warts or verrucae. They also occur around the genitals and in women can predispose to cervical dysplasia (precancerous changes in the cervix). The development of warts, especially when several occur at a time, indicates lowered immunity, and it is important to treat the problem systemically as well as locally.

Treatment The most successful remedy is the fresh juice of Greater celandine (*Chelidonium majus*) applied twice daily. The white juice from the fresh Dandelion, fresh Elderberry juice, Aloe vera juice, fresh Lemon balm, Garlic or Ginger or Olive leaf can also be applied to the warts.

Also recommended are immune-enhancing and antiviral herbs such as Lemon balm, Wild indigo, St John's wort, Pau d'arco, Cat's claw, Aloe vera, Barberry, Garlic, Echinacea and Olive leaf for internal use.

Burdock, Cleavers, Dandelion root, Blue flag, Red clover and Poke root help clear toxins from the system and are indicated in all skin problems.

Caution Seek medical attention if a wart grows or suddenly changes, as it may indicate skin cancer.

Greater celandine encourages the skin to heal, and its enzymes dissolve warts.

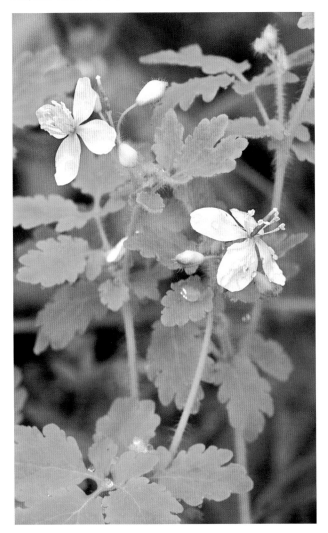

Psoriasis

A complex autoimmune skin problem, psoriasis speeds up the normal growth and renewal of skin cells by five to ten times and produces the build-up of scaly patches that can appear almost anywhere on the body. It can affect fingernails, leaving them discoloured, pitted or split, and is sometimes associated with polyarthritis. It may be hereditary or triggered by excess alcohol, sunburn, skin injury, a streptococcal throat infection, stress or shock, and can be improved by sunlight and visits to the Dead Sea. Food allergies, incomplete protein digestion, dysbiosis, poor liver function and nutritional deficiencies can also play a part.

Treatment Herbs containing psoralens such as Angelica, Wild carrot, Wild celery seed and Fennel help clear the skin, especially in combination with sunbathing. Antioxidant herbs like Oregon grape, Barberry, Golden seal or Red grape seed extract reduce free radical damage to the skin and decrease inflammation. Alkaloids in Oregon grape root slow proliferation of skin cells. Milk thistle and Forskohlii can also slow down the growth of skin cells. Sarsaparilla, Honeysuckle, Frankincense, raw Rehmannia root, Neem, Turmeric, Evening primrose oil and Peony are other good anti-inflammatories.

To aid the liver in its detoxifying work, use Burdock, Yellow dock, Red clover, Turmeric or Dandelion. Guggulu is also excellent.

Externally, creams containing Chamomile, Liquorice, Turmeric, Lavender oil, Evening primrose oil, Aloe vera juice, Oregon grape, capsaicin from Cayenne pepper or Wild oats can help clear the skin.

Other measures Supplements of omega-3 essential fatty acids, vitamin A and zinc are recommended.

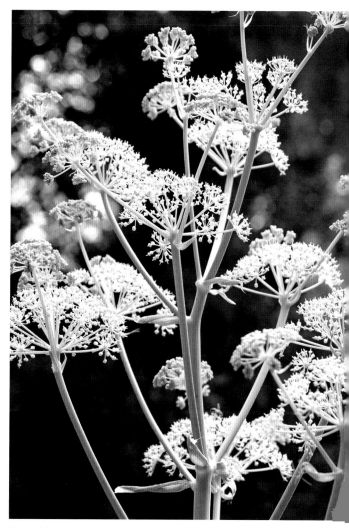

Fennel has a clarifying effect on skin conditions and is an anti-inflammatory herb.

Mouth and gum problems

Good oral hygiene and a healthy immune system will generally keep at bay infections that can develop from the many micro-organisms that generally inhabit the mouth. Lowered immunity from poor diet, chronic illness such as diabetes, digestive problems, dysbiosis, food allergies, alcohol, smoking, stress, tiredness and mercury fillings can predispose to infections and inflammatory problems, including bleeding gums and mouth ulcers.

Treatment Antimicrobial and anti-inflammatory herbs such as Echinacea, Cat's claw, Myrrh, Sage, Thyme, Marigold, Chamomile, Golden seal or Peppermint can be used as mouthwashes to combat infections in the mouth and taken internally to improve immunity and to remedy gut problems and dysbiosis. Bitter, detoxifying herbs Burdock, Dandelion, Milk thistle, Guduchi, Amalaki or Yellow dock can be added to support the work of the liver.

Astringent herbs like Plantain, Thyme, Marigold, Agrimony, Rose, Vervain, Periwinkle and Yarrow make good mouthwashes for strengthening gums and stopping bleeding, while antioxidants taken internally, such as Guduchi, Blueberry/Bilberry, Hawthorn, Cat's claw, Selfheal, Common grape vine and Sweet marjoram, will help to protect blood vessels from free radical damage.

Other measures As preventative measures, it is important to floss and rinse the mouth daily with herbal antiseptics.

The eyes

Often described as the 'gateway to the soul', the eyes are one of the sense organs and express emotions such as joy, excitement and happiness, as well as fear, anxiety, anger, grief and suffering. As such, they convey much to others about our state of health, both physical and mental.

The white opaque part of the eye, the sclera, protects the eye and serves as an attachment for muscles that move the eye. Light passes through the transparent cornea – the dome at the front of the eye – to the iris and pupil. The iris, the coloured part, comprises muscles that govern the amount of light entering the eye; the pupil is the hole that lets light pass to the back of the eye. The acqueous humour is found between the lens and cornea and the vitreous humour is the fluid in the major part of the eye. The crystalline lens behind the pupil focuses light onto the retina, which is composed of thousands of tiny structures known as rods and cones responsible for conveying messages via the optic nerve to the brain, resulting in vision.

Light influences our physical, mental and emotional health. Sunlight entering the eye stimulates the secretion of opiate-like endorphins by the pineal gland, giving a feeling of wellbeing. The many hours of darkness in a northern-hemisphere winter can predispose to SAD (seasonal affective disorder) and reduced resistance to infection, so it is important to spend time outside in sunlight even on a dull day.

The eyes are responsible for producing tears, which contain endorphins that help us release emotional pain and calm us down when we cry. Tiny amounts of tears constantly wash across the eyes, protecting them from damage and clearing debris. The inner and outer surfaces of the eyes are covered with delicate conjunctiva, and these are lubricated by tears that drain into channels passing into the nose. The eyelids also protect the eyes.

Protective nutrients and herbs

Certain nutrients are vital to eye health. Antioxidant carotenoids lutein and zeaxanthin protect the eyes from oxidative stress and high-energy light; they are found in dark green, leafy vegetables like spinach, kale, peas and broccoli, marigolds, squash, corn and eggs. Lutein is present in the macula, a small area of retina responsible for central vision, and a lutein-rich diet helps prevent

cataracts and macular degeneration as we age, as do high levels of antioxidant vitamins A, C and E. Essential fatty acids including omega-3s from oily fish, walnuts, soya beans and flax seeds are also vital. Copper found in nuts, sunflower seeds, liver, beans and lentils is another good antioxidant for the eyes. Zinc from oysters, nuts, beans, red meat and poultry helps maintain good vision through healthy macular function.

Elderberries and Blueberries/Bilberries are rich in antioxidant anthocyanosides, which contain or boost the action of gluthione an antioxidant in the acqueous humour, helping prevent cataracts. Anthocyanidins protect blood vessels in the eye, preventing poor night vision and retinal disorders. Herbs with a similar action include Astragalus root, Milk thistle, Turmeric and Garlic. Chamomile, Marigold, Marshmallow and Elderflower are used to treat problems of the eyelids and conjunctiva.

The eye Each eye is protected by an eyebrow, eyelashes and eyelid, while tear ducts produce a fluid that keeps the eye moist and free from infection. The eye's movement is controlled by three pairs of extrinsic eye muscles.

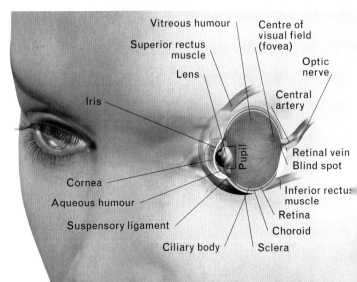

Vitreous humour
Centre of visual field (fovea)
Superior rectus muscle
Optic nerve
Lens
Central artery
Iris
Retinal vein
Blind spot
Pupil
Cornea
Inferior rectus muscle
Aqueous humour
Retina
Suspensory ligament
Choroid
Ciliary body
Sclera

Conjunctivitis, blepharitis and styes

In conjunctivitis the lining of the eye becomes irritated either by infection, allergy such as hay fever and rhinitis, dust or pollution in the atmosphere, and the eye becomes red and inflamed, often weepy. In blepharitis, the eyelids become red and inflamed, often indicating depleted immunity, a toxic system or allergy. Styes result from inflammation or infections of the glands at the base of the eyelashes and tend to occur when run-down or tired.

Treatment To soothe irritated and inflamed eyes, infusions of astringent and antiseptic herbs Eyebright, Marigold, Chamomile, Elderflower and Rose can be taken internally and used to bathe the eyes.

Black tea is a useful remedy to bathe the eyes, or lay a warm Chamomile tea bag over each eye and leave in place for 10–15 minutes. Warm infusions of Eyebright, Chamomile, Elderflower, Plantain or Marigold can be applied as compresses.

Antimicrobial herbs Echinacea, Golden seal, Pau d'arco, Burdock, Red clover or Liquorice can be taken to combat infection, boost immunity and detoxify the system. Chamomile, Nettle, Lemon balm, Yarrow, Feverfew and Baikal skullcap have antihistamine actions, which help relieve allergic eye conditions.

For chronic conjunctivitis and blepharitis, take supplements of Borage seed oil or Evening primrose oil.

Other measures Chronic conjunctivitis and blepharitis often respond well to omitting dairy products, tea and coffee from the diet and taking supplements of vitamin C and B.

Caution Always use a sterilized eyebath and don't use the same solution for both eyes. All teas used to bathe eyes should be prepared as decoctions and simmered for 10 minutes to ensure they are sterilized.

Eye disorders

The tendency to eye problems, including cataracts, glaucoma and macular degeneration, increases with age, largely due to free radical damage. This is increased by smoking, stress and drugs such as steroids. Damage to the retina associated with diabetes and atherosclerosis, and inflammatory eye conditions including episcleritis and iritis, can respond to herbal treatment.

Treatment Antioxidant herbs include Blueberry/Bilberry, Elderberry, Hawthorn berries, Rosemary, Thyme, Sage, Sweet marjoram, Bladderwrack, Selfheal, Rehmannia,

Shatavari, Amalaki, Ashwagandha, Ginkgo, Cat's claw and Red grape seed. They strengthen blood vessels within the eye and inhibit macular degeneration and diabetic retinopathy. Forskohlii increases circulation within the eye and decreases intraocular pressure in glaucoma.

Rosemary, Ginkgo, Eyebright, Vervain and Peppermint increase circulation to and from the eye.

Pasque flower and Chamomile are recommended for painful inflammatory eye conditions such as scleritis and iritis. Turmeric, Peony root, Frankincense, Gentian, Dandelion root and Amalaki are also helpful. Tepid Chamomile tea bags laid on the eyes for 10–15 minutes can swiftly relieve pain.

Other measures Foods containing vitamins A, B and C and supplements of antioxidants including lutein protect against free radical damage and help prevent macular degeneration and cataracts.

Caution Seek medical attention immediately if you experience eye pain or sudden changes in vision.

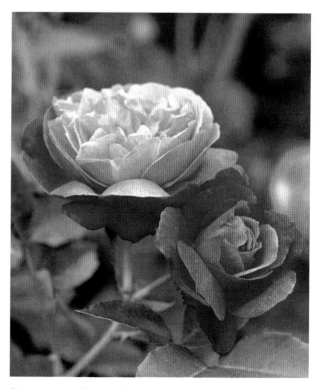

Rose, prepared as an infusion, makes a soothing eyebath for sore or inflamed eyes.

The hormonal system

The hormonal or endocrine system is a system of chemical messaging. Its purpose is the communication between and coordination of many different functions of the body that enable homeostasis – the maintenance of a stable state within the body, which is vital for health. These include tissue function, metabolism and the production of energy, reproduction, mood, growth and development.

These huge feats are accomplished via a network of endocrine glands and organs that produce, store and secrete hormones as they are required by the body. This hormonal network works in conjunction with the nervous system, reproductive system, kidneys, gut, liver and pancreas. Hormones are special chemicals that are manufactured by one cell or a group of cells and carried in the bloodstream to specific targets, which may be organs, tissues or cells. Different types of hormone cause different effects on other cells or tissues of the body. Endocrine glands are located in many regions of the body and include the hypothalamus, which controls the pituitary or master gland, which in turn controls all the other hormone-producing glands, such as the thyroid, parathyroid, thymus and adrenal glands, pancreas, ovaries and testes.

Hormonal imbalances

For healthy functioning of our endocrine system, the glands need to work correctly, the blood needs to carry hormones efficiently to their target points and the receptor sites on the target cells need to respond properly for the hormones to enter the cells and do their work. Too much or too little of any of the hormones secreted by these glands can cause disruption in the body. For example, too much growth hormone from the pituitary gland will mean that you grow excessively tall; too little and you will be very short. Too little insulin from the pancreas causes diabetes. Excess thyroid hormones cause an increase in metabolism, which imposes a strain on the nervous system and heart, while low thyroid function causes lethargy and weight problems. Imbalances of reproductive hormones cause a wide range of menstrual, sexual and gynaecological problems, and influence fertility. Such hormonal imbalances may be caused by problems with cell receptor sites or in regulating the

hormones in the bloodstream, or the body may have difficulty controlling hormone levels through inadequate breakdown and excretion of hormones from the body due to reduced liver or kidney function.

For our hormonal system to function well, we need to eat a healthy diet containing plenty of essential fatty acids, minerals (particularly magnesium), trace elements and antioxidant nutrients including betacarotene, zinc, selenium and vitamins B, C and E. Stress, excess coffee and alcohol and nutritional deficiencies can significantly disrupt hormonal balance.

Herbs such as Liquorice and Echinacea support the thymus gland in its immune work; Bladderwrack and Ashwagandha influence the thyroid; Chaste tree helps to regulate the pituitary gland; Liquorice, Wild yam, Ginseng and Borage influence the adrenals; Wild yam, Black cohosh, Chaste tree, Shatavari, Ashwagandha and Ginseng all help regulate reproductive hormones. Bitter herbs such as Dandelion root, Milk thistle and Burdock aid the liver's breakdown of hormones so that they are excreted from the body once they have done their work.

The endocrine system
The endocrine glands produce hormones, the 'chemical messengers', and release them into the bloodstream. Endocrine glands include the pituitary, thyroid, parathyroid and adrenal glands, as well as the ovaries, the testes, part of the pancreas and the placenta.

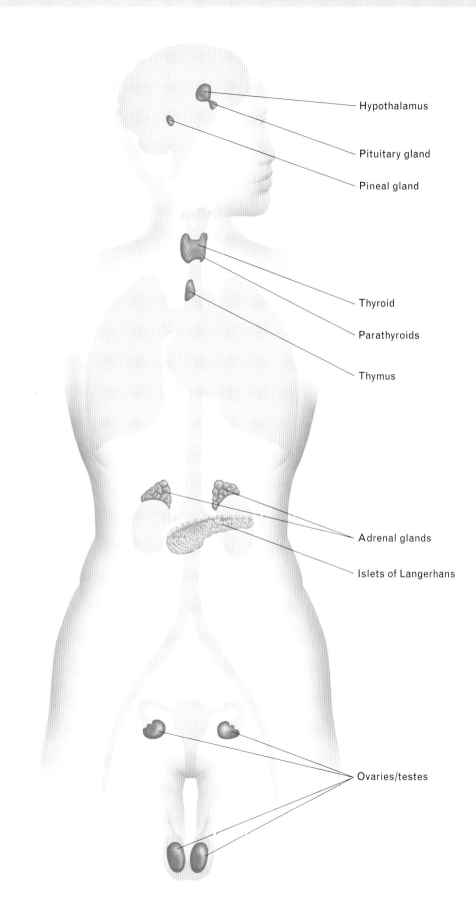

Hypothalamus

Pituitary gland

Pineal gland

Thyroid

Parathyroids

Thymus

Adrenal glands

Islets of Langerhans

Ovaries/testes

Premenstrual syndrome (PMS)

The familiar physical, mental and emotional symptoms of PMS in the second half of the cycle are generally linked to excess oestrogen in relation to progesterone. Environmental toxins from plastics, polychlorinated biphenyls (PCBs) and pesticides that mimic oestrogen in the body as well as oestrogen residues in tap water and meat, and the liver's inability to break down oestrogen, disrupt normal hormone balance. Deficiencies of nutrients, particularly magnesium, B-complex vitamins, zinc and essential fatty acids, are often also responsible.

Treatment Chaste tree is the best-known herb to increase progesterone and is generally taken as tincture, ½ teaspoon 30 minutes before breakfast. Adaptogenic herbs Wild yam, Liquorice, Ashwagandha, Shatavari, Chinese angelica and Black cohosh, are rich in steroidal saponins and increase resilience to stress and balance hormones. Nervines help to stabilize emotions and include Wild oats, Skullcap, Chamomile, Gotu kola, Bhringaraj and Motherwort.

Liver herbs such as Burdock, Dandelion, Guduchi, Milk thistle, Barberry and Yellow dock are important to help the breakdown of hormones.

Diuretic herbs Cleavers, Dandelion, Corn silk, Fennel, Coriander, Wild celery and Wild carrot help relieve fluid retention, bloating and breast discomfort.

A supplement of Evening primrose oil is also recommended for easing PMS symptoms.

Other measures Supplements of calcium, magnesium, vitamin B-complex and E can significantly relieve PMS symptoms.

Menstrual problems

These are largely due to hormone imbalances and nutritional deficiencies. Irregular or absent periods are associated with intense exercise, nutritional deficiency, sudden weight loss, drugs and psychological stress or shock. Other endocrine disorders can be involved. Painful periods are related to poor circulation, stress, overwork and muscular tension, lack of exercise, bad posture and caffeine. Heavy periods can be caused by fibroids, polyps, thyroid problems, uterine congestion and perimenopause.

Treatment To regulate hormones, use Chaste tree, Wild yam, Chinese angelica or Shatavari with Liquorice and Evening primrose oil. You can combine these with liver herbs like Burdock, Holy thistle, Oregon grape or Dandelion to aid the breakdown of hormones.

For intense cramps with scanty bleeding, Cramp bark, Black haw, Motherwort, Pasque flower and Black cohosh are excellent taken every 2 hours when necessary. For associated tension, add Valerian, Passion flower, Chamomile or Hops. Rubbing oils of Chamomile, Lavender or Rosemary gently into the abdomen helps relieve pain.

For heavy bleeding, astringent herbs such as Beth root, Yarrow, Periwinkle, Lady's mantle, Agrimony, Bearberry, Chinese Foxglove, Bayberry and Rose can be taken 3–6 times daily as required.

Iron-containing foods and herbs, such as Nettle, Coriander leaf, Codonopsis, Amalaki, Bladderwrack and Yellow dock, help combat anaemia.

Other measures Avoid caffeine, alcohol and refined and junk foods, and take supplements of vitamins B-complex and C, as well as zinc and magnesium. Also take regular exercise.

Chaste tree is renowned for its ability to balance hormones through its action on the pituitary or master gland.

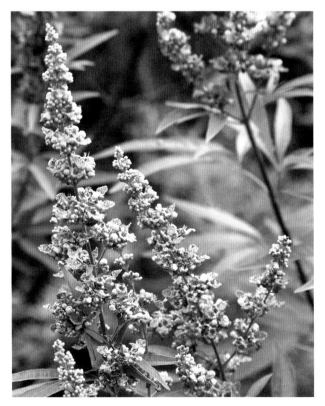

Benign breast problems

Benign mammary dysplasia (BMD), also known as fibrocystic breast disease or cyclical mastalgia, is characterized by breast lumps, swelling and tenderness, and fluctuates through the menstrual cycle but is usually worst premenstrually. It is related to oestrogen, prolactin, thyroid hormone and insulin levels and deficiencies of selenium, and is aggravated by methlyxanthines in coffee, tea, chocolate and cola. Thyroid hormones help the liver's metabolism of oestrogen, and low thyroid levels are related to high blood oestrogen levels. Excess dietary fat, dairy produce, refined carbohydrates, constipation and stress are also contributory factors. Mastitis involves infection in the breast that can occur when breast-feeding.

Treatment Hormone-balancing Chaste tree, Wild yam, Chinese angelica, Saw palmetto, Shatavari and Liquorice can normalize breast tissue. Liver remedies Burdock, Dandelion, Holy thistle, Milk thistle and Gentian aid the liver's metabolism of oestrogen. Cleavers, Dandelion root, Blue flag, Marigold and Poke root stimulate lymphatic drainage from the breast and reduce lumps and infection. If breasts are particularly painful, add analgesic and hormone balancer Black cohosh.

To regulate the thyroid gland, Bladderwrack and Guggulu are recommended. A supplement of Evening primrose oil is helpful.

Use dilute oils of Lavender, Fennel or Rose, or castor oil for daily breast massage. Reduction of dietary fat and avoidance of caffeine can be helpful.

Other measures Supplements of magnesium and vitamins B6, B12 and E are also helpful.

Caution It is important to investigate further any breast problems.

Vaginal infections

The delicate environment of pH and flora of the vagina can be disturbed by hormonal imbalances, antibiotics, stress, poor diet, the contraceptive pill, pregnancy, post-menopausal changes and diabetes, and become susceptible to inflammation and infection. Yeast infections (thrush) are most common and tend to be related to gut dysbiosis. Trichomonas, gardnerella, human papillomavirus (HPV), or vaginal warts, herpes and bacterial vaginiosis (common after the menopause) can also occur.

Treatment Antiseptic herbs to combat infection include Marigold, Golden seal, Thyme, Chamomile, Lavender, Pau d'arco, Neem, Turmeric, Echinacea and Sweet

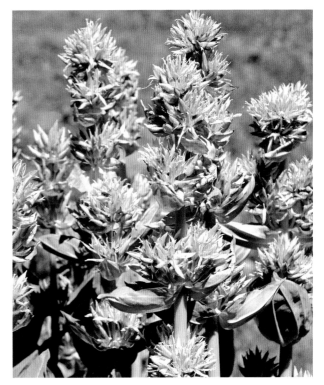

Gentian stimulates the gall bladder and liver, and helps the liver process oestrogen.

marjoram, which can be taken internally and used in creams, douches and sitz baths, and in lotions in which tampons can be soaked and inserted for 30 minutes morning and night.

Garlic is a great antimicrobial for internal and external use, active against bacterial, viral and fungal infections like thrush. Peel a clove carefully without nicking it, wrap it in clean gauze and insert for 6 consecutive nights. Alternatively, add 5 ml (1 teaspoon) of fresh garlic juice to a few tablespoons of live yogurt, soak a tampon in it or use as a douche twice daily. If the area is sore and inflamed, sitting in a bowl of Chamomile tea is wonderfully relieving.

The above herbs will resolve infection in the vagina and more systemic problems of toxicity and dysbiosis. Immune-enhancing herbs like Ashwagandha, Shatavari, Guduchi, Amalaki and Schisandra can be taken after infection to prevent further problems.

Hormone-balancing Chaste tree, Sage and Wild yam can be used for post-menopausal infections.

Caution Seek medical attention if you suspect sexually transmitted infection.

Endometriosis

This is the abnormal growth of tissue similar to that lining the uterus. It is generally found within the pelvic cavity and rarely in the lungs and even the nose. It grows and bleeds through the cycle just like the uterine wall. Symptoms can include sharp pain before periods and with intercourse, and heavy bleeding. Adhesions may form between the womb and bowel and inhibit conception, leading to infertility. Causes include hormone imbalances, retroverted menstruation linked to the use of tampons and intrauterine devices (IUDs), stress and immune problems caused by oestrogen-mimicking pollutants as in plastics and pesticides.

Treatment Chaste tree, Ashwagandha, Chinese angelica, Wild yam, Shatavari, Peony, Liquorice and Black cohosh help balance hormones.

Cramp bark, Pasque flower, Black cohosh and Passion flower help relieve pain and can be taken in acute doses. Massage with sesame or castor oil with 2 drops of Lavender, Rosemary, Rose, Chamomile or Ginger oil per 5 ml (1 teaspoon) can be helpful.

Hawthorn, Ginger, Gotu kola and Prickly ash improve

Ashwagandha enhances resilience to stress and has a balancing effect on the hormones.

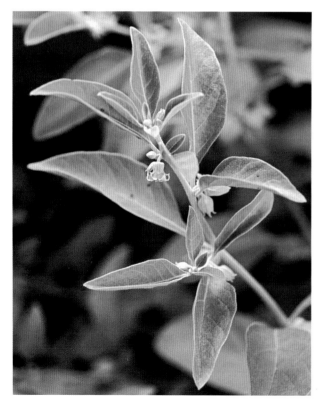

circulation to the uterus and relieve pelvic congestion, while Ashwagandha, Skullcap, Siberian ginseng, Shatavari and Wild oats increase resilience to stress.

Astringent herbs Beth root, Yarrow, Periwinkle, Lady's mantle, Agrimony, Rehmannia, Bayberry and Rose help reduce heavy bleeding.

To help the breakdown and excretion of hormones, take liver herbs Burdock, Milk thistle, Holy thistle and Dandelion. A supplement of Evening primrose oil is also recommended.

Other measures Supplements of magnesium, vitamins B and E, zinc and calcium are also helpful. It is important to avoid caffeine, alcohol and refined and junk foods, and to take regular exercise.

Menopausal problems

Low libido, hot flushes, night sweats, mood swings, 'mid-life crises', depression and insomnia are some of the symptoms that can characterize the menopause, when levels of oestrogen and progesterone decline to the point where menstruation ceases. The adrenal glands take over production of similar hormones, but stress and adrenal exhaustion can impair their ability to do so adequately, triggering the familiar symptoms. Subsequent health problems include increased risk of osteoporosis and heart and arterial disease.

Treatment Several plants contain isoflavones, similar in structure to oestrogen, called phytoestrogens. They occur in Shatavari, Red clover, Chinese angelica, Wild yam, Wild indigo, Siberian ginseng, Liquorice and Black cohosh. These herbs also support the adrenals, increase resilience to stress and are very helpful for relieving menopausal symptoms.

Chaste tree, Motherwort, Sage, Chamomile, Hops, Lady's mantle, Aloe vera, Hawthorn, Fennel, Sarsaparilla and Rehmannia will also reduce menopausal symptoms. Burdock, Dandelion, Holy thistle and Milk thistle aid the liver's metabolism of hormones, while relaxants Chamomile, Pasque flower, Motherwort, Vervain, Wild oats and Lemon balm are calming where anxiety is aggravating symptoms.

Supplements of Borage seed oil or Evening primrose oil are also helpful.

Other measures Supplements of vitamin E, calcium and magnesium are recommended.

Low sex drive/impotence

Lack of sexual interest in men and women and erectile dysfunction in men are increasingly common problems. Hormone imbalances, stress, depression, pain, obesity, poor health, low energy, marital problems, diabetes, high blood pressure, circulatory problems and the effects of drugs and smoking are all contributory factors. Low libido is frequently experienced by women around the menopause, and male impotence can also be related to environmental toxins and particularly the oestrogenic effects of plastics, pesticides and hormones used in animal rearing.

Treatment Herbs for balancing hormones and increasing sexual energy and performance include Ashwagandha, Shatavari, Astragalus, Chinese angelica, Schisandra, Liquorice and Korean and Siberian ginseng. These adaptogenic remedies also increase resilience to stress and counter the effects of anxiety and depression.

Wild oats, Rose, Rosemary, Gotu kola, Vervain and Skullcap are good relaxants.

Black cohosh, Wild yam, Sage, Motherwort and Chaste tree balance hormones during the menopause, while Sarsaparilla, Saw palmetto and Damiana support production of male hormones. Gingko, Ginger, Cinnamon, Hawthorn and Gotu kola can help circulatory problems.

Detoxifying remedies including Burdock, Nettle, Yellow dock and Milk thistle can be taken to support the liver and clear the side effects of drugs.

Infertility and low sperm count

Infertility is reaching epidemic proportions, related largely to the effect of environmental toxins and residues of the contraceptive pill in water supplies, which are causing widespread hormonal imbalances. Men and women are both affected, problems in men accounting for approximately one-third of problems. Hernia surgery, tubule infection, chlamydia, diabetes, drugs, mumps, stress, smoking, toxic metals and nutritional deficiencies may all affect sperm count. It takes 100 days for sperm to develop, so treatment needs to be continued over several months.

Treatment Detoxifying herbs such as Bladderwrack, Burdock, Andrographis, Globe artichoke, Shiitake and Reishi mushrooms, Guduchi, Milk thistle and Nettle can be taken to support the liver's breakdown of drugs and toxins.

Hormone-balancing and adaptogenic herbs to enhance fertility are Ashwagandha, Shatavari, Chaste tree, Wild yam, Astragalus, Chinese angelica, Schisandra,

Liquorice and Korean and Siberian ginseng. They also increase resilience to stress and counter the effects of anxiety and depression.

Black cohosh, Motherwort, Evening primrose oil and Rose can also be used for menstrual problems.

Other measures Supplements of vitamins B-complex and E, zinc, omega-3 and -6 oils and coenzyme Q10 are recommended. Pesticides are designed to disrupt the reproductive cycle of the insect, fungus or weed it is trying to kill, so eat organic produce.

CASE STUDY **INFERTILITY**

CLIENT PROFILE

Jenny, aged 42, had been trying to conceive with Peter for five years – unsuccessfully – and this was causing them considerable stress. Their doctor had carried out exhaustive tests: Peter's sperm count was excellent, and nothing could be found in Jenny's results except a small uterine fibroid. Jenny had a fairly large frame and was a little overweight. She suffered from water retention and painful breasts before her period, and a dragging-down sensation and feeling of general heaviness with the first two days of bleeding, which tended to be heavy.

THE HERBAL TREATMENT

Jenny's prescription consisted of hormone-balancing herbs and herbs to clear uterine congestion and reduce fibroids. It included Chaste tree, Motherwort, Kelp, Chinese angelica, Liquorice, Lady's mantle and Raspberry leaf, plus Burdock and Milk thistle to aid the liver's metabolism of oestrogen. I also recommended that she should take a formula called Kanchanar guggulu, which is specific for fibroids.

I advised that Jenny ensure her diet was excellent, with plenty of nourishing foods such as whole grains, nuts and seeds, but a minimum of fatty fried food, and that she avoid caffeine, alcohol and junk foods. I suggested drinking herbal teas of Rose, Nettle, Cinnamon and Ginger and some Dandelion coffee, and supplements of vitamin C, B complex, Evening primrose, zinc and magnesium. I reminded her to take regular exercise.

After four months of treatment Jenny conceived, and now the couple has a baby boy.

Fibroids

These are benign growths consisting of smooth muscle tissue that develop in the uterine wall. There may be a single fibroid or, more commonly, several. They are related to excess dietary fats, excess oestrogen, overuse of the contraceptive pill, uterine congestion, overweight and stress, and shrink after the menopause. Methylxanthines, which are present in coffee, also stimulate their growth. Approximately one in three women have fibroids, but they are so small that they are symptomless. Large fibroids cause heavy periods, clots, enlarged abdomen, pressure symptoms in the bladder, constipation and anaemia. They tend to grow in pregnancy and may cause miscarriage.

Treatment Hormone-balancing Chaste tree, Wild yam, Motherwort, Peony, Saw palmetto and Liquorice can normalize oestrogen levels. Liver remedies such as Burdock, Dandelion, Holy thistle, Milk thistle, Yellow dock and Gentian aid the liver's metabolism of oestrogen and help reduce tumours.

Astringent herbs like Beth root, Raspberry leaf, Yarrow, Periwinkle, Lady's mantle, Agrimony, Bearberry, Rehmannia, Bayberry or Rose reduce heavy bleeding.

Iron-containing foods and herbs, such as Nettle,

Peony helps to regulate female hormones and is highly regarded in Traditional Chinese Medicine.

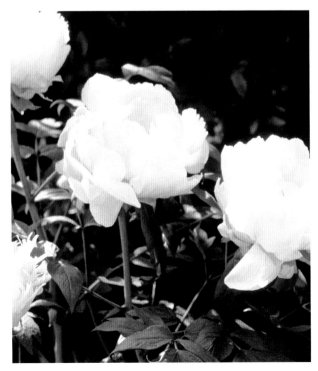

Coriander leaf, Codonopsis, Amalaki, Bladderwrack and Yellow dock, help combat anaemia. Poke root and Guggulu are also specific for reducing fibroid growths.

Siberian ginseng, Ashwagandha and Schisandra enhance resilience to stress. A supplement of Evening primrose oil is helpful.

Other measures Avoid caffeine, alcohol and fatty and junk foods, and take regular exercise. Take supplements of vitamin C, B-complex vitamins, zinc and magnesium.

Ovarian cysts

These are fluid-filled sacs on or near the ovaries that cause no symptoms if small but if large or numerous (polycystic) cause abdominal swelling, pain with intercourse, pressure on the bladder, hormone imbalances, irregularity or absence of periods, infertility and risk of miscarriage. Lack of dietary fibre and excess fats and junk foods combined with overburdening of the liver from toxins is linked to the rise of ovarian cysts. Pelvic congestion from poor circulation and lack of exercise are also implicated. Polycystic ovarian syndrome (PCOS) is a metabolic problem related to excess testosterone, raised blood sugar or insulin levels and insulin resistance. It is associated with overweight, acne, hirsutism, sugar cravings and mood swings.

Treatment Chinese angelica, Peony, Liquorice, Chaste tree and Saw palmetto with Evening primrose oil or Borage seed oil are recommended to balance hormones. Liver herbs such as Milk thistle, Barberry, Dandelion root, Burdock, Agrimony or Holy thistle help the breakdown and excretion of hormones and the re-establishment of normal hormone levels by increasing production of sex hormone-binding globulins (SHBGs), which bind free testosterone and reduce its effects, such as acne and hirsutism.

Gymnema, Fenugreek, Neem, Turmeric and Goat's rue help to regulate blood sugar and reduce insulin resistance.

Other measures Losing weight can have dramatic results. Avoiding tea, coffee and fatty and refined foods and taking supplements of chromium, vitamins B-complex, E and C, bioflavonoids, zinc, coenzyme Q10 and magnesium are recommended.

Caution Cysts can be cancerous, so seek medical attention to confirm diagnosis.

Thyroid problems

The thyroid gland works in conjunction with the pituitary gland, which produces thyroid-stimulating hormone (TSH) to make the hormones T3 and T4, which play a vital role in metabolism. Hypothyroidism, when the thyroid is underactive, is more common after menopause and causes slow metabolism, low energy, weight gain, fluid retention and dry skin and hair. Hyperthyroidism, when it is overactive (commonly related to autoimmune disease as in Hashimoto's disease, or to a cyst on the thyroid) causes goitre, weight loss, anxiety, heat intolerance and palpitations. Thyroid imbalances are complex and linked to poor diet, excess sugar, stress, adrenal exhaustion, hormonal changes, viruses, environmental toxins, food allergies and dysbiosis.

Forskohlii contains forskolin, which stimulates the release of hormones from the thyroid gland.

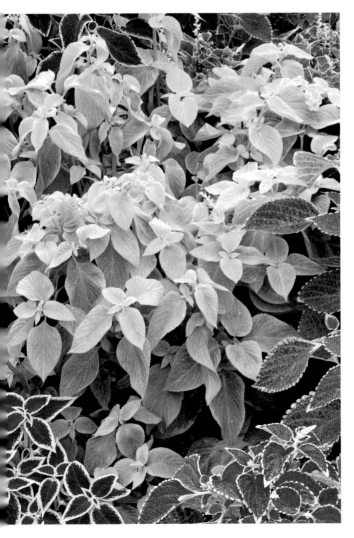

Treatment Forskohlii, Guggulu and Bladderwrack increase the production of thyroid hormones and regulate the thyroid. For autoimmune problems, detoxifying herbs that help metabolism include Oregon grape, Dandelion root, Gentian, Yellow dock, Horsetail and Barberry. They can be combined with adaptogens Ashwagandha, Bacopa, Gotu kola, Wild oats, Polygonum and Siberian ginseng, which are high in antioxidants, to regulate thyroid activity, enhance immunity and increase resilience to stress. To calm an overactive thyroid, try Meadowsweet, Motherwort and Lemon balm.

Other measures Supplements of selenium, zinc and vitamin E and B6 help conversion of T4 to T3.

Diabetes

Diabetes is a widespread problem, particularly among obese people, that involves lack of insulin production by the pancreas or resistance of the cell wall to insulin (known as insulin resistance), meaning that glucose being carried in the bloodstream cannot enter the cell to produce energy. Type 2 diabetes can be greatly improved by weight loss, changes in diet and using herbs and supplements that help to balance blood sugar by supporting the pancreas and decreasing insulin resistance. These can help prevent complications including circulatory problems, atherosclerosis, nerve damage, retinopathy and cataracts.

Treatment Gymnema, Turmeric and Fenugreek can reduce blood sugar and the need for insulin. Gymnema is thought to regenerate pancreatic cells and increase insulin receptors. Other herbs, including Garlic, Nettle, Guggulu, Pau d'arco, Cat's claw, Damiana, Goat's rue, Neem, Blueberry/Bilberry and Ginkgo, help prevent complications by improving circulation, strengthening blood-vessel walls and preventing oxidative damage.

Dandelion and Agrimony promote liver function, which is involved in maintaining normal sugar levels.

Adaptogens like Holy basil, Liquorice, Siberian ginseng, Amalaki and Guduchi improve resilience to stress, including free radical damage, which can contribute to diabetes.

Other measures Weight loss, a low-fat diet, avoidance of refined carbohydrates, regular exercise and taking supplements of chromium, zinc, magnesium and B-complex vitamins are recommended.

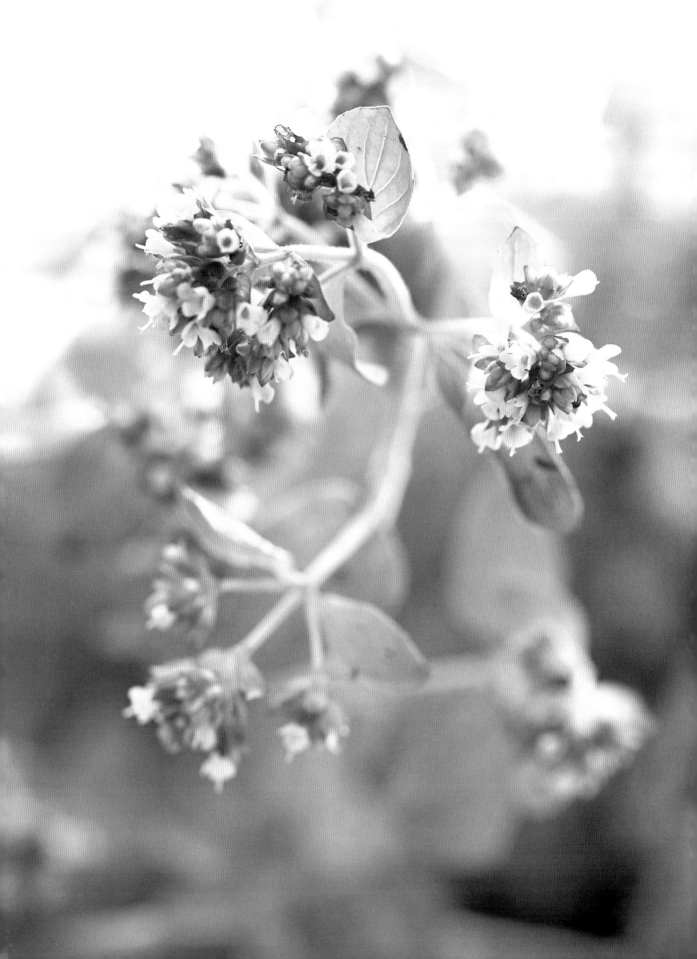

Growing, harvesting and storing herbs

There's no better way to be sure of the provenance of your herbs than growing them yourself; then you will be sure of their identity, be reassured of their organic status and be able to harvest them at the most potent time for their active ingredients. Many herbs are easy to grow – indeed some are considered invasive weeds by some – and instructions on preparing the soil, sowing and propagating, harvesting and preserving herbs to retain their maximum therapeutic properties are included in this chapter.

Growing herbs

Herbs are greatly rewarding plants to grow. Providing they have suitable soil and shelter from prevailing winds, most medicinal herbs grow easily in temperate climates, with no specialist knowledge or skills needed. Any herbs that originate from tropical regions will require a little more care, only being safe outdoors after the last frosts have gone and needing to be taken indoors in the autumn.

A herb garden can be as large or small, or as formal or informal, as you like. Whatever space you have available can be adapted to growing herbs. They can be intermingled with flowers and shrubs in large or small herbaceous borders, adding interest and beauty with their attractive foliage and architectural shapes, not to mention their delicious scents. Alternatively, they can be planted in specially designed herb gardens, in corners of vegetable gardens or intermingled with the vegetables, where they can work well as companion plants to deter pests. If you have less space, you can plant herbs in pots on a patio or even on your windowsill and in windowboxes. Both the planning and the practical laying out of a herb garden can bring many hours of pleasure and satisfaction.

Medicinal herbs consist of a mixture of annuals, biennials, perennials, shrubs and even trees. Annual herbs include Dill, Coriander, Basil, German and Roman chamomile, Borage and Marigold, and these can easily be grown from seed. Once cultivated, they may self-seed fairly freely and either be left to grow where they are or seedlings can be transplanted to their preferred site in the garden in springtime. Biennials take two summers to come into flower, usually producing an attractive rosette of leaves in the first year. They include Burdock, Angelica, Mullein and Evening primrose, all of which also self-seed freely. Herbaceous perennials continue from one year to the next, dying down in autumn and reappearing in spring the following year. They can mostly be grown from seed, but may be easier to grow using other methods of propagation, such as root division, cuttings or offsets.

Many common herbs can be bought in nurseries or garden centres and more unusual herbs can be found in specialist herb nurseries. Pot herbs can be planted at most times of the year, except when the ground is frozen or covered with snow, and provided they are healthy they will establish themselves with very little trouble. Try to avoid planting new pot herbs in dry, hot weather. Keep the plants thoroughly watered in dry weather until well established. Always ensure that you choose strong, healthy-looking plants, free from disease or insects, and avoid straggly plants and those whose roots are escaping from the bottom of the pot. Make sure the plants are clearly labelled to avoid confusion later. If you want your herb garden to look established quickly, buy two or three of each herb to plant in groups. Some fast-growing perennials may have to be moved once they grow and need more space.

Specially designed raised beds make a feature of architectural perennials, such as Globe artichoke and Fennel.

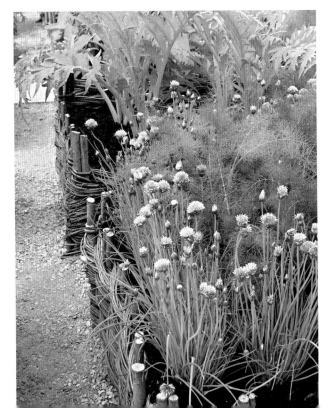

Planning your herb garden

Before planting your herbs, it is well worth making rough plans of your garden or the space you have available and a planting design on paper before approaching the practical side of planting. First, you need to decide where you will grow your herbs. Planting them near the house has its advantages, as it is easy to gather them, and harder to forget what you have and inadvertently let them grow beyond the optimum stage for harvesting before you notice them, which can be very annoying! You will also have more opportunity to appreciate them and their delicious scents the nearer you have them to the house. You also need to take into account your type of soil, and how much sun or shade you have in the space you have allocated for your herb garden.

Soil conditions and situations

Herbs are fairly easy to grow, as they are generally not fussy about where they grow and will tolerate most soils and situations. If your soil is deep, moist and rich, the plants will probably grow quickly with lots of lush foliage, but their flavour and smell will not be as strong as herbs grown in poorer, dry soil. Many of our favourite herbs, such as Rosemary, Sage, Lavender, Basil and Marjoram, are natives of the Mediterranean, where it is dry and the soil is hard and stony, so they are used to withstanding fairly adverse conditions. Plants grown in such soils do not look so vibrant and lushly attractive, but will taste and smell wonderful. Because they grow less fast than those grown on rich, moist soil, they cannot be harvested as frequently. The kind of soil that herbs tolerate least well is heavy, clay soil, which does not drain well in wet conditions and can become waterlogged. Many Mediterranean herbs will rot away in such damp situations. If your soil is wet and heavy, add plenty of organic matter and sharp sand to lighten it and aid drainage. If your soil is very light and sandy, dig in a small amount of organic matter, such as well-rotted manure, kitchen compost or seaweed, to make it more water retentive and able to retain nutrients in the soil.

Most herbs, particularly those that originate in warm climates, like to be grown in warm, sheltered and sunny positions, while some prefer light shade, so your herb-growing area should ideally include a shady area, which is often provided by a hedge or fence. A hedge or fence suitably placed for their protection will have another advantage in that it allows the delicate scents of aromatic herbs to linger on warm air, and not be blown away in a breezy, open position. However, if your garden is warm and sheltered, there is no need to be too concerned about enclosing it and herbs can be planted in the open.

HERBS FOR DIFFERENT SITES AND SOILS

Full sun
Lavender, Basil, Rosemary, Coriander, Sage, Hyssop, Thyme, Marjoram

Dappled shade
Angelica, Borage, Mint, Fennel, Lemon balm, Ground ivy

Shade
Comfrey, Valerian, Sweet violet

Moist loam
Angelica, Elecampane, Meadowsweet, Comfrey, Mint, Valerian, Lady's mantle, Lemon balm, Skullcap, Sweet violet

Well-drained loam
Lavender, Basil, Coriander, Marjoram, Wood betony, Hyssop, Rosemary, Burdock, Thyme, Sage, Dill, Fennel, Lady's mantle

Chalky soil
Hyssop, Lavender, Marjoram, Motherwort, Pasque flower, Rosemary

Light, sandy soil
Borage, Chamomile, Coriander, Evening primrose, Fennel, Lavender, Thyme, Wild carrot, Marjoram

Clay soil
Burdock, Comfrey, Mint, Wormwood
If there is adequate top soil with reasonable drainage and moist loam, other plants will grow well in clay.

Marshy ground
Horsetail, Mint, Iris, Marshmallow, Meadowsweet, Skullcap, Comfrey, Valerian, Angelica

Sowing seeds

You can buy herb seeds from specialist suppliers or save them from the previous year. For early plants, sow seed in pots or seed trays in a greenhouse or propagator in early spring. Using fresh seed compost, sow the seeds evenly and sparingly by sprinkling them over the firmed surface of the soil or in shallow drills. Cover the seeds lightly with a thin layer of compost or fine sand and water with a fine

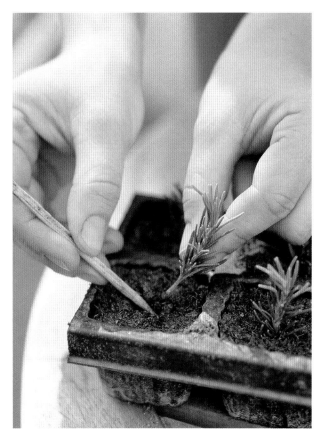

Prick out the seedlings once they have developed their first true leaves, transferring them into individual pots.

rose on your watering can. Label clearly. Cover the tray with a piece of glass or plastic, or a sheet of newspaper. Once the seeds have germinated, remove the newspaper, or once the seedlings reach the glass or plastic sheet remove it. When the seedlings are large enough to handle, you can thin them or transplant them to pots to encourage growth. Once they have become sturdy little plants, they are ready to plant outdoors in early summer. Alternatively, you can sow seeds directly into warmer soil in late spring or early summer once all sign of winter frosts has gone. Cover the seeds with soil, the depth of which can be measured by multiplying the diameter of the seeds two to three times.

Growing herbs from seed is both satisfying and fascinating, particularly if you are using seed that you have collected yourself. You may often find that your own seeds germinate more successfully than bought ones, particularly if they are fresh and sown immediately they are ripe and ready to drop. They can be sown in trays and left in a greenhouse or cold frame covered with a piece of glass or polythene until they germinate. They may not

germinate until the following spring, so you need to be fairly patient.

Many herbs self-seed freely if their seed heads are left alone, such as Elecampane, Lady's mantle, Chamomile, Coriander, Marigold and Motherwort. Seeds will germinate when conditions are right and will grow into strong, healthy plants. If they grow where you do not want them, they can easily be moved when ready.

Many variegated types of herb and decoratively coloured herbs such as Purple and Golden sages will not come true when grown from seed and so need to be propagated by other methods, such as cuttings or root division (see below).

Root division

Herbs that form good clumps are excellent candidates for root division; in fact, herbs such as Irises, Comfrey, Valerian, Lemon balm, Elecampane and Yarrow need to be divided every three to four years into smaller clumps for best results. Root division is best done in autumn or early spring. First, cut back the top growth and dig up the entire plant with a fork. Carefully divide the clump with your hands into several pieces, each retaining a good system of roots, and replant where you have chosen. If the clump is too solid to divide with your hands, you will need to use a garden fork. Dig the fork into the middle of the clump and lever it about, forcing the clump to separate into smaller pieces.

Taking cuttings

Taking cuttings from established plants is an easy way to propagate herbs and can be very rewarding. Softwood, semi-ripe and hardwood cuttings can be taken, depending on the plant. Softwood cuttings are generally successful with most herbaceous perennials, while semi-ripe and hardwood cuttings are suitable for shrubs and small trees.

When taking cuttings, gently tear a small side shoot off a stem so that it has a heal on it, or cut the shoot's stem just below a leaf joint using a sharp knife 5–10 cm (2–4 inches) long. Remove the lower leaves and insert into holes made with a pencil, stick or dibber around the edge of a pot of cutting compost, or a mixture of peat and sand. You may wish to dip the end into hormone rooting powder first if you would like to speed up the rooting process. Firm the soil around the cuttings and water in well.

Once you detect signs of new growth at the tip of the cutting, lift each cutting gently using your fingers or your dibber and plant up in individual pots, disturbing the new roots as little as possible.

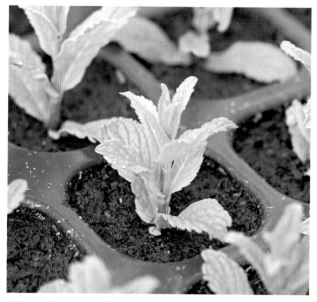

Take soft wood cuttings just below a leaf joint, remove the lower leaves and insert into cutting compost.

Softwood cuttings

These are best taken in spring and early summer from healthy looking plants. Once inserted around the edge of your pot or tray, the cuttings should be sprayed with water using a plant spray and covered with a plastic propagator lid, a sheet of polythene or an inflated plastic bag to retain the moisture. Roots develop quickly on softwood cuttings, generally within three to six weeks, but it can be just a few days in warm conditions. Root development stimulates leaf growth, so you will know that the roots have formed when you see tiny new leaves shooting at the growing tip. Once the root system has had a chance to establish itself, the cutting can be gently lifted and potted up in an individual pot or planted in a nursery bed. Generally speaking, cuttings are best kept in pots in a sheltered area, a greenhouse or plastic tunnel in cold areas during their first winter and planted out in their positions the following spring.

Semi-ripe cuttings

These are taken in summer when stems are harder, as they ripen at the base but are still flexible. Side shoots are taken off the new growth, torn away from the main stem to leave a little heel of older wood. Once inserted in pots or trays and watered in, they are also best covered with plastic or polythene to retain moisture, but it is not absolutely vital, as they are more resilient than softwood cuttings. Keep in pots in a cold frame or a sheltered area of the garden out of direct sunlight until growth starts the following spring, as rooting takes considerably longer than with softwood cuttings.

Hardwood cuttings

These are taken from shrubby herbs or trees such as Witch hazel, Rosemary, Hawthorn and Cramp bark in autumn once the plant is dormant. Take a side shoot of the current year's growth up to 30 cm (12 inches) long, remove the lower leaves and insert half their length in light soil in the garden in a sheltered position. Firm the soil around the cutting and water well. Leave in position for around a year until a good root system has developed.

Root cuttings or offsets

This is the ideal method of propagation for herbs that have running roots or that send up side shoots around the main plant, such as Yarrow, Chamomile, Comfrey, Elecampane and Mint. Cut the spreading roots or runners from the parent plant at the end of summer or early autumn. Cut the root into small pieces approximately 5 cm (2 inches) long and put them flat on top of compost with a little sand in a seed tray. Cover with a plastic bag or plastic sheet and leave in a cold frame, greenhouse, plastic tunnel or sheltered part of the garden. Once new shoots appear, remove the plastic bag or sheet and plant the cuttings out.

Layering

Low-growing and shrubby herbs such as Sage, Thyme, Lavender and Periwinkle can be propagated by layering. Take a low-growing branch and fix it with a peg or a stone in contact with the soil. If you nick the underside of the branch, it will root more readily. Once a root has developed, you can separate the newly formed plant, dig it up and replant it.

Mounding

Spreading herbs such as Chamomile, Thyme and Marjoram can be partially covered with soil in their centre, thus bringing many different parts of the plant in contact with the soil, so that, once rooted, lots of new plants can be separated off.

Harvesting herbs

When harvesting herb plants, it is important to establish first which part of the plant you need – the leaves, flowers, roots, rhizomes or seeds – and when the best time is to harvest that required part. Choose plants that look as healthy and vibrant as possible, free from disease and infestation.

Make sure plants are growing well away from areas that have been sprayed or polluted by traffic, industry or animals. Only pick the amount of herb that you need at any one time, as it will easily spoil and be wasted otherwise. Harvest just a few leaves and flowers from each plant, to avoid threatening the health or survival of any one plant.

Leaves and flowers

Aromatic leaves of herbs such as Basil, Thyme, Sage, Mint and Lemon balm are best harvested when the flowers are about to open, as the essential oil content is highest at that period. Flowers and flowering tops such as St John's wort, Agrimony, Goldenrod, Yarrow, Skullcap and Hyssop are best picked as they are about to burst into bloom. A flat basket is the best vessel to collect herbs in, as it makes it easier to avoid bruising or crushing leaves or flowers. They should be collected on a dry day once the dew has dried. During the growing season, leaves and flowers are best gathered and used fresh, ideally straight from the garden. At the same time, harvest some extra ones for drying or freezing to last through the winter months, as the growing time for herbs is relatively short. Herbs that are particularly worth storing are those that could be useful for treating winter colds and coughs, such as Hyssop, Thyme, Marjoram, Ground ivy and Mullein, and fevers, like Chamomile, Yarrow and Elderflower. Herbs for use fresh in the kitchen can be picked throughout the growing season, for example Coriander leaves, Mint, Sage, Marjoram, Rosemary, Basil and Fennel.

Seeds

Seeds such as Dill, Coriander and Fennel need to be caught when ripe, before they drop. You can cut off the whole flower head when harvesting them, tie it up in muslin or a paper bag with string or an elastic band and hang it upside down in a well-ventilated, dry room. As the flower head dries, the seeds will conveniently drop into the bag. Store the seeds in envelopes, foil or small boxes with well-fitting lids, and label clearly with the herb name and harvest date.

Roots and rhizomes

The roots and rhizomes of herbs such as Valerian, Dandelion, Elecampane and Burdock are best harvested when the aerial parts have died down in autumn or before growing recommences in spring, as they are richest in stored food at that time.

Flowering tops such as Elderflower are best harvested just as the flowers are about to burst into bloom.

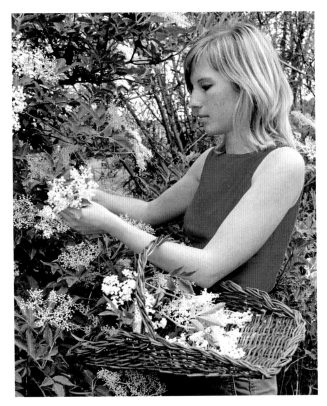

Preserving herbs

The object of the drying process is to eliminate the moisture in the herb quickly before it starts to die so that it can be stored for a few months without deteriorating and retains its therapeutic properties.

Harvesting and preparation

When harvesting flowers and leaves for storage, make sure they are dry from rain or dew and pick them in the morning before the heat of the day reaches its peak. Use your fingers/hands to pick, unless stalks (such as Agrimony or Yarrow) are very tough, in which case you will need scissors. Pick gently, taking care not to bruise the plant.

When lifting roots, dig them up with a garden fork, trying not to puncture the outer skin. Wash the soil off the roots and cut off any remaining leaves. Chop the roots up into sections or slices to speed drying and lie them out to dry. If bark is needed, as from Witch hazel or Cramp bark, it is best to peel the bark off whole branches that have been pruned rather than shaving bark off branches on the living tree, as it may harm the tree.

Drying

Provided that herbs are dried properly, those dried at home are often of a much higher quality than shop-bought herbs in terms of colour, flavour and healing properties. Drying needs to occur as quickly and evenly as possible. Shade, air and constant warmth are all essential for this.

The best places for drying herbs are a shaded, well-ventilated room or garden shed or barn, free from moisture or condensation. It is vital to avoid the kitchen, bathroom, utility room and sheds or garages if they are steamy or damp, as the herbs will not dry properly and will deteriorate. A steady temperature of about 32°C (90°F) is ideal, such as an airing cupboard, above an enclosed stove or in a low oven with the door left open to allow water to evaporate and the circulation of air. If the atmosphere is too cold (below 22°C/72°F), the plants will reabsorb moisture from the air and take too long to dry.

You can loosely tie aerial parts of herbs in small bunches by their stems, and hang them from a beam or a hook indoors. In warm, dry climates, bunches of herbs can be hung up out of doors in the shade or from a high ceiling in a warm room with the windows open. This may be rather an unpredictable way to dry herbs, as the temperature varies so much through 24 hours. More reliable results may be obtained by spreading sprigs of herbs or pieces of bark or root or seeds evenly over a tray, wire netting, box lid, fruit tray, drying frame, sheets of paper or muslin. Drying frames can be made fairly easily by stretching muslin or fine netting over a wooden frame, and are excellent for drying, as they allow free circulation of air. Spread out the herbs so that there is plenty of space between them and turn them frequently – once or twice on the first day, and once daily after that. Large-leaved herbs such as Borage or Comfrey will dry more quickly if the leaves are stripped from their fleshy stems and the stems discarded. Always dry herbs separately – never mix species.

Before storing herbs, check that they are properly dry by seeing if they are brittle and rustle, crumble or snap easily between your fingers and thumb. If herbs are stored before they are completely dry, they will reabsorb moisture from the atmosphere and deteriorate. It takes roughly three to seven days for most herbs to dry.

Freezing

Some herbs, particularly those with soft leaves such as Marjoram, Borage, Comfrey, Coriander, Fennel, Lemon balm, Basil and Mint, are ideal for freezing. Pick the leaves or flowers, wash them and then place them in small plastic bags to freeze.

Storing

Dried herbs are best stored in airtight, dark containers, wooden or cardboard boxes, paper bags or jars – glass jars are ideal kept in a dark cupboard, as exposure to light will cause deterioration of the medicinal constituents of the herbs. Never store dried herbs in plastic, as it encourages condensation. Be sure to label the herbs clearly with their name and harvest date. Remove stalks and twigs from aerial parts of plants, and break roots, rhizomes and barks into small pieces before storing. Store seeds in packets in the refrigerator or in airtight jars.

Growing conditions

Achillea millefolium
Yarrow is a perennial native to the northern hemisphere that thrives in partial shade to full sun on well-drained soil.

Aesculus hippocastanum
Horse chestnut is native to mountain woods from the Balkans through western Asia to the Himalayas. It prefers well-drained, moist soil in full sun to partial shade.

Agathosma/Barosma betulina
A hardy perennial native to South Africa, where it is widely cultivated on the hillsides. It is also grown in parts of South America. It is raised from cuttings in late summer and requires well-drained soil and plenty of sun.

Agrimonia eupatoria
Native to Eurasia, Agrimony grows in all types of soil, but prefers sunny slopes, sandy terrain and poor pastureland.

Agropyron/Triticum/Elymus repens
Couch grass is an invasive weed found in Europe, the Americas, northern Asia and Australia. It likes disturbed ground, gardens, fields and riverbanks.

Alchemilla vulgaris
Lady's mantle grows in damp soils in meadows, pastures, shrubland, forest paths and ditches throughout Europe.

Allium sativum
Garlic is native to central Asia but cultivated worldwide, and naturalizes in sandy soils.

Aloe barbadensis
Aloe vera is a perennial succulent native to tropical Africa. It prefers full sun, moderate water and well-drained soil and needs to stay indoors in temperate climates.

Althea officinalis
Marshmallow is found in coastal areas of eastern Europe and western Asia, growing in moist ground and salt marshes or on loamy soils.

Andrographis paniculata
A hardy perennial native to the Indian subcontinent, Kalamegha grows in thickets and forests throughout south Asia. It can be an annual or perennial shrub.

Anemone pulsatilla
Native to Europe, Pasque flower thrives in dry grassland in central and northern parts of the continent, preferring chalky soil.

Anethum graveolens
Dill is native to southern Europe and Central and South Asia, growing in wild, open areas. It is widely cultivated, notably in England, Germany and North America, and likes rich, well-drained soil and full sun in a sheltered position. Grow away from fennel, as they easily cross-pollinate.

Angelica archangelica
Angelica is native to Syria and Europe and prefers rich, moist soil and light shade, especially near running water. The seeds benefit from exposure to frost.

Angelica polymorph var. sinensis
Chinese angelica is a perennial native to the mountain forests of China. It requires a deep, moist fertile soil in dappled shade or full sun. This species is not fully hardy in colder areas. Plants are reliably perennial if they are prevented from setting seed.

Apium graveolens
Wild celery is believed to be native to the Mediterranean region, but has widely naturalized. It prefers deep, damp, well-manured soil and not too much sun.

Arctium lappa
Burdock grows on wasteland and along waysides, fences, railway lines and riverbanks in Europe and Asia.

Arctostaphylos uva ursi
Bearberry is native to Asia, Europe and North America. It is often found growing in woodlands at elevations of up to 30,000 metres (100,000 feet) in coarse, gravely soil.

Artemisia absinthium
Wormwood is native to western Asia, Europe and North Africa, but has naturalized in North America. It requires full sun, but will tolerate varying soil and moisture conditions, including drought.

Artemisia annua
Sweet Annie/Qing-hao is native to Asia and Eastern Europe, but has dispersed throughout temperate and subtropical regions of the world. It is an easily grown plant, succeeding in a well-drained circumneutral or slightly alkaline loamy soil, preferring a sunny position. Plants are longer lived, more hardy and more aromatic when they are grown in a poor, dry soil.

Asclepias tuberosa
Native to the southern USA, Pleurisy root is a hardy perennial, upright herb growing to 1 metre (3 feet) in height with spikes of numerous orange or yellow flowers. The root is unearthed in spring.

Asparagus racemosus
Shatavari is a hardy perennial. A thorny, shrub-like climbing plant, it is found growing in eastern Asian lowland jungle, woods and shaded hillsides.

Astragalus membranaceous
Native to Mongolia and China, Astragalus grows along forest margins and in open woodland and grassy areas. It is a perennial, upright plant propagated from seed in spring or autumn and thrives in sandy, well-drained soil with plenty of sun. The roots of four-year-old plants are harvested in autumn.

Azadirachta indica
Native to Iran, Pakistan, India and Sri Lanka, Neem is found throughout the subcontinent in forests and along roads, planted for shade. It grows in tropical, semi-arid places.

Bacopa monnieri/Herpestis monniera
Believed to be native to India, Bacopa grows throughout tropical regions of the world. It prefers muddy shores and wetland areas.

Baptisia tinctoria
Wild indigo is native to eastern parts of North America and grows from North Carolina to southern Canada in dry, hilly woods. This perennial with purplish blue flowers thrives in poor, dry soil and grows to 1 metre (3 feet).

Berberis/Mahonia aquifolium
Oregon grape is a hardy evergreen herb native to North America. Drought resistant, it will tolerate even poor soil and shady or sunny conditions.

Berberis vulgaris
Native to Europe, Barberry is naturalized in North America and grows in forest margins, hedgerows and open pine forests. It is cultivated as a garden plant and medicinal herb. The bark is gathered in spring and autumn and the berries in autumn.

Borago officinalis
Borage is native to Eurasia and North Africa. It thrives in poor soil, in full sun to partial shade, and although an annual, it self-seeds easily.

Boswellia serrata
Native to North Africa, the Frankincense tree is small, deciduous and usually found growing in full sun in hot, dry conditions. It grows in dry, hilly regions of central and northern India.

Calendula officinalis
Marigold is native to Eurasia, but grows worldwide. It prefers open, sunny areas and, like sunflowers, its flowers often turn to face the path of the sun. It flourishes in almost all soils.

Capsicum minimum/frutescens
Cayenne is native to the Americas. In the garden, it enjoys full sun and can tolerate dry conditions.

Carduus/Cnicus benedictus
Holy thistle is believed to be native to the Mediterranean and Eurasia. An annual, it often grows in wasteland areas. It flourishes on dry, stony ground in open areas.

Carduus/Silybum marianum
Native to the Mediterranean, Milk thistle grows wild throughout Europe and is widely naturalized in California and Australia. It thrives in open areas. Cultivated as an ornamental, it likes a sunny site and self-seeds.

Cassia senna/Senna alexandrina
Native to southern India, North Africa and parts of the Middle East, Senna does well in partial shade to full sun. It can tolerate drought, but thrives in a moist soil.

Centella/Hydrocotyle asiatica
Gotu kola is native to India and southern USA, and prefers marshy areas and riverbanks and can be grown as an annual in temperate zones.

Cimicifuga/Actaea racemosa
Native to North America, Black cohosh is a hardy perennial that prefers moist or dry woodland environments.

Cinnamomum zeylanicum/cassia
Native to Sri Lanka, this variety of Cinnamon grows best in almost pure sand in tropical countries.

Codonopsis pilosula
Codonopsis is a hardy perennial twining vine native to Central and East Asia. It is propagated from seed in spring or autumn. The root is harvested in autumn once the aerial parts have died down.

Coleus forskohlii/Plectranthus barbatus
Forskohlii grows on the dry slopes of the Indian plains and in the foothills of the Himalayas. It is also found in subtropical and warm temperate areas, including Nepal, Sri Lanka, Burma and parts of East Africa. It flourishes in well-drained soil in sun or partial shade. Both root and leaves are harvested in autumn.

Commiphora molmol/myrrha
Myrrh is native to north-eastern Africa, especially Somalia, but is now also found in Ethiopia, Saudi Arabia, India, Iran and Thailand. It grows in thickets and likes well-drained soil in the sun.

Commiphora mukul
Guggulu is native to Asia and Africa, and thrives in the dry, semi-arid and desert environments of the Indian subcontinent.

Coriandrum sativum
Native to Southern Europe and western Asia, Coriander is cultivated throughout the world. It can be found on wasteland, disturbed ground and in fields on nutrient-rich soils.

Crataegus monogyna
Hawthorn is a small tree native to northern Asia, Europe and temperate America. It grows by streams and in meadows, forests and open spaces. It prefers full sun to partial shade and moist, well-drained soil, but will tolerate drought.

Curcuma longa
Turmeric is a perennial native to South Asia. It requires a warm, frost-free climate, light shade and moderate water.

Cynara scolymus
Native to the Mediterranean region, Globe artichoke thrives in rich soil in warm temperate climates.

Daucus carota
Wild carrot is native to Europe. Cultivated subspecies are grown around the world. The root is harvested in late summer, and the seeds are gathered in late summer or early autumn. Propagate by sowing seeds in spring in light, sandy soil and full sun.

Dioscorea villosa
Wild yam is native to North and Central America, but has now become naturalized in tropical, semi-tropical and temperate climates around the world. It is propagated from seed in spring or from sections of tubers or by root division in spring or autumn. It thrives in sunny conditions and rich soil. The root and tuber are harvested in autumn.

Echinacea angustifolia
Echinacea is a hardy perennial native to North America, and prefers full sun, has low water requirements and will grow in a variety of soil conditions.

Elettaria cardamomum
Cardamom is native to southern India and Sri Lanka where it grows well in forests above sea level. It needs a shady position and rich, moist, well-drained soil and is hardy to about 32°F.

Eleutherococcus senticosus
Siberian ginseng is a hardy perennial native to eastern Russia, China, Korea and Japan, and prefers a cool climate. Plants grow in full sun to light shade and need a moist, rich, well-drained soil. It can be grown from seed, but is a difficult plant to germinate.

Equisetum arvense
Native to Europe, North Africa, northern Asia and the Americas, Horsetail is a hardy perennial, preferring damp soil.

Eschscholzia californica
California poppy is native to south-western United States, and grows wild in sunny areas. It is widely cultivated as a garden annual, preferring sandy soils.

Eupatorium perfoliatum
Boneset is a Native American hardy perennial, growing in low, moist areas. It is found in meadows and marshland.

Eupatorium purpureum
Gravel root is a hardy perennial native to the meadows, woodlands and lowlands of Europe and eastern North America. The root is unearthed in autumn.

Euphrasia officinalis
Eyebright is a small annual herb native to Europe. It is semiparasitic, in that its roots attach to those of grasses. It does best in open areas, such as pastures.

Filipendula ulmaria
Native to Europe, Meadowsweet is a hardy perennial and grows easily in damp places, preferring ditches and river and stream banks.

Foeniculum vulgare
Native to the Mediterranean region, Fennel is a hardy perennial found growing in temperate regions around the world. It prefers full sun and low to moderate amounts of water, and does best in well-worked, well-drained soil.

Fucus vesiculosus
Bladderwrack is native to North Atlantic shores and the western Mediterranean, and is harvested all year. It is commonly attached to submerged rocks between the high and low tidemarks.

Galega officinalis
Native to Asia and Continental Europe, and naturalized in Britain, Goat's rue grows in almost any soil. It is harvested in summer.

Galium aparine
Common throughout Europe and North America, Cleavers is found in many other temperate regions, including Australia. It grows prolifically in gardens and along roadsides, and is gathered when it is just about to flower in late spring.

Ganoderma lucidum
Native to China, Reishi is a fungus that grows on decaying hardwood in moist, shady conditions. Nowadays it is more likely to be cultivated than found growing in the wild.

Gentiana lutea
Gentian is a hardy perennial native to the Eurpoean Alps. It prefers moist soil in full sun to partial shade.

Ginkgo biloba
This large, deciduous tree is native to China. Ginkgo trees are grown on large plantations in China, France and South Carolina. It prefers rich, sandy soil.

Glechoma/Nepeta hederacea
Native to Europe and western Asia, Ground ivy thrives on the margins of woods and along paths and hedges.

Glycyrrhiza glabra
Liquorice grows wild in south-eastern Europe and south-western Asia, and is now extensively cultivated. It prefers full sun to partial shade, moderate amounts of water and well-drained, sandy soil. It fixes nitrogen and can be cultivated and turned into the soil to enrich it.

Gymnema sylvestre
Gymnema is native to the tropical forests of southern and central India, East Asia, Australia and West and South Africa. It prefers loamy soils.

Hamamelis virginiana
Witch hazel is a deciduous shrub native to North America. It most often grows in damp woods on acidic soils and flowers in winter/early spring.

Harpagophytum procumbens
Devil's claw is native to South and East Africa, and is found most commonly on the veldt of the Transvaal. It thrives in clay or sandy soils, preferring roadsides and wasteground. Propagated from seed in spring, the young tubers are unearthed in autumn and cut into short lengths.

Humulus lupulus
Hops are indigenous to Europe and Asia, and flourish on dumps and roadsides. They are grown commercially in northern Europe.

Hydrastis canadensis
Golden seal grows wild in moist mountainous woodland areas of North America and prefers soil that is well covered with dead leaves. It is propagated by root division. Rhizomes from three-year-old plants are dug up in the autumn and dried in the open on cloth.

Hypericum perforatum
St John's wort thrives in temperate regions worldwide. It prefers a sunny site and well-drained, chalky soil. It can be grown from seed or by root division.

Hyssopus officinalis
Native to Southern Europe, Hyssop is a hardy perennial and grows wild in Mediterranean countries, especially in the Balkans and Turkey. It prefers sunny, dry sites and is a common garden herb. It prefers full sun to partial shade, has low water requirements and does well in sandy, well-drained soil.

Inula helenium
Elecampane is a hardy perennial native to Europe and northern Asia. It can be found growing in ditches and other wasteland areas.

Iris versicolor
Blue flag is native to North America, preferring damp and marshy areas in the wild. It is also widely cultivated as a garden plant.

Juglans regia
Walnut is a deciduous tree native to the Balkans, south-west and central Asia, to the Himalayas and south-west China. It is widely cultivated in temperate zones. *Juglans nigra* is native to North America. Both benefit from mild protection and are drought hardy. They grow in most well-drained soils.

Lactuca virosa
Common throughout Europe, Wild lettuce grows in open areas and along roadsides. It grows best in moist soil with plenty of sunshine.

Lavandula spp.
Lavender is a small, hardy perennial shrub, native to the Mediterranean region, which prefers dry soil and full sun.

Lentinula edodes
Native to China, Shiitake mushroom is a light amber fungi with ragged gills. It grows on fallen broadleaved trees such as Beech, Chestnut, Oak, Maple, Walnut and Mulberry.

Leonurus cardiaca
Motherwort is a hardy perennial native to Europe and western Asia. It prefers partial shade to full sun and moist, light, sandy soil, but will tolerate even poor soil conditions.

Marrubium vulgare
White horehound is a hardy perennial native to Europe, Asia and North Africa. In the garden, it will tolerate poor soil and prefers dry conditions and full sun.

Melissa officinalis
Lemon balm is a hardy perennial native to Europe, preferring to grow in undisturbed areas and open woods. It thrives in full sun to partial shade, needs only moderate watering and prefers well-drained soil.

Mentha spp.
There are about 20 true mints. Mints thrive in partial shade to full sun and like moderate to high amounts of water, but are not particular about what kind of soil they grow in. They are hardy perennials and tend to grow in colonies. Plant Mint where you don't mind it spreading, as it can be invasive.

Myrica cerifera
Bayberry is a hardy perennial evergreen shrub found in coastal regions of eastern and southern USA as far west as Texas. It grows in dry woods, fields and thickets near sandy swamps.

Myristica fragrans
Native to the Indonesian Molucca Islands, the Nutmeg tree is an evergreen. The tree thrives in hot, humid climates with well-drained soil and in partial shade.

Ocimum sanctum
Holy basil is indigenous to India and other tropical regions of Asia. A prolific shrub, it prefers full sun and moderate amouts of water and can be grown as an annual in temperate zones.

Oenothera biennis
Native to North America, Evening primrose is now commonly found in many temperate zones around the world. A hardy perennial, it thrives in open areas, especially in sand dunes and sandy soil.

Olea europaea
Olive trees are evergreens native to Africa, Southern Europe and western Asia. They need a long, hot growing season, full sun and well-drained soil, and can survive dry conditions.

Origanum spp.
Sweet marjoram is a perennial in warmer climates, native to North Africa, Europe and Asia. Cultivated worldwide, it will grow in almost any kind of soil and thrives in dry conditions with lots of sun.

Paeonia lactiflora/officinalis/suffruticosa
Peonies are ornamental hardy perennials famed for their aromatic hermaphroditic flowers. The plants prefer moderately alkaline soil, whether dry or moist, and partial shade to full sun. Many can live for 50 years or longer.

Panax ginseng
This hardy perennial grows in shady hardwood forests of North America and temperate regions of Asia. It is native to north-eastern China, eastern Russia and North Korea, but is now extremely rare in the wild. Cultivation requires great skill. Propagated from seed in spring, it requires rich, moist but well-drained soil. The plant takes at least four years to mature.

Passiflora incarnata
A deciduous vine native to North America, Passion flower prefers rich soil and full sun. It is propagated from seed in spring and is hardy.

Phytolacca decandra
Native to North America, Poke root is now naturalized in the Mediterranean region and thrives in damp woodland and open areas. It can be grown in most soils with plenty of moisture and in full sun to partial shade.

Piper longum
Long pepper flourishes in rich, well-drained loamy soil. It requires a hot, moist climate and an elevation between 100 and 1,000 metres (330 and 3,300 feet) for its cultivation. In its natural habitat the plant is found growing as an under shrub.

Plantago major/minor/lanceolata/psyllium
Native to Eurasia, Plantain's habitats include lawns, fallow fields and roadsides. A hardy perennial it likes full sunlight and grows in most soils.

Polygonum multiflorum
Ho shou wu is a hardy perennial climber, growing to 4.5 metres (15 feet), native to China. The plant will grow in light, sandy or heavy, clay soils but requires moist conditions, in semi-shade, light woodland or in full sun.

Prunella vulgaris
Selfheal is a hardy perennial that thrives in damp soil in full sun or in light shade. It will grow thicker in a semi-shaded environment.

Rehmannia glutinosa
Chinese Foxglove is a hardy perennial native to China and prefers well-drained yet moist light (sandy) or medium (loamy) soils. It can grow in semi-shade or full sun.

Rhodiola rosea
This hardy perennial succulent grows in the high mountains of Europe, northern Asia and North America. It thrives in well-drained soil, can tolerate drought once established and requires lots of sun.

Rosa spp.
Rose suckers freely from roots and underground stems. Roses do best in full sun and will not tolerate much shade and prefer medium, slightly acidic, well-drained soil.

Rosmarinus officinalis
Native to Europe, Rosemary is a semi-hardy perennial and prefers a light, sandy soil of medium to low fertility. As long as it is not waterlogged, it will tolerate most growing conditions.

Rubus idaeus
Native to Europe and temperate Asia, Raspberry is a hardy shrub and will grow in full sun or semi-shade in well-drained, rich soil.

Rumex spp.
Dock are found throughout the world thriving in fields, roadsides and waste ground. The roots are harvested in autumn.

Salix alba/nigra
White willow grows in damp conditions in Europe, North Africa and central Asia, while Black willow is native to eastern North America. Willows will grow in full sun to light shade and are tolerant of a wide range of soil types and conditions.

Salvia officinalis
Sage is native to Southern Europe and the Mediterranean. In the garden, it does best in full sun and well-drained soil, with low to moderate amounts of water.

Sambucus nigra
A hardy perennial native to Europe. Although tolerant of many growing conditions, Elder does best in deep, moist soil and partial shade.

Schisandra chinensis
Native to China, Schisandra grows in woods in rich, loose soil, preferring a cool climate.

Scutellaria baicalensis
Baikal skullcap is a small perennial native to Siberia, Russia, North China, Mongolia and Japan. It prefers a well-drained soil and sun or part shade.

Scutellaria lateriflora
Native to North America, Skullcap will grow in light, sandy, medium, loamy and heavy, clay soils, but requires moist conditions. It cannot grow in the shade.

Serenoa repens
Saw palmetto is native to North America. It requires well-drained but moist soil and lots of sunshine.

Smilax ornata
Sarsaparilla is a climbing vine found in tropical rainforests and in temperate regions in Asia and Australia.

Solidago virgaurea
Native to North America, Goldenrod, a hardy perennial, prefers open areas and hillsides. It will grow in just about any place that receives a good amount of sunshine, whether in dry or moist conditions.

Stachys betonica/Betonica officinalis
Native to Europe, Wood betony grows in shady woods where lime is present in the soil.

Stellaria media
Chickweed is a hardy perennial native to Eurasia, and will grow in partial or full sun and in a fairly fertile loam or clay-loam soil.

Symphytum officinale
Comfrey is native to Europe and western Asia and thrives in moist, marshy places, growing in open woods or along streams and meadows. In the garden, it can be invasive and difficult to eradicate.

Tabebuia impetiginosa
Indigenous to South America, Pau d'arco is a tree that grows well in mountainous terrains. In Peru and Argentina it is found growing high up in the Andes. It is also found in low-lying areas in Paraguay and Brazil.

Tanacetum parthenium syn. Pyrethrum parthenium/Chrysanthemum parthenium
Feverfew was originally indigenous to south-eastern Europe, but is now common throughout Europe. It requires well-drained soil and sun.

Taraxacum officinale
Dandelion grows wild in most parts of the world, and is cultivated in Germany and France.

Thymus vulgaris
Thyme is native to the Mediterranean, and prefers light, warm, well-drained and dry soil, along with full sun. It requires little care in the garden but dislikes damp soil.

Tilia spp.
Native to Europe, western Asia and North America, Lime trees favour a good, loamy soil, although they can be found growing on sandy, infertile soils as well.

Tinospora cordifolia
Guduchi is a creeper found in the forests of India. Those growing up Neem (*Azadirachta indica*) trees are said to be the best, as the synergy between these two bitter plants enhances Guduchi's efficacy.

Trifolium pratense
Red clover is found growing wild and can be found growing in grassy areas ranging from lawns to roadsides. It prefers full sun to partial shade and moderate amounts of water, and thrives in a wide variety of soils.

Trigonella foenum-graecum
Native to the Mediterranean, Ukraine and India, Fenugreek thrives in dry, fertile soil. To grow, sow the seeds thickly in the spring in an area that will receive full sun. Avoid cold, wet soil, otherwise the seeds will rot before germinating.

Trillium erectum
Beth root is a hardy perennial native to North America, and grows in moist but well-drained, deep, humus-rich soil in full or partial shade.

Turnera aphrodisiaca/diffusa
Damiana is a small deciduous shrub native to south-west America, Mexico and the West Indies. It thrives in any good soil if given a sunny location.

Tussilago farfara
Coltsfoot is a perennial native to Eurasia, but has become widely naturalized, growing in zinc-rich, clay soils in wasteland and along roadsides.

Ulmus fulva/rubra
The deciduous Slippery elm tree grows in open areas in full sun to partial shade and where the soil is moist and firm.

Uncaria tomentosa
Cat's claw, a climbing vine, is native to the Amazon, where it can be found in old second-growth forests, especially in Peru.

Urtica dioica/urens
Nettles can adapt to light conditions ranging from full sun to partial shade, loves soil that is high in organic matter and enjoys moderate to high amounts of water.

Vaccinium myrtillus
Blueberry/Bilberry is found in damp, acidic soils throughout the temperate and sub-Arctic regions of the world.

Valeriana officinalis
Valerian is native to Europe, Asia and North America. In the garden, it requires a moist soil and full sun. It stimulates earthworm activity and the growth of nearby plants.

Verbascum thapsus
Mullein is native to Europe, Asia and North Africa. In the garden, it thrives in full sun and well-drained soil, with low to moderate amounts of water.

Verbena officinalis
Vervain is native to Europe, but can be found growing wild in many parts of the world. It requires moist soil and full sun to partial shade.

Viburnum opulus
Cramp bark grows in woodlands, hedges and thickets in Europe and eastern North America. It does best on moist and moderately alkaline soils, although it tolerates most soil types well.

Viburnum prunifolium
Native to central and southern North America, Black haw grows in woodland. It prefers moist, well-drained soils of average fertility in full sun, but is adaptable to poor soils of various pH, moist soils, dry soils, drought and pollution.

Vinca major/minor
Greater and Lesser periwinkle are adapted to mild climates and will tolerate a wide range of soil types. They usually require part shade and ample moisture, but will cope with full sun if it is adequately watered.

Viola odorata
Native to much of Europe and Asia, Sweet violet is a common wayside plant also found along roadsides and in woodland. It prefers full to partial shade, soil that is rich in organic matter and moderate to high amounts of water.

Viola tricolor
Wild pansy is native to Europe, North Africa and temperate regions of Asia, and has become naturalized in the Americas. It thrives in many habitats, from grassy mountainous areas to coastal sites, and is cultivated as a garden plant.

Viscum album
Mistletoe is an evergreen, semi-parastic plant native to Europe, Asia and North Africa. It grows on Apple and other fruit trees, Poplar, Chestnut, Pine and Spruce trees, among others. It is harvested in autumn.

Vitex agnus castus
Chaste tree is a deciduous shrub native to the coast of North Africa, western Asia and Europe. It is cultivated in subtropical areas around the world, and has become naturalized in many regions. It likes riverbanks and damp ground.

Vitis vinifera
Native to the Mediterranean, Central Europe and South West Asia. Common grape vine will grow in full sun or partial shade and tolerates a variety of soil types.

Withania somniferum
Native to India, Ashwagandha grows well in sandy loam or light red soil with good drainage and prefers warm dry climates. It can be grown in temperate zones and taken in during winter.

Zanthoxylum americanum
Prickly ash is a shrub native to North America. It requires a well-drained, alkaline soil, moderate moisture and full sun to partial shade.

Zea mays
Sweet corn is native to the Andes and Central America, possibly originating in Peru. It prefers slightly acidic soil, plenty of sunshine and moisture.

Zingiber officinale
Native to South Asia, Ginger thrives in partial shade in fertile, moist, well-drained soils. In gardens in temperate climates, the plant will need to be brought indoors when the cold weather begins.

References

The chemistry of herbs

1 Pengelly, A., *The Constituents of Medical Plants*, CABI Publishing, Oxon, UK, 2004.
2 *Ibid*.
3 Huang, K., *The Pharmacology of Chinese Herbs*, CRC Press, Boca Raton, 1993.
4 Pengelly, A., *The Constituents of Medical Plants*, CABI Publishing, Oxon, UK, 2004.
5 Hoffman, D., *Therapeutic Herbalism*
6 Tillotson, A.K., Tillotson, Y.B. and Robert, A. Jr, *The One Earth Herbal Sourcebook*, Kensington Publishing Corps, New York, USA, 2001.
7 Pengelly, A., *The Constituents of Medical Plants*, CABI Publishing, Oxon, UK, 2004.

The materia medica

1 Candan, F., Unlu, M. and Tepe, B., et al., *Antioxidant and antimicrobial activity of the essential oil and methanol extracts of Achillea Millefolium Ethno-Pharmacol*, August; 87 (2–3): 215–220, 2003.
2 Foster, S. and Johnson, R., *Desk Reference to Nature's Medicine*, National Geographic Society, Washington DC, USA, 2006.
3 *Ibid*.
4 Chow, J., 'Probiotics and prebiotics: a brief overview', *Journal of Renal Nutrition*, April 2002; 12(2)76-86.
5 Ankri, S. and Mirelman, D., 'Antimicrobial properties of allicin from garlic', *Microbes and Infection*, February 1999; 1(2)125-9.
6 Banerjee, S.K., Mukherjee P.K., Maulik S.K., 'Garlic as an antioxidant the good, the bad and the ugly', *Phytother Res.*, 2003 Feb; 17(2)97-10676.
7 Thomson, M. and Ali, M., 'Garlic, a review of its potential use as an anticancer agent', *Current Cancer Drug Targets*, February 2003; 3(1)67-81.
8 Menzies-Trull, C., *Keys to Physiomedicalism Including Pharmacopoeia*, FPHM, Staffordshire, UK, 2003.
9 Kuhn, M. and Winston, D., *Herbal Therapy and Supplements*, Lippincott, Philadelphia, USA, 2001.
10 Pole, S., *Ayurvedic Medicine*, Elsevier, Philadelphia, USA, 2006.
11 *Ibid*.
12 Bone, K., *The Ultimate Herbal Compendium*, Phytotherapy Press, Queensland, Australia, 2007.
13 Kuhn, M. and Winston, D., *Herbal Therapy and Supplements*, Lippincott, Philadelphia, USA, 2001.
14 Pole, S., *Ayurvedic Medicine*, Elsevier, Philadelphia, USA, 2006.
15 Kuhn, M. and Winston, D., *Herbal Therapy and Supplements*, Lippincott, Philadelphia, USA, 2001.
16 Amroyan, 1999, cited in Pole, S., *Ayurvedic Medicine*, Elsevier, Philadelphia, USA, 2006.
17 WHO monograph 1999, cited in Pole, S., *Ayurvedic Medicine*, Elsevier, Philadelphia, USA, 2006.
18 Singh, G., Kapoor, I.P., Pandey, S.K., Singh, U.K. and Singh, R.K., 'Studies on essential oils part 10; antibacterial activity of volatile oils of some spices', *Phytotherapy Research*, November 2002; 16(7)680-2.
19 Jirovetz, L., Buchbauer, G., Stoyanova, A.S., Georgiev, E.V. and Damianova, S.T., 'Composition, quality control and antimicrobial activity of the essential oil of long-time stored dill (*Anethum graveolens L*) seeds from Bulgaria', *Journal of Agriculture and Food Chemistry*, 18 June 2003; 51(13)3854-7.
20 Foster, S. and Johnson, R., *Desk Reference to Nature's Medicine*, National Geographic Society, Washington DC, USA, 2006.
21 Skidmore-Roth, L., *Mosby's Handbook of Herbs and Natural Supplements*, Mosby, Inc, St Louis, USA, 2001.
22 Newall, C., Anderson, L. and David Phillipson, J., 1996, *Herbal Medicines: A Guide for Health Care Professionals*, The Pharmaceutical Press, London, UK, 1996.
23 Flickinger, E.A., Hatch, T.F. and Wofford, R.C., 'In vitro fermentation properties of selected fructooligosaccharide-containing vegetables and in vivo colonic microbial populations are affected by the diets of healthy human infants', *Journal of Nutrition*, August 2002; 132(8)2188-94.
24 Skidmore-Roth, L., *Mosby's Handbook of Herbs and Natural Supplements*, Mosby, Inc, USA, 2001.
25 *Ibid*.
26 Menzies-Trull, C., *Keys to Physiomedicalism Including Pharmacopoeia*, FPHM, Staffordshire, UK, 2003.
27 *Ibid*.
28 Chang, H.M. and But, P.P., 1987, cited in Bone, K., *Clinical Applications of Ayurvedic and Chinese Herbs*, Phytotherapy Press, Queensland, Australia, 1996.
29 Foster, S. and Chongxi, Y., *Herbal Emissaries*, Healing Arts Press, Vermont, USA, 1992.
30 Foster, S. and Johnson, R., *Desk Reference to Nature's Medicine*, National Geographic Society, Washington DC, USA, 2006.
31 Willard, T., *Textbook of Modern Herbology*, Wild Rose College of Natural Healing Ltd, Alberta, Canada, 1993.
32 Bartram, T., *Bartram's Encyclopedia of Herbal Medicine*, Constable and Robinson Ltd, London, UK, 1998.
33 Chopra, D. and Simon, D., *The Chopra Centre Herbal Handbook*, Rider, London, UK, 2000.
34 Mandal, S.C., Nandy, A., Pal, M. and Saha, B.P., 'Evaluation of antibacterial activity of *Asparagus racemosus* wild root', *Phytotherapy Research*, March 2000; 14(2)118-9.
35 Chopra, D. and Simon, D., *The Chopra Centre Herbal Handbook*,

Rider, London, UK, 2000.

36 Foster, S. and Johnson, R., *Desk Reference to Nature's Medicine*, National Geographic Society, Washington DC, USA, 2006.

37 Barnett, R., *Tonics*, HarperCollins, New York, USA, 1997.

38 Foster, S. and Johnson, R., *Desk Reference to Nature's Medicine*, National Geographic Society, Washington DC, USA, 2006.

39 *Ibid*.

40 Upton et al., 1999, cited in Kuhn, M. and Winston, D., *Herbal Therapy and Supplements*, Lippincott, Philadelphia, USA, 2001.

41 Skidmore-Roth, L., *Mosby's Handbook of Herbs and Natural Supplements*, Mosby, Inc, USA, 2001.

42 Sankla, R., Singh S. and Bhandari, C.R., 'Preliminary clinical trials on antidiabetic actions of *Azadirachta indica*',1973, Medicine, Surgery 1311

43 Fabry, W., Okemo, P.O. and Ansorg, R., 'Antibacterial activity of East African medicinal plants', *Journal of Ethnopharmacol*, 1998; 6079-84 and 'Fungistatic and fungicidal activity of East African medicinal plants', *Mycoses, Journal of Ethnophamacol*, 1996; 3967-70.

44 Mackinnon, S., Durst, T. and Arnason, J.R. et al., 'Antimalarial activity of tropical Meliaceae extracts and Gedunin derivatives', *Journal of Natural Products*, 1997; 60(4)336.

45 Skidmore-Roth, L., *Mosby's Handbook of Herbs and Natural Supplements*, Mosby, Inc, St Louis, USA, 2001.

46 Mars, B., *The Desktop Guide to Herbal Medicine*, Basic Health Publications, California, USA, 2007.

47 *Ibid*.

48 *Ibid*.

49 *Ibid*.

50 Kuhn, M. and Winston, D., *Herbal Therapy and Supplements*, Lippincott, Philadelphia, USA, 2001.

51 Skidmore-Roth, L., *Mosby's Handbook of Herbs and Natural Supplements*, Mosby, Inc, St Louis, USA, 2001.

52 Ryzhikova et al., *Determination of four alkaloids in Berberis plants by HPLC*, 1999.

53 Kutchan, 1996, and Leung and Foster, 1996, cited in Kuhn, M. and Winston, D., *Herbal Therapy and Supplements*, Lippincott, Philadelphia, USA, 2001.

54 Kuhn, M. and Winston, D., *Herbal Therapy and Supplements*, Lippincott, Philadelphia, USA, 2001.

55 *Ibid*.

56 Pole, S., *Ayurvedic Medicine*, Elsevier, Philadelphia, USA, 2006.

57 Kuhn, M. and Winston, D., *Herbal Therapy and Supplements*, Lippincott, Philadelphia, USA, 2001.

58 Tillotson, 2001, and Bone, 2003, cited in Pole, S., *Ayurvedic Medicine*, Elsevier, Philadelphia, USA, 2006.

59 Foster, S. and Johnson, R., *Desk Reference to Nature's Medicine*, National Geographic Society, Washington DC, USA, 2006.

60 *Ibid*.

61 Kuhn, M. and Winston, D., *Herbal Therapy and Supplements*, Lippincott, Philadelphia, USA, 2001.

62 *Ibid*.

63 Bone, K., *The Ultimate Herbal Compendium*, Phytotherapy Press, Queensland, Australia, 2007.

64 Curi-Pedrosa, R. and Creczynski-Pasa, T.B., 'Protective properties of butanolic extract of the *Calendula officinalis* L. (marigold) against lipid peroxidation of rat liver microsomes and action as free radical scavenger', *Redox Report*, 2002; 7(2)95-102.

65 Wagner, H., 'The immune-stimulating polysaccharides and heteroglycans of higher plants. A preliminary communication', *Arzneimittelforschung*, 1984; 34 (6)659-661.

66 Dumenil, G., Chemli, R., Balansard, G., Guirand, H. and Lallemand, M., 'Evaluation of antibacterial properties of marigold flowers and homeopathic mother tincture of *Calendula officinalis*', *Annales Pharmaceutiques Françaises*, 1980; 36(6)493-9.

67 Boucaud-Maitre, Y., Algernon, O. and Raynaud, J., 'Cytotoxic and antihumoral activity of *Calendula officinalis* extracts', *Pharmazie*, 1988; 43221-222.

68 Mars, B., *The Desktop Guide to Herbal Medicine*, Basic Health Publications, California, USA, 2007.

69 *Ibid*.

70 Kuhn, M. and Winston, D., *Herbal Therapy and Supplements*, Lippincott, Philadelphia, USA, 2001.

71 Foster, S. and Johnson, R., *Desk Reference to Nature's Medicine*, National Geographic Society, Washington DC, USA, 2006.

72 Mars, B., *The Desktop Guide to Herbal Medicine*, Basic Health Publications, California, USA, 2007.

73 Bone, K., *The Ultimate Herbal Compendium*, Phytotherapy Press, Queensland, Australia, 2007.

74 Mars, B., *The Desktop Guide to Herbal Medicine*, Basic Health Publications, California, USA, 2007.

75 Cesarone, M.R., Laurora, G. and De Sanctis, M.T. et al., 'The microcirculatory activity of *Centella asiatica* in venous insufficiency. A double-blind study', *Minerva Cardioangiol*, June 1994; 42(6)299-304.

76 Rao, M.V.R., Srinivasan, K. and Rao, K.T., 'Effect of mandukaparni on general mental ability of mentally retarded children', *Journal of Research Indian Medicine*, 1973; 8,9.

77 Sampson, J.H., Raman, A. and Karlsen, G. et al., 'In vitro keratinocyte antiproliferant effect of *Centella asiatica* extract and triterpenoid saponins', *Phytomedicine*, May 2001; 8(3)230-5.

78 Tenni, R., Zanaboni, G. and De Agostini M.P. et al., 'Effect of the triterpenoid fraction of *Centella asiatica* on macromolecules of the connective matrix in human skin fibroblast cultures', *Italian Journal of Biochemistry*, March–April 1988; 37(2)69-77.

79 Roberts, A. and Williams, J.M., 'The effect of olfactory stimulation on fluency, vividness of imagery and associated mood a preliminary study', *British Journal of Medical Psychology*, 1992; 65(2)197-199.

80 Carle, R. and Isaac, 0., *Z Phytother*,

1987; 8 67-77.

81 Foster, S. and Chongxi, Y., *Herbal Emissaries*, Healing Arts Press, Vermont, USA, 1992.

82 Barnett, R., *Tonics*, HarperCollins, New York, USA, 1997.

83 Foster, S. and Chongxi, Y., *Herbal Emissaries*, Healing Arts Press, Vermont, USA, 1992.

84 *Ibid.*

85 *Ibid.*

86 Foster, S. and Chongxi, Y., *Herbal Emissaries*, Healing Arts Press, Vermont, USA, 1992 and Barnett, R., *Tonics*, HarperCollins, New York, USA, 1997.

87 Bone, K., *The Ultimate Herbal Compendium*, Phytotherapy Press, Queensland, Australia, 2007.

88 Foster, S. and Chongxi, Y., *Herbal Emissaries*, Healing Arts Press, Vermont, USA, 1992.

89 *Ibid.*

90 Bone, K., *The Ultimate Herbal Compendium*, Phytotherapy Press, Queensland, Australia, 2007.

91 Foster, S. and Johnson, R., *Desk Reference to Nature's Medicine*, National Geographic Society, Washington DC, USA, 2006.

92 *Ibid.*

93 Mishra, L.C., *Scientific Basis for Ayurvedic Therapies*, CRC Press, New York, USA, 2003.

94 Foster, S. and Johnson, R., *Desk Reference to Nature's Medicine*, National Geographic Society, Washington DC, USA, 2006.

95 Bone, K., *Clinical Applications of Ayurvedic and Chinese Herbs*, Phytotherapy Press, Queensland, Australia, 1996.

96 Bone, K., *The Ultimate Herbal Compendium*, Phytotherapy Press, Queensland, Australia, 2007.

97 Kuhn, M. and Winston, D., *Herbal Therapy and Supplements*, Lippincott, Philadelphia, USA, 2001.

98 Foster, S. and Johnson, R., *Desk Reference to Nature's Medicine*, National Geographic Society, Washington DC, USA, 2006.

99 Bone, K., *The Ultimate Herbal Compendium*, Phytotherapy Press, Queensland, Australia, 2007.

100 Pole, S., *Ayurvedic Medicine*, Elsevier, Philadelphia, USA, 2006.

101 *Ibid.*

102 Foster, S. and Johnson, R., *Desk Reference to Nature's Medicine*, National Geographic Society, Washington DC, USA, 2006.

103 Pole, S., *Ayurvedic Medicine*, Elsevier, Philadelphia, USA, 2006.

104 Foster, S. and Johnson, R., *Desk Reference to Nature's Medicine*, National Geographic Society, Washington DC, USA, 2006.

105 *Ibid.*

106 Pole, S., *Ayurvedic Medicine*, Elsevier, Philadelphia, USA, 2006.

107 Foster, S. and Johnson, R., *Desk Reference to Nature's Medicine*, National Geographic Society, Washington DC, USA, 2006.

108 Pole, S., *Ayurvedic Medicine*, Elsevier, Philadelphia, USA, 2006.

109 Kuhn, M. and Winston, D., *Herbal Therapy and Supplements*, Lippincott, Philadelphia, USA, 2001.

110 Mester et al., 1979, cited in Pole, S., *Ayurvedic Medicine*, Elsevier, Philadelphia, USA, 2006.

111 Kuhn, M. and Winston, D., *Herbal Therapy and Supplements*, Lippincott, Philadelphia, USA, 2001.

112 Pole, S., *Ayurvedic Medicine*, Elsevier, Philadelphia, USA, 2006.

113 *Ibid.*

114 Kuhn, M. and Winston, D., *Herbal Therapy and Supplements*, Lippincott, Philadelphia, USA, 2001.

115 Mars, B., *The Desktop Guide to Herbal Medicine*, Basic Health Publications, California, USA, 2007.

116 Pole, S., *Ayurvedic Medicine*, Elsevier, Philadelphia, USA, 2006.

117 *Ibid.*

118 Kuhn, M. and Winston, D., *Herbal Therapy and Supplements*, Lippincott, Philadelphia, USA, 2001.

119 Pole, S., *Ayurvedic Medicine*, Elsevier, Philadelphia, USA, 2006.

120 Foster, S., *Herbal Renaissance*, Gibbs-Smith, Salt Lake City, USA, 1993.

121 Kuhn, M. and Winston, D., *Herbal Therapy and Supplements*, Lippincott, Philadelphia, USA, 2001.

122 Mars, B., *The Desktop Guide to Herbal Medicine*, Basic Health Publications, California, USA, 2007.

123 Chopra, D. and Simon, D., *The Chopra Centre Herbal Handbook*, Rider, London, UK, 2000.

124 Srivastava. R. et al., 'Prostaglandins Leukot Essent Fatty Acids', 1995; 52, 223-227.

125 Kuttan, R., Sudheeran, P.C. and Joseph, C.D., 'Turmeric and curcumin as topical agents in cancer therapy', *Tumori*, 1987; 73, 29-31, and Nagabhusham et al., 1992.

126 Kuttan, R., Sudheeran, P.C. and Joseph, C.D., 'Turmeric and curcumin as topical agents in cancer therapy', *Tumori*, 1987; 73, 29-31.

127 Kuhn, M. and Winston, D., *Herbal Therapy and Supplements*, Lippincott, Philadelphia, USA, 2001.

128 Mills and Bone, 1999, cited in Kuhn, M. and Winston, D., *Herbal Therapy and Supplements*, Lippincott, Philadelphia, USA, 2001.

129 Kuhn, M. and Winston, D., *Herbal Therapy and Supplements*, Lippincott, Philadelphia, USA, 2001.

130 Foster, S. and Johnson, R., *Desk Reference to Nature's Medicine*, National Geographic Society, Washington DC, USA, 2006.

131 Chevallier, A., *Encyclopedia of Herbal Medicine*, DK Publishing Inc, New York, USA, 2000.

132 Kuhn, M. and Winston, D., *Herbal Therapy and Supplements*, Lippincott, Philadelphia, USA, 2001.

133 *Ibid.*

134 Wildfeuer, A. and Mayerhofer, D., 'The effects of plant preparations on cellular functions in body defence', *Arzneimittelforschung*, March 1994; 44(3) 361-6 and Barrett, B., 'Medicinal properties of *Echinacea*, a critical review', *Phytomedicine*, January 2003; 10(1)66-86.

135 Binns, S.E., Hudson, J., Merali, S. and Arnason, J.T., 'Antiviral activity of characterized extracts from *Echinacea* spp. against herpes simplex virus', *Planta Medica*, September, 2002; 68(9)780-3.

136 Clifford, L.J., Nair, M.G., Rana, J. and Dewitt, D.L., 'Bioactivity of alkamides isolated from *Echinacea purpurea*', *Phytomedicine*, April, 2002; 9(3)249-53.

137 Mullins, R.J. and Heddle, R., 'Adverse reactions associated with *Echinacea*: the Australian experience', *1 Annals of Allergy, Asthma and Immunology*, January, 2002; 88(1)42-51.

138 Dixit, S.P. and Achar, M.P., 'Bhringaraj in the treatment of infective hepatitis', *Curremt Medical Practice*, 1979; 236, 237-242.

139 Chopra, D. and Simon, D., *The Chopra Centre Herbal Handbook*, Rider, London, UK, 2000.

140 Winston, D. and Maimes, S., *Adaptogens*, Healing Arts Press, Rochester, Vermont, USA, 2007.

141 Mars, B., *The Desktop Guide to Herbal Medicine*, Basic Health Publications Inc, Laguna Beach, USA, 2007.

142 Chevallier, A., *Encyclopedia of Herbal Medicine*, DK Publishing Inc, New York, USA, 2000.

143 *Ibid.*

144 Mars, B., *The Desktop Guide to Herbal Medicine*, Basic Health Publications Inc, Laguna Beach, USA, 2007.

145 Chevallier, A., *Encyclopedia of Herbal Medicine*, DK Publishing Inc, New York, USA, 2000.

146 Mars, B., *The Desktop Guide to Herbal Medicine*, Basic Health Publications Inc, Laguna Beach, USA, 2007.

147 *Ibid.*

148 *Ibid.*

149 Williamson, P.M., *Potter's Herbal Cyclopaedia*, C.W. Daniel Company Limited, Essex, UK, 2003.

150 Mars, B., *The Desktop Guide to Herbal Medicine*, Basic Health Publications Inc, Laguna Beach, USA, 2007.

151 *Ibid.*

152 Bone, K., *The Ultimate Herbal Compendium*, Phytotherapy Press, Queensland, Australia, 2007.

153 Chevallier, A., *Encyclopedia of Herbal Medicine*, DK Publishing Inc, New York, USA, 2000.

154 Mars, B., *The Desktop Guide to Herbal Medicine*, Basic Health Publications Inc, Laguna Beach, USA, 2007.

155 Bone, K., *The Ultimate Herbal Compendium*, Phytotherapy Press, Queensland, Australia, 2007.

156 Kuhn, M. and Winston, D., *Herbal Therapy and Supplements*, Lippincott, Philadelphia, USA, 2001.

157 *Ibid.*

158 *Ibid.*

159 Bone, K., *The Ultimate Herbal Compendium*, Phytotherapy Press, Queensland, Australia, 2007.

160 Mars, B., *The Desktop Guide to Herbal Medicine*, Basic Health Publications Inc, Laguna Beach, USA, 2007.

161 *Ibid.*

162 Williamson, P.M., *Potter's Herbal Cyclopaedia*, C.W. Daniel Company Limited, Essex, UK, 2003.

163 Chevallier, A., *Encyclopedia of Herbal Medicine*, DK Publishing Inc, New York, USA, 2000.

164 Williamson, P.M., *Potter's Herbal Cyclopaedia*, C.W. Daniel Company Limited, Essex, UK, 2003.

165 Chevallier, A., *Encyclopedia of Herbal Medicine*, DK Publishing Inc, New York, USA, 2000.

166 Mars, B., *The Desktop Guide to Herbal Medicine*, Basic Health Publications Inc, Laguna Beach, USA, 2007.

167 Bone, K., *The Ultimate Herbal Compendium*, Phytotherapy Press, Queensland, Australia, 2007.

168 Mars, B., *The Desktop Guide to Herbal Medicine*, Basic Health Publications Inc, Laguna Beach, USA, 2007.

169 Yan, X.J., Chuda, Y., Suzuki, M. and Nagata, T., *Bioscience, Biotechnology and Biochemistry*, 1999; 63(3) 605-607.

170 Chevallier, A., *Encyclopedia of Herbal Medicine*, DK Publishing Inc, New York, USA, 2000.

171 Moro, C.O. and Basile, G., 'Obesity and medicinal plants', *Fitoterapia*, 2000; 71 S73-S82.

172 Bone, K., *The Ultimate Herbal Compendium*, Phytotherapy Press, Queensland, Australia, 2007.

173 Mars, B., *The Desktop Guide to Herbal Medicine*, Basic Health Publications Inc, Laguna Beach, USA, 2007.

174 Foster, S. and Johnson, R., *Desk Reference to Nature's Medicine*, National Geographic Society, Washington DC, USA, 2006.

175 Bone, K., *The Ultimate Herbal Compendium*, Phytotherapy Press, Queensland, Australia, 2007.

176 Foster, S. and Johnson, R., *Desk Reference to Nature's Medicine*, National Geographic Society, Washington DC, USA, 2006.

177 *Ibid.*

178 *Ibid.*

179 Bone, K., *The Ultimate Herbal Compendium*, Phytotherapy Press, Queensland, Australia, 2007.

180 Kuhn, M. and Winston, D., *Herbal Therapy and Supplements*, Lippincott, Philadelphia, USA, 2001.

181 Barnett, R., *Tonics*, HarperCollins, New York, USA, 1997.

182 *Ibid.*

183 Kuhn, M. and Winston, D., *Herbal Therapy and Supplements*, Lippincott, Philadelphia, USA, 2001.

184 Barnett, R., *Tonics*, HarperCollins, New York, USA, 1997.

185 Kuhn, M. and Winston, D., *Herbal Therapy and Supplements*, Lippincott, Philadelphia, USA, 2001.

186 Bone, K., *The Ultimate Herbal Compendium*, Phytotherapy Press, Queensland, Australia, 2007.

187 Barnett, R., *Tonics*, HarperCollins, New York, USA, 1997.

188 Kuhn, M. and Winston, D., *Herbal Therapy and Supplements*, Lippincott, Philadelphia, USA, 2001.

189 *Ibid.*

190 Winston, D. and Maimes, S., *Adaptogens*, Healing Arts Press, Rochester, Vermont, USA, 2007.

191 Boon, H. and Smith, M., *50 Most Common Medical Herbs*, Robert Rose Inc, Canada, 2004.

192 *Ibid.*

193 Bone, K., *The Ultimate Herbal*

Compendium, Phytotherapy Press, Queensland, Australia, 2007.

194 Winston, D. and Maimes, S., *Adaptogens*, Healing Arts Press, Rochester, Vermont, USA, 2007.

195 Baker, M.E. et al., 'Liquorice and enzymes other than 11 beta-hydroxysteroid dehydrogenase an evolutionary perspective', *Steroids*, February, 1994; 59(2) 136-41.

196 Tillotson, A.K. et al., *The One Earth Herbal Sourcebook*, Kensington Publishing Corps, New York, USA, 2001.

197 *Ibid.*

198 Numazake, K. et al., 'Effect of glycyrrhizin in children with liver dysfunction associated with cytomegalovirus infection', *The Tohoku Journal of Experimental Medicine*, February 1994; 172(2) 147-53.

199 Pompei, R. et al., 'Antiviral activity of glycyrrhizic acid', *Experimentia*, March 15, 1980; 36(3).

200 Mars, B., *The Desktop Guide to Herbal Medicine*, Basic Health Publications Inc, Laguna Beach, USA, 2007.

201 Kuhn, M. and Winston, D., *Herbal Therapy and Supplements*, Lippincott, Philadelphia, USA, 2001.

202 *Ibid.*

203 Bone, K., *The Ultimate Herbal Compendium*, Phytotherapy Press, Queensland, Australia, 2007.

204 *Ibid.*

205 Pole, S., *Ayurvedic Medicine*, Elsevier, Philadelphia, USA, 2006.

206 *Ibid.*

207 Kuhn, M. and Winston, D., *Herbal Therapy and Supplements*, Lippincott, Philadelphia, USA, 2001.

208 Masaki, H., Sakaki, S., Atsumi, T. and Sakurai, H., 'Active-oxygen scavenging activity of plant extracts', *Biological Pharmaceutical Bulletin*, January 1995; 18(1) 162-6.

209 Foster, S. and Johnson, R., *Desk Reference to Nature's Medicine*, National Geographic Society, Washington DC, USA, 2006.

210 Bone, K., *The Ultimate Herbal Compendium*, Phytotherapy Press, Queensland, Australia, 2007.

211 Foster, S. and Johnson, R., *Desk Reference to Nature's Medicine*, National Geographic Society, Washington DC, USA, 2006.

212 Chrubasik et al.,1996, cited in Kuhn, M. and Winston, D., *Herbal Therapy and Supplements*, Lippincott, Philadelphia, USA, 2001.

213 Foster, S. and Johnson, R., *Desk Reference to Nature's Medicine*, National Geographic Society, Washington DC, USA, 2006.

214 Bone, K., *The Ultimate Herbal Compendium*, Phytotherapy Press, Queensland, Australia, 2007.

215 Foster, S. and Johnson, R., *Desk Reference to Nature's Medicine*, National Geographic Society, Washington DC, USA, 2006.

216 Kuhn, M. and Winston, D., *Herbal Therapy and Supplements*, Lippincott, Philadelphia, USA, 2001.

217 Chevallier, A., *Encyclopedia of Herbal Medicine*, DK Publishing Inc, New York, USA, 2000.

218 Zava et al., 1998, cited in Kuhn, M. and Winston, D., *Herbal Therapy and Supplements*, Lippincott, Philadelphia, USA, 2001.

219 Foster, S. and Johnson, R., *Desk Reference to Nature's Medicine*, National Geographic Society, Washington DC, USA, 2006.

220 *Ibid.*

221 *Ibid.*

222 Chevallier, A., *Encyclopedia of Herbal Medicine*, DK Publishing Inc, New York, USA, 2000.

223 Foster, S. and Johnson, R., *Desk Reference to Nature's Medicine*, National Geographic Society, Washington DC, USA, 2006.

224 *Ibid.*

225 *Ibid.*

226 Mars, B., *The Desktop Guide to Herbal Medicine*, Basic Health Publications Inc, Laguna Beach, USA, 2007.

227 Mars, B., *The Desktop Guide to Herbal Medicine*, Basic Health Publications Inc, Laguna Beach, USA, 2007.

228 *Ibid.*

229 *Ibid.*

230 Larrondo, J.V. et al., 'Antimicrobial activity of essences from labiates', *Microbios*, 1995; 82(332) 171-2.

231 Holmes, C. et al., 'Lavender oil as a treatment for agitated behaviour in severe dementia; a placebo-controlled study', *International Journal of Geriatric Psychiatry*, April 2002; 17(4) 305-8.

232 Foster, S., *Herbal Renaissance*, Gibbs-Smith, Utah, USA, 1997; 116.

233 Cornwell, X. and Dale, A., 'Lavender oil and perineal repair', *Mod Midwife*, 1995; 531-33.

234 Mars, B., *The Desktop Guide to Herbal Medicine*, Basic Health Publications Inc, Laguna Beach, USA, 2007.

235 *Ibid.*

236 *Ibid.*

237 Jones, 1995, cited in Kuhn, M. and Winston, D., *Herbal Therapy and Supplements*, Lippincott, Philadelphia, USA, 2001.

238 Barnett, R., *Tonics*, HarperCollins, New York, 1997.

239 Kuhn, M. and Winston, D., *Herbal Therapy and Supplements*, Lippincott, Philadelphia, USA, 2001.

240 Bone, K., *The Ultimate Herbal Compendium*, Phytotherapy Press, Queensland, Australia, 2007.

241 Mars, B., *The Desktop Guide to Herbal Medicine*, Basic Health Publications Inc, Laguna Beach, USA, 2007.

242 Barnett, R., *Tonics*, HarperCollins, New York, 1997.

243 Kuhn, M. and Winston, D., *Herbal Therapy and Supplements*, Lippincott, Philadelphia, USA, 2001.

244 Mars, B., *The Desktop Guide to Herbal Medicine*, Basic Health Publications Inc, Laguna Beach, USA, 2007.

245 Barnett, R., *Tonics*, HarperCollins, New York, 1997.

246 Mars, B., *The Desktop Guide to Herbal Medicine*, Basic Health Publications Inc, Laguna Beach, USA, 2007.

247 Kuhn, M. and Winston, D., *Herbal*

Therapy and Supplements, Lippincott, Philadelphia, USA, 2001.

248 *Ibid.*

249 *Ibid.*

250 *Ibid.*

251 Nagasawa et al., 1992, cited in Kuhn, M. and Winston, D., *Herbal Therapy and Supplements*, Lippincott, Philadelphia, USA, 2001.

252 Duke, J., *Green Pharmacy*, St Martins Press New York, 1997.

253 Mars, B., *The Desktop Guide to Herbal Medicine*, Basic Health Publications Inc, Laguna Beach, USA, 2007.

254 Ballard, C.G., O'Brien, J.T., Reichelt, K. and Perry, E.K., 'Aromatherapy as a safe and effective treatment for the management of agitation in severe dementia, the results of a double-blind, placebo-controlled trial with *Melissa*', *Journal of Clinical Psychiatry*, July 2002; 63(7)553-8.

255 Koytchev, R., Alken, R.G. and Dundarov, S., 'Balm mint extract (LO-701) for topical treatment of recurring herpes labialis', *Phytomedicine*, October 1999; 6(4)225-30.

256 Englberger, W., Hadding, V. and Etschenberg, E. et al., 'Rosmarinic acid; a new inhibitor of complement C3-convertase with anti-inflammatory activity', *International Journal of Immunopharmacology*, 1988; 10(6)729-37.

257 Imai, H., Osawa, K., Yasuda, H., Hamashima, H., Arai, T. and Sasatsu, M., 'Inhibition by the essential oils of peppermint and spearmint of the growth of pathogenic bacteria', *Microbios*, 2001; 106 Suppl 131-9.

258 Inoue, T., Sugimoto, Y., Masuda, H. and Kamei, C., 'Antiallergic effect of flavonoid glycosides obtained from *Mentha piperita*', *Biological and Pharmaceutical Bulletin*, February 2002; 25(2)256-9.

259 Kuhn, M. and Winston, D., *Herbal Therapy and Supplements*, Lippincott, Philadelphia, USA, 2001.

260 Mars, B., *The Desktop Guide to Herbal Medicine*, Basic Health Publications Inc, Laguna Beach, USA,

2007.

261 *Ibid.*

262 Williamson, P.M., *Potter's Herbal Cyclopaedia*, C.W. Daniel Company Limited, Essex, UK, 2003.

263 Chevallier, A., *Encyclopedia of Herbal Medicine*, DK Publishing Inc, New York, USA, 2000.

264 Williamson, P.M., *Potter's Herbal Cyclopaedia*, C.W. Daniel Company Limited, Essex, UK, 2003.

265 Mars, B., *The Desktop Guide to Herbal Medicine*, Basic Health Publications Inc, Laguna Beach, USA, 2007.

266 Williamson, P.M., *Potter's Herbal Cyclopaedia*, C.W. Daniel Company Limited, Essex, UK, 2003.

267 Bone, K., *The Ultimate Herbal Compendium*, Phytotherapy Press, Queensland, Australia, 2007.

268 Tillotson, A.K. et al., *The One Earth Herbal Sourcebook*, Kensington Publishing Corps, New York, USA, 2001.

269 Singh, R.H., Khosa K.L. and Upadhyaya, B.B., 'Antibacterial activity of some Ayurvedic drugs', *Journal of Research into Indian Medicine*, 1974; 9(2)65.

270 Reddy, P., Srinivas, J., Jamil K, et al., 'Antibacterial activity of isolates from *Piper longum* and *Taxus baccata*', *Pharmaceutical Biology*, 2001; 39(3) 236.

271 Gogte, V.V.M., *Ayurvedic Pharmacology and Therapeutic Uses of Medicinal Plants*, Bharatiya Vidya Bhavan, Mumbai, India, 2000.

272 Ebringerova, A., Kardosova, A., Hromadkova, Z. and Hri-balova, V.V., 'Mitogenic and comitogenic activities of polysaccharides from some European herbaceous plants', *Fitoterapia*, February 2003; 74(1-2)52-61.

273 Chiang, L.C., Chiang, W., Chang, M.Y., Ng, L.T. and Lin, C.C., 'Antiviral activity of *Plantago* major extracts and related compounds in vitro', *Antiviral Research*, July 2002; 55(1)53-62.

274 Winston, D. and Maimes, S., *Adaptogens*, Healing Arts Press, Rochester, Vermont, USA, 2007.

275 Bone, K., *The Ultimate Herbal Compendium*, Phytotherapy Press, Queensland, Australia, 2007.

276 *Ibid.*

277 Winston, D. and Maimes, S., *Adaptogens*, Healing Arts Press, Rochester, Vermont, USA, 2007.

278 *Ibid.*

279 Zheng, M., 'Experimental study of 472 herbs with antiviral action against the herpes simplex virus', *Zhong Xi Yi Jie He Za Zhi*, January 1990; 10(1)39-41, 6 and Yamasaki, K., Otake, T., Mori, H., Morimoto, M., Ueba, N., Kurokawa, Y., Shiota, K. and Yuge, T., 'Screening test of crude drug extract on anti-HIV activity', *Yakugaku Zasshi*, November 1993; 113(11)818-24.

280 Markova, H., Sousek, J. and Ulrichova, J., '*Prunella vulgaris L.* – a rediscovered medicinal plant', *Ceska Slov Farm*, April 1997; 46(2)58-63.

281 Lamaison, J.L., Petitjean-Freytet, C. and Carnat, A., 'Medicinal Lamiaceae with antioxidant properties, a potential source of rosmarinic acid', *Pharmaceutica Acta Helvetiae*, 1991; 66(7)185-8.

282 Lee, H. and Lin, J.Y., 'Antimutagenic activity of extracts from anticancer drugs in Chinese medicine', *Mutat Res.*, February 1988; 204(2)229-34.

283 Foster, S. and Johnson, R., *Desk Reference to Nature's Medicine*, National Geographic Society, Washington DC, USA, 2006.

284 Winston, D. and Maimes, S., *Adaptogens*, Healing Arts Press, Rochester, Vermont, USA, 2007.

285 Bone, K., *Clinical Applications of Ayurvedic and Chinese Herbs*, Phytotherapy Press, Queensland, Australia, 1996.

286 *Ibid.*

287 Bone, K., *The Ultimate Herbal Compendium*, Phytotherapy Press, Queensland, Australia, 2007.

288 *Ibid.*

289 Foster, S. and Johnson, R., *Desk Reference to Nature's Medicine*, National Geographic Society, Washington DC, USA, 2006.

290 *Ibid.*

291 *Ibid.*

292 *Ibid.*

293 Bone, K., *The Ultimate Herbal Compendium*, Phytotherapy Press, Queensland, Australia, 2007.

294 *Ibid.*

295 Yesilada, E., Ustun, O., Sezik, E., Takaishi, Y., Ono,Y. and Honda, G., 'Inhibitory effects of Turkish folk remedies on inflammatory cytokines interleukin-1alpha, interleukin-1beta and tumor necrosis factor alpha', *Journal of Ethnopharmacology*, September 1997; 58(1)59-73.

296 Rossnagel, K. and Willich, S.N., 'Value of complementary medicine exemplified by rose-hips', *Gesundheitswesen*, June 2001; 63(6)412-6.

297 Moss, M., Cook, J., Wesnes, K., Duckett P. 'Aromas of rosemary and lavender essential oils differentially affect cognition and mood in healthy adults', *International Journal of Neuroscience*, January 2003;113(1)15-38.

298 Aqel, M.B., 'Relaxant effect of the volatile oil of *Rosmarinus officinalis* on tracheal smooth muscle', *Journal of Ethnopharmacology*, May–June 1991; 33(1-2)57-62.

299 Mangena, T. and Muyima, N.Y., 'Comparative evaluation of the antimicrobial activities of essential oils of *Artemisia afra*, *Pteronia incana* and *Rosmarinus officinalis* on selected bacteria and yeast strains', *Letters in Applied Microbiology*, April 1999; 28(4)291-6.

300 Barnett, R. *Tonics*, HarperCollins, New York, USA, 1997.

301 Barak, V., Birkenfeld, S., Halperin, T. and Kalickman, I., 'The effect of herbal remedies on the production of human inflammatory and anti-inflammatory cytokines', *Israel Medical Association Journal*, November 2002; 4(11 Suppl)919-22.

302 Zakay-Rones, Z., Varsano, N., Zlotnik, M., Manor, O., Regev, L., Schlesinger, M. and Mumcuoglu, M., 'Inhibition of several strains of influenza virus in vitro and reduction of symptoms by an elderberry extract (*Sambucus nigra L.*) during an outbreak of influenza B Panama', *Journal of Alternative and Complementary Medicine*, winter 1995; 1(4)361-9.

303 Kuhn, M. and Winston, D., *Herbal Therapy and Supplements*, Lippincott, Philadelphia, USA, 2001.

304 *Ibid.*

305 Mars, B., *The Desktop Guide to Herbal Medicine*, Basic Health Publications Inc, Laguna Beach, USA, 2007.

306 Kuhn, M. and Winston, D., *Herbal Therapy and Supplements*, Lippincott, Philadelphia, USA, 2001.

307 Mars, B., *The Desktop Guide to Herbal Medicine*, Basic Health Publications Inc, Laguna Beach, USA, 2007.

308 Kuhn, M. and Winston, D., *Herbal Therapy and Supplements*, Lippincott, Philadelphia, USA, 2001.

309 *Ibid.*

310 *Ibid.*

311 Chevallier, A., *Encyclopedia of Herbal Medicine*, DK Publishing Inc, New York, USA, 2000.

312 *Ibid.*

313 Williamson, P.M., *Potter's Herbal Cyclopaedia*, C.W. Daniel Company Limited, Essex, UK, 2003.

314 Mars, B., *The Desktop Guide to Herbal Medicine*, Basic Health Publications Inc, Laguna Beach, USA, 2007.

315 Bone, K., *The Ultimate Herbal Compendium*, Phytotherapy Press, Queensland, Australia, 2007.

316 *Ibid.*

317 *Ibid.*

318 Williamson, P.M., *Potter's Herbal Cyclopaedia*, C.W. Daniel Company Limited, Essex, UK, 2003.

319 Mars, B., *The Desktop Guide to Herbal Medicine*, Basic Health Publications Inc, Laguna Beach, USA, 2007.

320 Bone, K., *The Ultimate Herbal Compendium*, Phytotherapy Press, Queensland, Australia, 2007.

321 Foster, S. and Johnson, R., *Desk Reference to Nature's Medicine*, National Geographic Society, Washington DC, USA, 2006.

322 Mars, B., *The Desktop Guide to Herbal Medicine*, Basic Health Publications Inc, Laguna Beach, USA, 2007.

323 Kuhn, M. and Winston, D., *Herbal Therapy and Supplements*, Lippincott, Philadelphia, USA, 2001.

324 Foster, S. and Johnson, R., *Desk Reference to Nature's Medicine*, National Geographic Society, Washington DC, USA, 2006.

325 Mars, B., *The Desktop Guide to Herbal Medicine*, Basic Health Publications Inc, Laguna Beach, USA, 2007.

326 Guiraud et al., cited in Kuhn, M. and Winston, D., *Herbal Therapy and Supplements*, Lippincott, Philadelphia, USA, 2001.

327 Foster, S. and Johnson, R., *Desk Reference to Nature's Medicine*, National Geographic Society, Washington DC, USA, 2006.

328 Bradley, P. (Ed), *British Herbal Compendium, Vol 1*, Dorset British Herbal Medicine Association, UK, 1992.

329 Bisset, N., *Herbal Drugs and Phytopharmaceutical*, Scientific Publishers, Stuttgart, Germany, 1996.

330 Wagner, H., Wierer M. and Bauer, R., 'In vitro inhibition of prostaglandin biosynthesis by essential oils and phenolic compounds', *Planta Medica*, June 1986; (3)184-7.

331 Kuhn, M. and Winston, D., *Herbal Therapy and Supplements*, Lippincott, Philadelphia, USA, 2001.

332 Kuhn, M. and Winston, D., *Herbal Therapy and Supplements*, Lippincott, Philadelphia, USA, 2001.

333 Kuhn, M. and Winston, D., *Herbal Therapy and Supplements*, Lippincott, Philadelphia, USA, 2001.

334 Mars, B., *The Desktop Guide to Herbal Medicine*, Basic Health Publications Inc, Laguna Beach, USA, 2007.

335 Kuhn, M. and Winston, D., *Herbal Therapy and Supplements*, Lippincott, Philadelphia, USA, 2001.

336 *Ibid.*

337 Mars, B., *The Desktop Guide to*

Herbal Medicine, Basic Health Publications Inc, Laguna Beach, USA, 2007.

338 Foster, S. and Johnson, R., *Desk Reference to Nature's Medicine*, National Geographic Society, Washington DC, USA, 2006.

339 Bone, K., *The Ultimate Herbal Compendium*, Phytotherapy Press, Queensland, Australia, 2007.

340 Foster, S. and Johnson, R., *Desk Reference to Nature's Medicine*, National Geographic Society, Washington DC, USA, 2006.

341 *Ibid.*

342 *Ibid.*

343 *Ibid.*

344 Mars, B., *The Desktop Guide to Herbal Medicine*, Basic Health Publications Inc, Laguna Beach, USA, 2007.

345 Mabey, R., *The New Age Herbalist*, Gaia Books Ltd, London, UK, 2004.

346 Menzies-Trull, C., *Keys to Physiomedicalism Including Pharmacopoeia*, FPHM, Staffordshire, UK, 2003.

347 *Ibid.*

348 *Ibid.*

349 Mabey, R., *The New Age Herbalist*, Gaia Books Ltd, London, UK, 2004.

350 *Ibid.*

351 Menzies-Trull, C., *Keys to Physiomedicalism Including Pharmacopoeia*, FPHM, Staffordshire, UK, 2003.

352 Kuhn, M. and Winston, D., *Herbal Therapy and Supplements*, Lippincott, Philadelphia, USA, 2001.

353 *Ibid.*

354 Foster, S. and Johnson, R., *Desk Reference to Nature's Medicine*, National Geographic Society, Washington DC, USA, 2006.

355 Skidmore-Roth, L., *Mosby's Handbook of Herbs and Natural Supplements*, Mosby, Inc, St Louis, USA, 2001.

356 Mars, B., *The Desktop Guide to Herbal Medicine*, Basic Health Publications Inc, Laguna Beach, USA, 2007.

357 Menzies-Trull, C., *Keys to Physiomedicalism Including Pharmacopoeia*, FPHM, Staffordshire, UK, 2003.

358 *Ibid.*

359 Mars, B., *The Desktop Guide to Herbal Medicine*, Basic Health Publications Inc, Laguna Beach, USA, 2007.

360 *Ibid.*

361 Menzies-Trull, C., *Keys to Physiomedicalism Including Pharmacopoeia*, FPHM, Staffordshire, UK, 2003.

362 Mars, B., *The Desktop Guide to Herbal Medicine*, Basic Health Publications Inc, Laguna Beach, USA, 2007.

363 *Ibid.*

364 *Ibid.*

365 Mabey, R., *The New Age Herbalist*, Gaia Books Ltd, London, UK, 2004.

366 Bartram, T., *Bartram's Encyclopedia of Herbal Medicine*, Constable and Robinson Ltd, London, 1998.

367 Skidmore-Roth, L., *Mosby's Handbook of Herbs and Natural Supplements*, Mosby, Inc, St Louis, USA, 2001.

368 Mabey, R., *The New Age Herbalist*, Gaia Books Ltd, London, UK, 2004.

369 Skidmore-Roth, L., *Mosby's Handbook of Herbs and Natural Supplements*, Mosby, Inc, St Louis, USA, 2001.

370 *Ibid.*

371 *Ibid.*

372 Mars, B., *The Desktop Guide to Herbal Medicine*, Basic Health Publications Inc, Laguna Beach, USA, 2007.

373 *Ibid.*

374 Foster, S. and Johnson, R., *Desk Reference to Nature's Medicine*, National Geographic Society, Washington DC, USA, 2006.

375 Mars, B., *The Desktop Guide to Herbal Medicine*, Basic Health Publications Inc, Laguna Beach, USA, 2007.

376 *Ibid.*

377 *Ibid.*

378 Foster, S. and Johnson, R., *Desk Reference to Nature's Medicine*, National Geographic Society, Washington DC, USA, 2006.

379 *Ibid.*

380 Mars, B., *The Desktop Guide to Herbal Medicine*, Basic Health Publications Inc, Laguna Beach, USA, 2007.

381 Kuhn, M. and Winston, D., *Herbal Therapy and Supplements*, Lippincott, Philadelphia, USA, 2001.

382 *Ibid.*

383 Mars, B., *The Desktop Guide to Herbal Medicine*, Basic Health Publications Inc, Laguna Beach, USA, 2007.

384 *Ibid.*

385 Kuhn, M. and Winston, D., *Herbal Therapy and Supplements*, Lippincott, Philadelphia, USA, 2001.

386 *Ibid.*

387 *Ibid.*

388 Mars, B., *The Desktop Guide to Herbal Medicine*, Basic Health Publications Inc, Laguna Beach, USA, 2007.

Treatment of common ailments

1 Landis and Khalsa, 1997. 0357.

Index

Page numbers in italic refer to the illustrations

Acknowledgements

Executive Editor Jessica Cowie

Senior Editor Charlotte Macey

Executive Art Editor Penny Stock

Designer Leigh Jones

Production Controller Linda Parry

Picture Researchers Roland and Sarah Smithies

Special Photography:
© Octopus Publishing Group/Ruth Jenkinson

Other Photography:
Alamy/Arco Images GmbH 75 picture 1 (clockwise from top left), 93 picture 1 (clockwise from top left), 96 picture 3 (clockwise from top left), 238; /Peter Arnold, Inc. 228; /blickwinkel 201; /Bon Appetit 95 picture 2 (clockwise from top left); /Cleuna (Medicinal Plants) 84 picture 6 (clockwise from top left); /Adrian Davies 186; /Robert Francis 12 top; /Bob Gibbons 220; /Mike Goldwater 34; /Steffen Hauser/botanikfoto 197; /Interfoto 15; /Geoffrey Kidd 74 picture 6 (clockwise from top left), 79 picture 4 (clockwise from top left), 81 picture 4 (clockwise from top left), 98 picture 7 (clockwise from top left); /kpzfoto 193; /McPhoto 227; /Natural Visions 91 picture 2 (clockwise from top left); /Nikreates 231; /outis 81 picture 5 (clockwise from top left); /Photofrenetic 221; /Phototake Inc. 79 picture 6 (clockwise from top left); /rabh images 207; /WILDLIFE GmbH 217.
Bridgeman Art Library/National Museums of Scotland 21; /Private Collection 22; /Private Collection/The Stapleton Collection 6.
ChinaFotoPress 10.
Corbis/Paul Almasy 11; /Envision 187; /David Forman/Eye Ubiquitous 25; /Gerd Ludwig 39; /Ken Seet 33; /Keren Su 28; /Luca Tettoni 24;
DK Images 74 picture 5; /Andy Crawford/Steve Gorton 93 picture 3 (clockwise from top left), 98 picture 6 (clockwise from top left); /Neil Fletcher 75 picture 8 (clockwise from top left), 86 picture 2 (clockwise from top left); /Neil Fletcher/Matthew Ward 73 picture 4 (clockwise from top left), 82 picture 7 (clockwise from top left), 82 picture 1 (clockwise from top left), 83 picture 3 (clockwise from top left), 83 picture 4 (clockwise from top left), 89 picture 3 (clockwise from top left), 90 picture 5 (clockwise from top left), 96 picture 4 (clockwise from top left), 99 picture 2 (clockwise from top left); /Steve Gorton 73 picture 3 (clockwise from top left), 74 picture 2 (clockwise from top left), 75 picture 2 (clockwise from top left), 75 picture 7 (clockwise from top left), 82 picture 6 (clockwise from top left), 86 picture 1 (clockwise from top left), 92 picture 2 (clockwise from top left), 95 picture 4 (clockwise from top left), 96 picture 2 (clockwise from top left), 97 picture 3 (clockwise from top left), 98 picture 2 (clockwise from top left); /Frank Greenaway 92 picture 3 (clockwise from top left); /Derek Hall 99 picture 1 (clockwise from top left); /Dave King 73 picture 8 (clockwise from top left), 80 picture 2 (clockwise from top left), 83 picture 2 (clockwise from top left), 86 picture 4 (clockwise from top left), 96 picture 5 (clockwise from top left); /Roger Phillips 73 picture 7 (clockwise from top left); /David Murray 93 picture 7 (clockwise from top left); /Matthew Ward 81 picture 1 (clockwise from top left), 84 picture 5 (clockwise from top left), 85 picture 2 (clockwise from top left), 85 picture 6 (clockwise from top left).
Fotolia/adisa 199; /Martina Berg 200; /Alison Bowden 42; /Pavel Davidenko 196; /Dmitry 89 picture 4; /ExQuisine 92 picture 1 (clockwise from top left); /leafy 91 picture 3 (clockwise from top left); /mtsyri 73 picture 2 (clockwise from top left); /Olga Shelego 183; /jerome whittingham 216.
GAP Photos/Heather Edwards 237; /Dianna Jazwinski 29; /Friedrich Strauss 236.
Getty Images/Dinodia Photos 89 picture 6 (clockwise from top left); /Neil Fletcher and Matthew Ward 89 picture 2 (clockwise from top left); /John Kelly 52; /Stock Montage/Hulton Archive 13; /Lew Robertson 93 picture 6 (clockwise from top left).
Natural Visions/Heather Angel 38.
Octopus Publishing Group 14; /Michael Boyes 180; /Philip Dorell 71 to 99 (unless otherwise stated); /William Lingwood 53; /Russell Sadur 54; /David Sarton/Design: del Buono Gazerwitz 234; /George Wright 31.
Photolibrary/Gerrit Buntrock 213; /Carole Drake 181; /Pablo Galan Cela 206; /Garden Picture Library 230; /Georgianna Lane 202; /imagebroker 93 picture 4 (clockwise from top left); /Andrea Jones 203; /Roel Loopers 35; /Antonio Molero 191; /Photononstop 19 right; /Pixtal Images 190; /Isabelle Plasschaert 40; /Radius Images 41; /Howard Rice 223; /Gerhard Schulz 12 bottom; /Luca Invernizzi Tettoni 23; /The Print Collector 18; /Mark Turner 43, 210, 226.
Photoshot/World Illustrated 17.
Pukka Herbs Ltd. **(www.pukkaherbs.com)** 19 left, 71 picture 1 (clockwise from top left), 74 picture 7 (clockwise from top left), 182.
Science Photo Library/Annabella Bluesky/Acumedic 49; /Jerry Mason 81 picture 3 (clockwise from top left); /TH Foto-Werbung 84 picture 1 (clockwise from top left).
Stockfood/Ottmar Diez 86 picture 6 (clockwise from top left), 86 picture 7 (clockwise from top left).
The Art Archive/Private Collection/Gianni Dagli Orti 27.
TopFoto/The Granger Collection 30.
Wellcome Library, London 7, 26, 48.